# Hearing Disorders: Diagnosis, Management, and Future Opportunities

# Hearing Disorders: Diagnosis, Management, and Future Opportunities

Editor

**George Psillas**

MDPI • Basel • Beijing • Wuhan • Barcelona • Belgrade • Manchester • Tokyo • Cluj • Tianjin

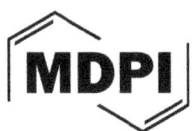

*Editor*
George Psillas
Aristotle University of Thessaloniki,
AHEPA Hospital
Greece

*Editorial Office*
MDPI
St. Alban-Anlage 66
4052 Basel, Switzerland

This is a reprint of articles from the Special Issue published online in the open access journal *Journal of Clinical Medicine* (ISSN 2077-0383) (available at: https://www.mdpi.com/journal/jcm/special_issues/hearing_disorders).

For citation purposes, cite each article independently as indicated on the article page online and as indicated below:

LastName, A.A.; LastName, B.B.; LastName, C.C. Article Title. *Journal Name* **Year**, *Volume Number*, Page Range.

**ISBN 978-3-0365-5715-1 (Hbk)**
**ISBN 978-3-0365-5716-8 (PDF)**

© 2022 by the authors. Articles in this book are Open Access and distributed under the Creative Commons Attribution (CC BY) license, which allows users to download, copy and build upon published articles, as long as the author and publisher are properly credited, which ensures maximum dissemination and a wider impact of our publications.

The book as a whole is distributed by MDPI under the terms and conditions of the Creative Commons license CC BY-NC-ND.

# Contents

George Psillas, Grigorios George Dimas, Christos Savopoulos and Jiannis Constantinidis
Autoimmune Hearing Loss: A Diagnostic Challenge
Reprinted from: *J. Clin. Med.* **2022**, *11*, 4601, doi:10.3390/jcm11154601 . . . . . . . . . . . . . . . . . 1

Hwa-Sung Rim, Myung-Gu Kim, Dong-Choon Park, Sung-Soo Kim, Dae-Woong Kang, Sang-Hoon Kim and Seung-Geun Yeo
Association of Metabolic Syndrome with Sensorineural Hearing Loss
Reprinted from: *J. Clin. Med.* **2021**, *10*, 4866, doi:10.3390/jcm10214866 . . . . . . . . . . . . . . . . . 5

Minna Kraatari-Tiri, Maria K. Haanpää, Tytti Willberg, Pia Pohjola, Riikka Keski-Filppula, Outi Kuismin, Jukka S. Moilanen, Sanna Häkli and Elisa Rahikkala
Clinical and Genetic Characteristics of Finnish Patients with Autosomal Recessive and Dominant Non-Syndromic Hearing Loss Due to Pathogenic *TMC1* Variants
Reprinted from: *J. Clin. Med.* **2022**, *11*, 1837, doi:10.3390/jcm11071837 . . . . . . . . . . . . . . . . . 17

Marlin Johansson, Eva Karltorp, Kaijsa Edholm, Maria Drott and Erik Berninger
A Prospective Study of Etiology and Auditory Profiles in Infants with Congenital Unilateral Sensorineural Hearing Loss
Reprinted from: *J. Clin. Med.* **2022**, *11*, 3966, doi:10.3390/jcm11143966 . . . . . . . . . . . . . . . . . 27

Yuan Jin, Xiaozhou Liu, Sen Chen, Jiale Xiang, Zhiyu Peng and Yu Sun
Analysis of the Results of Cytomegalovirus Testing Combined with Genetic Testing in Children with Congenital Hearing Loss
Reprinted from: *J. Clin. Med.* **2022**, *11*, 5335, doi:10.3390/jcm11185335 . . . . . . . . . . . . . . . . . 45

Ghizlene Lahlou, Hannah Daoudi, Evelyne Ferrary, Huan Jia, Marion De Bergh, Yann Nguyen, Olivier Sterkers and Isabelle Mosnier
Candidacy for Cochlear Implantation in Prelingual Profoundly Deaf Adult Patients
Reprinted from: *J. Clin. Med.* **2022**, *11*, 1874, doi:10.3390/jcm11071874 . . . . . . . . . . . . . . . . . 53

Attila Ovari, Lisa Hühnlein, David Nguyen-Dalinger, Daniel Fabian Strüder, Christoph Külkens, Oliver Niclaus and Jens Eduard Meyer
Functional Outcomes and Quality of Life after Cochlear Implantation in Patients with Long-Term Deafness
Reprinted from: *J. Clin. Med.* **2022**, *11*, 5156, doi:10.3390/jcm11175156 . . . . . . . . . . . . . . . . . 67

So Young Jeon, Dae Woong Kang, Sang Hoon Kim, Jae Yong Byun and Seung Geun Yeo
Prognostic Factors Associated with Recovery from Recurrent Idiopathic Sudden Sensorineural Hearing Loss: Retrospective Analysis and Systematic Review
Reprinted from: *J. Clin. Med.* **2022**, *11*, 1453, doi:10.3390/jcm11051453 . . . . . . . . . . . . . . . . . 83

Dae-Woong Kang, Seul Kim and Woongsang Sunwoo
Correlation of Neutrophil-to-Lymphocyte Ratio and the Dilation of the Basilar Artery with the Potential Role of Vascular Compromise in the Pathophysiology of Idiopathic Sudden Sensorineural Hearing Loss
Reprinted from: *J. Clin. Med.* **2022**, *11*, 5943, doi:10.3390/jcm11195943 . . . . . . . . . . . . . . . . . 93

Maria-Del-Carmen Moleon, Estrella Martinez-Gomez, Marisa Flook, Andreina Peralta-Leal, Juan Antonio Gallego, Hortensia Sanchez-Gomez, Maria Alharilla Montilla-Ibañez, Emilio Dominguez-Durán, Andres Soto-Varela, Ismael Aran, Lidia Frejo and Jose A. Lopez-Escamez
Clinical and Cytokine Profile in Patients with Early and Late Onset Meniere Disease
Reprinted from: *J. Clin. Med.* **2021**, *10*, 4052, doi:10.3390/jcm10184052 . . . . . . . . . . . . . . . . . 105

**Yi Zhang, Chenyi Wei, Zhengtao Sun, Yue Wu, Zhengli Chen and Bo Liu**
Hearing Benefits of Clinical Management for Meniere's Disease
Reprinted from: *J. Clin. Med.* **2022**, *11*, 3131, doi:10.3390/jcm11113131 . . . . . . . . . . . . . . . . **119**

**Ioanna Sfakianaki, Paris Binos, Petros Karkos, Grigorios G. Dimas and George Psillas**
Risk Factors for Recurrence of Benign Paroxysmal Positional Vertigo. A Clinical Review
Reprinted from: *J. Clin. Med.* **2021**, *10*, 4372, doi:10.3390/jcm10194372 . . . . . . . . . . . . . . . . **133**

**George Psillas, Ioanna Petrou, Athanasia Printza, Ioanna Sfakianaki, Paris Binos, Sofia Anastasiadou and Jiannis Constantinidis**
Video Head Impulse Test (vHIT): Value of Gain and Refixation Saccades in Unilateral Vestibular Neuritis
Reprinted from: *J. Clin. Med.* **2022**, *11*, 3467, doi:10.3390/jcm11123467 . . . . . . . . . . . . . . . . **153**

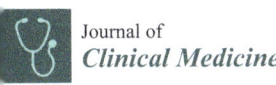

*Editorial*

# Autoimmune Hearing Loss: A Diagnostic Challenge

George Psillas [1,*], Grigorios George Dimas [2], Christos Savopoulos [2] and Jiannis Constantinidis [1]

1. 1st Otolaryngology Department, School of Medicine, Faculty of Health Sciences, Aristotle University of Thessaloniki, AHEPA Hospital, 54636 Thessaloniki, Greece
2. 1st Propedeutic Department of Internal Medicine, Faculty of Health Sciences, Aristotle University of Thessaloniki, AHEPA Hospital, 54636 Thessaloniki, Greece
* Correspondence: psill@otenet.gr; Tel.: +30-2310-994-762; Fax: +30-2310-994-916

Autoimmune hearing loss (AIHL) is a clinical disease and may involve the deposition of immune complexes in the labyrinth vessels, the activation of the complement system, the functional alteration in T-cell subpopulations, or an inflammation process in the inner ear [1]. The diagnosis AIHL is still unclear and there are no serologic or radiologic criteria for its identification. When initially described, AIHL was recognized as always being both bilateral and progressive [2]; however, AIHL may involve only one ear [3] and a significant proportion of patients with AIHL may experience a sudden onset of symptoms [4,5]. Moreover, positive response to steroid administration was considered as a clinical prerequisite for AIHL [2]; nevertheless, less than half of patients respond favorably to steroid therapy [5,6] and, over time, a progression of hearing loss has been observed.

Different pure-tone audiogram shapes in patients with AIHL have been recorded, including down-sloping (which is the most frequent), up-sloping, flat, cookie-bite, and inverse cookie-bite shapes; almost half of cases have moderate hearing loss [1,5]. AIHL is a long-standing disease with relapses and is more commonly observed after unilateral or bilateral sudden hearing loss [7].

Immunologic laboratory tests should be performed in every patient with suspected AIHL, such as complete blood count, erythrocyte sedimentation rate, antinuclear antibodies (ANA), antineutrophil cytoplasmic antibodies (ANCA), anticardiolipine/antiphospholipid antibodies, rheumatoid factor, immunoglobulines IgG, IgM, IgA, complement factors C3, C4, and anti-cochlin/anti-β-tubulin antibodies [8].

Genetic factors such as the human leukocyte antigen (HLA) system should also be investigated for AIHL. The haplotypes HLA B27, B35, B51, C4, C7, and A1-B8-DR3 have been reported as prognostic markers for the development of AIHL [9,10]. In a recent study [11], HLA DRB1*04 alleles were recorded at higher proportions compared with the healthy control group; HLA–DRB1*04 alleles were found to be strongly associated with Vogt–Koyanagi–Harada disease, which is an autoimmune disease that also affects the inner ear [12]. Moreover, HLA–DRB1*04 alleles, such as DRB1*0401, DRB1*0404, DRB1*0405, and DRB1*0408, have been reported to be highly expressed in patients suffering from rheumatoid arthritis [13]; finally, HLA DRB1*04, as a poor prognostic marker, was found at high frequency in patients with sudden sensorineural hearing loss and no satisfactory response to steroid treatment [14].

Presence of other autoimmune diseases should be investigated as potential clinical clues for AIHL in patients who have complained of progressive hearing loss or recurrent sudden hearing loss. Hashimoto's thyroiditis is an autoimmune disorder that can cause hypothyroidism and in which significant increases in thyroid peroxidase antibody (anti-TPO) and thyroglobuline antibody (anti-Tg) have been found in a patient with AIHL [15]. In our study [5], we noted that Hashimoto's thyroiditis was very commonly associated with patients suffering from AIHL; 13 (24.5%) out of 53 patients with AIHL had concomitant Hashimoto's thyroiditis. It has been shown that, in Hashimoto's thyroiditis, the number of T-regulatory (Treg) cells are reduced, and their function is defective, resulting in their limited downregulating effect against the ongoing autoimmune process and leading to extensive defects in the inner ear [16]. Close monitoring of hearing is recommended in the treatment of these patients with Hashimoto's thyroiditis using a thorough audiometric test battery at least once a year.

In conclusion, this Special Issue gives new insight into the immune-mediated pathophysiologic mechanisms involving the inner ear. Specialized laboratory tests and an extended audiological test battery to identify underlying autoimmune process will be reported. Management of AIHL associated with other systemic autoimmune disorders will be discussed and new therapeutic protocols will be evaluated. Multicentric studies and collaboration are required to establish diagnostic criteria and therapeutic guidelines. Assessing the current knowledge and elucidating the effect of autoimmunity on the cochlea will help us to promote our understanding of this complex clinical disorder.

**Author Contributions:** Conceptualization, G.P.; methodology, G.P. and G.G.D.; investigation, data curation, and visualization, G.P.; project administration, G.P., C.S.; resources, G.P.; supervision, G.P. and J.C.; writing—original draft preparation, G.P.; writing—review and editing, G.P., G.G.D., C.S. and J.C. All authors have read and agreed to the published version of the manuscript.

**Funding:** This research did not receive any specific grant from funding agencies in the public, commercial, or not-for-profit sectors.

**Data Availability Statement:** The data presented in this study is available upon request from the corresponding author.

**Conflicts of Interest:** The authors declare no conflict of interest.

# References

1. Ralli, M.; D'Aguanno, V.; Di Stadio, A.; de Virgilio, A.; Croce, A.; Longo, L.; Greco, A.; de Vincentiis, M. Audiovestibular symptoms in systemic autoimmune diseases. *J. Immunol. Res.* **2018**, *2018*, 5798103. [CrossRef] [PubMed]
2. McCabe, B.F. Autoimmune sensorineural hearing loss. *Ann. Otol. Rhinol. Laryngol.* **1979**, *88*, 585–589. [CrossRef] [PubMed]
3. Atturo, F.; Colangeli, R.; Bandiera, G.; Barbara, M.; Monini, S. Can unilateral, progressive or sudden hearing loss be immune-mediated in origin? *Acta Otolaryngol.* **2017**, *137*, 823–828. [CrossRef] [PubMed]
4. Rossini, B.A.A.; Penido, N.O.; Munhoz, M.S.L.; Bogaz, E.A.; Curi, R.S. Sudden sensorineural hearing loss and autoimmune systemic diseases. *Int. Arch. Otorhinolaryngol.* **2017**, *21*, 213–223. [CrossRef] [PubMed]
5. Psillas, G.; Dimas, G.G.; Daniilidis, M.; Binos, P.; Tegos, T.; Constantinidis, J. Audiological Patterns in Patients with Autoimmune Hearing Loss. *Audiol. Neurootol.* **2022**, *27*, 336–346. [CrossRef] [PubMed]
6. Zeitoun, H.; Beckman, J.G.; Arts, H.A.; Lansford, C.D.; Lee, D.S.; El-Kashlan, H.K.; Telian, S.A.; Denny, D.E.; Ramakrishnan, A.; Nair, T.S.; et al. Corticosteroid response and supporting cell antibody in autoimmune hearing loss. *Arch. Otolaryngol. Head Neck Surg.* **2005**, *131*, 665–672. [CrossRef] [PubMed]
7. Mata-Castro, N.; García-Chilleron, R.; Gavilanes-Plasencia, J.; Ramírez-Camacho, R.; García-Fernández, A.; García-Berrocal, J.R. Analysis of audiometric relapse-free survival in patients with immune-mediated hearing loss exclusively treated with corticosteroids. *Acta Otorrinolaringol. Esp.* **2018**, *69*, 214–218. [CrossRef] [PubMed]
8. Agrup, C.; Luxon, L.M. Immune-mediated inner-ear disorders in neuro-otology. *Curr. Opin. Neurol.* **2006**, *19*, 26–32. [CrossRef] [PubMed]
9. Das, S.; Bakshi, S.S.; Seepana, R. Demystifying autoimmune inner ear disease. *Eur. Arch. Otorhinolaryngol.* **2019**, *276*, 3267–3274. [CrossRef] [PubMed]
10. Psillas, G.; Daniilidis, M.; Gerofotis, A.; Veros, K.; Vasilaki, A.; Vital, I.; Markou, K. Sudden Bilateral Sensorineural Hearing Loss Associated with HLA A1-B8-DR3 Haplotype. *Case Rep. Otolaryngol.* **2013**, *2013*, 590157. [CrossRef] [PubMed]
11. Psillas, G.; Binos, P.; Dimas, G.G.; Daniilidis, M.; Constantinidis, J. Human Leukocyte Antigen (HLA) Influence on Prognosis of Autoimmune Hearing Loss. *Audiol. Res.* **2021**, *11*, 31–37. [CrossRef] [PubMed]
12. Shi, T.; Lv, W.; Zhang, L.; Chen, J.; Chen, H. Association of HLA-DR4/HLA-DRB1*04 with Vogt-Koyanagi-Harada disease: A systematic review and meta-analysis. *Sci. Rep.* **2014**, *4*, 6887. [CrossRef] [PubMed]
13. Balandraud, N.; Picard, C.; Reviron, D.; Landais, C.; Toussirot, E.; Lambert, N.; Telle, E.; Charpin, C.; Wendling, D.; Pardoux, E.; et al. HLA-DRB1 genotypes and the risk of developing anti citrullinated protein antibody (ACPA) positive rheumatoid arthritis. *PLoS ONE* **2013**, *8*, e64108. [CrossRef] [PubMed]
14. Yeo, S.W.; Chang, K.H.; Suh, B.D.; Kim, T.G.; Han, H. Distribution of HLA-A, -B and -DRB1 alleles in patients with sudden sensorineural hearing loss. *Acta Otolaryngol.* **2000**, *120*, 710–715. [CrossRef] [PubMed]

15. Fayyaz, B.; Upreti, S. Autoimmune inner ear disease secondary to Hashimoto's thyroiditis: A case report. *J. Community Hosp. Intern. Med. Perspect.* **2018**, *8*, 227–229. [CrossRef] [PubMed]
16. Rodríguez-Valiente, A.; Álvarez-Montero, Ó.; Górriz-Gil, C.; García-Berrocal, J.R. l-Thyroxine does not prevent immunemediated sensorineural hearing loss in autoimmune thyroid diseases. *Acta Otorrinolaringol. Esp.* **2019**, *70*, 229–234. [CrossRef] [PubMed]

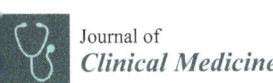 

## Article

# Association of Metabolic Syndrome with Sensorineural Hearing Loss

Hwa-Sung Rim [1], Myung-Gu Kim [2], Dong-Choon Park [3], Sung-Soo Kim [4], Dae-Woong Kang [1], Sang-Hoon Kim [1] and Seung-Geun Yeo [1,*]

[1] Department of Otolaryngology—Head & Neck Surgery, School of Medicine, Kyung Hee University, Seoul 02454, Korea; marslover@naver.com (H.-S.R.); kkang814@naver.com (D.-W.K.); hoon0700@naver.com (S.-H.K.)
[2] Department of Otorhinolaryngology, Samsung Changwon Hospital, Sungkyunkwan University School of Medicine, Changwon 51353, Korea; mgent.kim@samsung.com
[3] St. Vincent's Hospital, The Catholic University of Korea, Suwon 16247, Korea; dcpark@catholic.ac.kr
[4] Department of Biochemistry and Molecular Biology, School of Medicine, Kyung Hee University, Seoul 02447, Korea; sgskim@khu.ac.kr
* Correspondence: yeo2park@gmail.com; Tel.: +82-2-958-8980; Fax: +82-2-958-8470

**Abstract:** The prevalence of sensorineural hearing loss has increased along with increases in life expectancy and exposure to noisy environments. Metabolic syndrome (MetS) is a cluster of co-occurring conditions that increase the risk of heart disease, stroke and type 2 diabetes, along with other conditions that affect the blood vessels. Components of MetS include insulin resistance, body weight, lipid concentration, blood pressure, and blood glucose concentration, as well as other features of insulin resistance such as microalbuminuria. MetS has become a major public health problem affecting 20–30% of the global population. This study utilized health examination to investigate whether metabolic syndrome was related to hearing loss. Methods: A total of 94,223 people who underwent health check-ups, including hearing tests, from January 2010 to December 2020 were evaluated. Subjects were divided into two groups, with and without metabolic syndrome. In addition, Scopus, Embase, PubMed, and Cochrane libraries were systematically searched, using keywords such as "hearing loss" and "metabolic syndrome", for studies that evaluated the relationship between the two. Results: Of the 94,223 subjects, 11,414 (12.1%) had metabolic syndrome and 82,809 did not. The mean ages of subjects in the two groups were 46.1 and 43.9 years, respectively. A comparison of hearing thresholds by age in subjects with and without metabolic syndrome showed that the average pure tone hearing thresholds were significantly higher in subjects with metabolic syndrome than in subjects without it in all age groups. ($p < 0.001$) Rates of hearing loss in subjects with 0, 1, 2, 3, 4, and 5 of the components of metabolic syndrome were 7.9%, 12.1%, 13.8%, 13.8%, 15.5% and 16.3%, respectively, indicating a significant association between the number of components of metabolic syndrome and the rate of hearing loss ($p < 0.0001$). The odds ratio of hearing loss was significantly higher in subjects with four components of metabolic syndrome: waist circumference, blood pressure, and triglyceride and fasting blood sugar concentrations ($p < 0.0001$). Conclusions: The number of components of the metabolic syndrome is positively correlated with the rate of sensorineural hearing loss.

**Keywords:** metabolic syndrome; sensorineural hearing loss

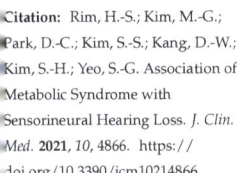

Citation: Rim, H.-S.; Kim, M.-G.; Park, D.-C.; Kim, S.-S.; Kang, D.-W.; Kim, S.-H.; Yeo, S.-G. Association of Metabolic Syndrome with Sensorineural Hearing Loss. *J. Clin. Med.* **2021**, *10*, 4866. https://doi.org/10.3390/jcm10214866

Academic Editor: George Psillas

Received: 26 September 2021
Accepted: 20 October 2021
Published: 22 October 2021

**Publisher's Note:** MDPI stays neutral with regard to jurisdictional claims in published maps and institutional affiliations.

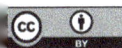

**Copyright:** © 2021 by the authors. Licensee MDPI, Basel, Switzerland. This article is an open access article distributed under the terms and conditions of the Creative Commons Attribution (CC BY) license (https://creativecommons.org/licenses/by/4.0/).

## 1. Introduction

Sensorineural hearing loss is an important public health problem whose prevalence has increased as life expectancy has become longer [1]. For example, the Global Burden of Disease Study reported that the prevalence of hearing loss increased from 14.33% in 1990 to 18.06% in 2015 and that hearing loss is the fifth most frequent cause of disability in both developed and developing countries [2]. Approximately 50% of people aged over 70 years and 80% of those aged over 85 years experience hearing loss, which affects their ability to communicate and their social lives [1]. The pathophysiological mechanisms of hearing loss are complex, although several risk factors have been reported to contribute to hearing loss, including genetic factors, inflammatory processes, systemic diseases, noise, medications, oxidative stress, and aging [3].

Metabolic syndrome is a disease that includes hypertension, central obesity, hyperlipidemia, and diabetes [4]. Metabolic syndrome was found to be associated with various clinical conditions, including stroke, myocardial infarction, death from cardiovascular disease, and diabetes [5,6]. Studies have recently reported that metabolic syndrome may be associated with hearing loss [3,7–12]. Using health examination data, this study therefore investigated the relationships between metabolic syndrome and hearing loss. In addition, studies published on this relationship were subjected to comparative analysis and a systematic review.

## 2. Materials and Methods

### 2.1. Study Population

This study included a total of 94,223 people, ranging in age from their 20s to their 70s, who underwent health checkups, including hearing tests, at a tertiary university hospital from January 2010 to December 2020. Height, weight, body mass index, waist circumference and blood pressure (both systolic and diastolic) were measured in all subjects, and all subjects underwent hearing and blood tests and pulmonary function tests (PFT). Subjects without hearing test results and those with a $\geq$ 20 dB difference between the two hearing thresholds, a history of surgery for otitis media, or suspected central disease were excluded. The study protocol was approved by the Institutional Review Board of Kyung Hee University Medical Center (KMC 2019-07-065).

### 2.2. Definition of Metabolic Syndrome

The criteria for metabolic syndrome were defined according to the revised National Cholesterol Education Program Adult Treatment Panel III: [13] (1) waist circumference (WC) > 90 cm for men or > 80 cm for women, (2) fasting blood sugar > 100 mg/dL or a diagnosis of diabetes, (3) BP >130/85 mmHg or a diagnosis of high blood pressure, (4) triglyceride concentration > 150 mg/dL, and (5) high-density lipoprotein-cholesterol (HDL-C) < 40 mg/dL for men or < 50 mg/dL for women. Subjects with three or more of these five factors were defined as positive for metabolic syndrome.

### 2.3. Hearing Test

Hearing threshold tests were performed at frequencies of 500, 1000, 2000, 3000, 4000, and 6000 Hz, measured in that order, followed by a retest at 1000 Hz, with air conduction measured at a frequency of 500 Hz. Pure tone audiometry was performed using the standard hexadecimal method, by measuring the air conduction values of each ear at four frequencies (500, 1000, 2000, and 4000 Hz) and calculating their sum using the equation: (500 Hz + 2 × 1000 Hz + 2 × 2000 Hz + 4000 Hz)/6 [14–17].

### 2.4. Research on Hearing Loss and Metabolic Syndrome

To systematically review the results of studies on the correlation between hearing loss and metabolic syndrome, the Scopus, Embase, PubMed, and Cochrane library databases were searched using the keywords "hearing loss" and "metabolic syndrome". A total of 1373 papers were identified initially, including 390, 612, 364, and seven, respectively, in these databases. Of these, 1300 papers were excluded due to lack of relevance in the title, and an additional 44 papers were excluded due to duplication of papers. Of the 29 papers reviewed in full, 17 were included in the systematic analysis (Table 1).

Table 1. Studies assessing the association between hearing loss and metabolic syndrome.

| Author (Year) | Study Design | N | Age (Years) | Associated Variables | Conclusions |
|---|---|---|---|---|---|
| Kang S.H. et al. (2015) [9] | Cross-sectional | 16,554 | 50.4 ± 16.6 (men) 49.2 ± 16.4 (women) | MetS or CKD/Hearing thresholds | MetS is associated with hearing thresholds in women; and CKD is associated with hearing thresholds in men and women. Subjects with MetS or CKD should be closely monitored for hearing impairment. |
| Sun Y.-S. et al. (2015) [3] | Cross-sectional | 2100 | ≤65 | MetS components/SNHL | Significant associations between the number of components of metabolic syndrome and hearing thresholds in US adults, with the strongest association between low HDL and hearing loss. |
| Kang S.H. et al. (2015) [18] | Cross-sectional | 8198 | 54.7 ± 9.9 | WHR/HL | WHR may be a surrogate marker for predicting the risk of hearing loss resulting from metabolic syndrome. |
| Bener A. et al. (2016) [19] | Cross-sectional | 459 | 20–59 | DM, HTN/HL | Adults with DM and hypertension showed greater hearing impairment in a highly endogamous population. Diabetic patients with hearing loss were likely to have high blood glucose and other risk factors like hypertension, retinopathy, nephropathy, and neuropathy. |
| Kim S.H. et al. (2016) [20] | Cross-sectional | 61,052 | 42.33 ± 7.49 (normal) 49.89 ± 9.32 (HL) | BMI/HL | Underweight and severe obesity were associated with an increased prevalence of hearing loss in a Korean population. |
| Kang S.H. et al. (2016) [21] | Cross-sectional | 7449 | 53.2 ± 10.7 56.7 ± 11.0 59.8 ± 10.8 | HbA1c/HL | HbA1c level was associated with hearing impairment in nondiabetic individuals. |
| Lee H.Y. et al. (2016) [22] | Retrospective | 16,779 | ≥19 | MetS components/SNHL | Metabolic syndrome itself was not an independent risk factor for hearing impairment. Among its individual components, only increased fasting plasma glucose was independently associated with hearing impairment. |
| Aghazadeh-Attari J. et al.(2017) [12] | Cross-sectional | 11,114 | 20–60 | MetS components/SNHL | Possible associations between different components of MetS (obesity, hypertension, hypertriglyceridemia, high fasting glucose levels, and waist circumference) and SNHL in a population of West Azerbaijan drivers. |
| Jung D.J. et al. (2017) [23] | Cross-sectional | 18,004 | >40 | TG/HDL ratio/SNHL | High TG/HDL-C ratio was associated with hearing impairment in a Korean population |
| Nwosu J. N. et al. (2017) [24] | Case-control | 416 | 26–80 years | DM/HL | High prevalence of hearing loss among diabetic adults at University of Nigeria Teaching Hospital, Enugu. Hearing loss was predominantly sensorineural and often mild to moderate in severity. |
| Lee Y. et al. (2017) [25] | Retrospective | 2602 | 57.6 ± 7.3 | Factors relevant abdominal fats (FRAs)/Age-related hearing loss (ARHL) | FRAs were associated with frequency-specific hearing losses according to sex. DM and visceral adipose tissue (VAT) are particularly important role for hearing. |

**Table 1.** Cont.

| Author (Year) | Study Design | N | Age (Years) | Associated Variables | Conclusions |
|---|---|---|---|---|---|
| Kim T.S. et al. (2017) [8] | Prospective | 1381 | >50 | MetS components/ age-related hearing impairment (ARHI) | MetS is associated with age-related hearing impairment in women aged ≥ 50 years. At 5-year follow-up, high-frequency hearing loss tended to be greater in women with than without MetS, suggesting the need for hearing evaluation in older women with MetS. |
| Han X. et al. (2018) [7] | Cross-sectional | 18,824 | $61.1 \pm 7.6$ $66.6 \pm 7.2$ $71.0 \pm 7.7$ | MetS components/SNHL | MetS, including its components central obesity, hyperglycemia, and low HDL-C levels, is positively associated with hearing loss. |
| Jung D.J. et al. (2019) [11] | Cross-sectional | 17,513,555 | >40 | MetS components/SNHL | Among the components of MetS, low HDL and high TG levels were especially associated with hearing loss. Rather than assessing MetS, each MetS component should be evaluated individually. |
| Shim H.S. et al. (2019) [10] | Cross-sectional | 28,866 | all age groups | MetS components/SNHL | MetS may be associated with hearing loss, especially in subjects who meet four or five of the diagnostic criteria for MetS. |
| Hu H. et al. (2020) [26] | Prospective cohort | 48,549 | 20–64 | BMI (w/o Waist circumference)/SNHL | Overweight and obesity are associated with an increased risk of hearing loss, with metabolically unhealthy status conferring an additional risk. |
| Kim J. et al. (2021) [27] | Cross-sectional | 10,356 | 40–80 | MetS components/HL | MetS is associated with high-frequency hearing loss in subjects exposed to noise. |

Abbreviations: MetS, metabolic syndrome; CKD, chronic kidney disease; SNHL, sensorineural hearing loss; HL, hearing loss; DM, diabetes mellitus; HTN, hypertension; BMI, body mass index; WHR, waist hip ratio; HDL, high density lipoprotein; TG, triglyceride.

*2.5. Statistics*

Subjects were divided into two groups, those with and without metabolic syndrome, for analysis of clinical results, and into six groups by age, 20s, 30s, 40s, 50s, 60s, and 70s and over, for analysis of average hearing threshold and degree of hearing loss. To evaluate risk factors related to hearing loss, subgroups were classified according to the number of factors corresponding to the diagnostic criteria for metabolic syndrome. Continuous variables were compared by t-tests and categorical variables by chi-square tests and Fisher's exact tests. Normal and adjusted odds ratios (ORs) of the relationships of hearing loss with age and number of factors of metabolic syndrome were analyzed by univariate and multivariate logistic regression analyses. All statistical analyses were performed using IBM SPSS version 22 (IBM Corp., Armonk, NY, USA), with $p$ values < 0.05 defined as statistically significant.

## 3. Results

Of the 94,223 subjects, 11,414 (12.1%) had metabolic syndrome and 82,809 (87.9%) did not. The mean ages of these two subgroups were 46.1 and 43.9 years, respectively. Of the 11,414 subjects with metabolic syndrome, 8255 (72.3%) were men, whereas, of the 82,809 subjects without metabolic syndrome, 45,200 (54.5%) were men, making the percentage of men significantly higher in subjects with metabolic syndrome ($p < 0.001$). Waist circumference, BP, and triglyceride and fasting blood glucose concentrations were all significantly higher in subjects with metabolic syndrome than in subjects without it. ($p < 0.001$) (Table 2).

**Table 2.** Demographic characteristics of study subjects.

|  |  | Non-MetS | | MetS | | p-Value |
|---|---|---|---|---|---|---|
|  |  | n or Mean | % or SD | n or Mean | % or SD |  |
| Age | | 43.91 | 9.42 | 46.12 | 9.30 | <0.0001 *,a |
| Sex | Male | 45,157 | (54.53%) | 8253 | (72.31%) | <0.0001 *,b |
|  | Female | 37,652 | (45.47%) | 3161 | (27.69%) |  |
| Waist circumference | | 82.00 | 7.86 | 93.40 | 8.15 | <0.0001 *,a |
| Systolic blood pressure | | 116.39 | 11.18 | 127.91 | 11.97 | <0.0001 *,a |
| Diastolic blood pressure | | 70.96 | 8.99 | 79.11 | 9.29 | <0.0001 *,a |
| HDL | | 61.84 | 15.62 | 45.79 | 11.83 | <0.0001 *,a |
| TG | | 107.12 | 64.92 | 233.77 | 141.82 | <0.0001 *,a |
| FPG | | 90.89 | 14.14 | 109.39 | 28.33 | <0.0001 *,a |
| BMI | | 23.26 | 3.00 | 27.50 | 3.24 | <0.0001 *,a |

Abbreviations: MetS, metabolic syndrome; Non-MetS, without metabolic syndrome; HDL, high density lipoprotein cholesterol; TG, triglyceride; FPG, fasting plasma glucose; BMI, body mass index. * p values between Non-MetS and MetS were tested using the t-test [a] and chi-square [b]. * Statistically significant. $p < 0.05$.

A comparison of hearing thresholds by age in subjects with and without metabolic syndrome showed that the average pure tone hearing thresholds were significantly higher in subjects with metabolic syndrome than in subjects without it in all age groups. ($p < 0.001$) (Figure 1). In addition, comparisons by age group confirmed that the percentages of subjects with hearing loss were higher in subjects with metabolic syndrome than in subjects without metabolic syndrome, and there was a significant statistical difference in the groups in their 30s, 40s, and 50s. ($p < 0.05$) (Table 3).

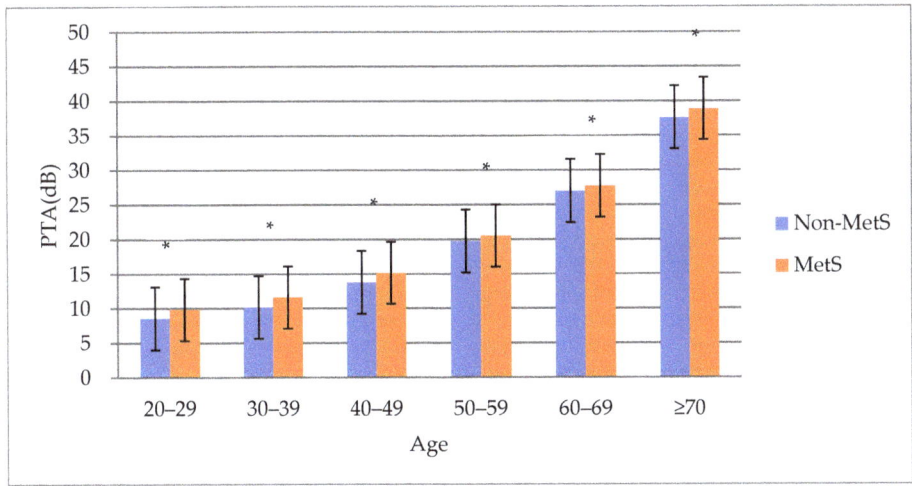

**Figure 1.** PTA threshold according to age. Abbreviations: MetS, metabolic syndrome; Non–MetS, without metabolic syndrome; PTA, pure tone audiometry. * Statistically significant. $p < 0.05$.

Subjects in this study were divided into subgroups according to the number of components belonging to the diagnostic criteria for metabolic syndrome, and the proportions of subjects diagnosed with hearing loss in each group were compared. Rates of hearing loss in subjects with 0, 1, 2, 3, 4, and 5 of the components of metabolic syndrome were 7.9%, 12.1%, 13.8%, 13.8%, 15.5%, and 16.3%, respectively, indicating a significant association between the number of components of metabolic syndrome and the rate of hearing loss. ($p < 0.0001$) (Table 4).

Table 3. Comparison of hearing by age groups in MetS and non-MetS subjects.

| Age (Years) | Non-MetS | | | | | MetS | | | | | p-Value [a] |
|---|---|---|---|---|---|---|---|---|---|---|---|
| | Normal | | Hearing Loss | | Total | Normal | | Hearing Loss | | Total | |
| 20–29 | 4645 | (99.06%) | 44 | (0.94%) | 4689 | 272 | (98.19%) | 5 | (1.81%) | 277 | 0.1943 |
| 30–39 | 20,996 | (97.78%) | 477 | (2.22%) | 21,473 | 2309 | (96.81%) | 76 | (3.19%) | 2385 | 0.0041 * |
| 40–49 | 32,068 | (92.98%) | 2422 | (7.02%) | 34,490 | 4465 | (91.48%) | 416 | (8.52%) | 4881 | 0.0002 * |
| 50–59 | 14,199 | (79.26%) | 3715 | (20.74%) | 17,914 | 2316 | (76.84%) | 698 | (23.16%) | 3014 | 0.0028 * |
| 60–69 | 1828 | (56.86%) | 1387 | (43.14%) | 3215 | 341 | (53.36%) | 298 | (46.64%) | 639 | 0.1064 |
| ≥70 | 197 | (29.1%) | 480 | (70.9%) | 677 | 40 | (23.53%) | 130 | (76.47%) | 170 | 0.1532 |

Abbreviations: MetS: metabolic syndrome; Non-MetS, without metabolic syndrome. * p values between Non-MetS and MetS were tested using the Fisher's exact test [a]. * Statistically significant. $p < 0.05$.

Table 4. Comparison of the groups of subjects with normal hearing and hearing loss.

| | Subject Group | | | | | | p-Value [a,b] |
|---|---|---|---|---|---|---|---|
| | Normal Hearing (n) | | | Hearing Loss (n) | | | |
| | n (%) | PTA(dB) | SD | n (%) | PTA(dB) | SD | |
| Non-MetS | 38,069 (92.0%) | 11.11 | 4.96 | 3293 (7.9%) | 38.70 | 15.44 | <0.0001 * |
| Non-MetS (1 factor) | 22,635 (87.9%) | 12.25 | 5.22 | 3109 (12.1%) | 38.72 | 14.75 | <0.0001 * |
| Non-MetS (2 factors) | 13,272 (86.2%) | 12.84 | 5.23 | 2123 (13.8%) | 38.16 | 13.83 | <0.0001 * |
| MetS (3 factors) | 6900 (86.2%) | 13.19 | 5.20 | 1098 (13.8%) | 37.79 | 13.56 | <0.0001 * |
| MetS (4 factors) | 2396 (84.5%) | 13.34 | 5.12 | 438 (15.5%) | 37.56 | 13.56 | <0.0001 * |
| MetS (5 factors) | 449 (83.7%) | 13.65 | 5.28 | 87 (16.3%) | 38.86 | 12.95 | <0.0001 * |

Results are reported as mean ± SD or as n (%). Abbreviations: MetS, metabolic syndrome; Non-MetS, without metabolic syndrome; PTA, pure tone audiometry. * p values between Normal hearing and Hearing loss were tested using the t-test [a] and chi-square [b]. * Statistically significant. $p < 0.05$.

To correct for the effects of age and gender on the relationship between BMI (Body Mass Indx) and hearing loss, multivariate analysis was performed to determine the normal and corrected odds ratios of hearing loss. The odds ratio of hearing loss was 1.89-fold higher in women than in men, and it was 1.13-fold higher as age increased by 1 year ($p < 0.0001$). Relative to subjects with 0 components of metabolic syndrome, the odds ratios of hearing loss in subjects with 3, 4, and 5 components of metabolic syndrome were 1.06 ($p = 0.1119$), 1.29 ($p < 0.0001$), and 1.21 ($p = 0.1410$), respectively (Table 5).

Table 5. Crude and adjusted odds ratios of hearing loss among subjects with metabolic syndrome.

| | Univariable Analysis | | | | Multivariable Analysis [a] | | | |
|---|---|---|---|---|---|---|---|---|
| | OR | 95% CI | | p-Value [a] | OR | 95% CI | | p-Value [b] |
| Sex | 1.97 | 1.89 | 2.06 | <0.0001 * | 1.89 | 1.80 | 1.99 | <0.0001 * |
| Age | 1.13 | 1.13 | 1.14 | <0.0001 * | 1.13 | 1.13 | 1.14 | <0.0001 * |
| MetS (3 factors) | 1.38 | 1.29 | 1.48 | <0.0001 * | 1.06 | 0.99 | 1.14 | 0.1119 |
| MetS (4 factors) | 1.59 | 1.43 | 1.76 | <0.0001 * | 1.29 | 1.15 | 1.44 | <0.0001 * |
| MetS (5 factors) | 1.68 | 1.34 | 2.12 | <0.0001 * | 1.21 | 0.94 | 1.56 | 0.1410 |

Abbreviations: MetS, metabolic syndrome; OR, odds ratio; CI, confidence interval. * p values were tested using univariate [a] and multivariate [b] logistic regression analyses. * Statistically significant. $p < 0.05$. [a] Including the variables age, sex, and metabolic syndrome.

When analyzing the influence of each component of metabolic syndrome, the odds ratio of hearing loss was significantly higher in the group with four factors: waist circumference, blood pressure and triglyceride, and fasting blood sugar concentrations ($p < 0.0001$) (Table 6).

**Table 6.** Association between hearing loss and metabolic syndrome.

| Risk Factors | Univariable Analysis | | | Multivariable Analysis | | | |
|---|---|---|---|---|---|---|---|
| | OR | 95% CI | | $p$-Value [a] | OR | 95% CI | | $p$-Value [b] |
| Waist circumference | 0.96 | 0.92 | 1.01 | 0.1003 | 1.09 | 1.04 | 1.15 | 0.0009 * |
| Systolic BP | 1.72 | 1.64 | 1.80 | <0.0001 * | 1.12 | 1.06 | 1.18 | <0.0001 * |
| Triglyceride level | 1.25 | 1.19 | 1.31 | <0.0001 * | 1.08 | 1.03 | 1.13 | 0.0037 * |
| HDL-C level | 1.20 | 1.13 | 1.28 | <0.0001 * | 1.05 | 0.98 | 1.12 | 0.1641 |
| FPG level | 2.14 | 2.05 | 2.24 | <0.0001 * | 1.14 | 1.09 | 1.20 | <0.0001 * |

Abbreviations: Systolic BP, systolic blood pressure; HDL-C, high density lipoprotein cholesterol; FPG, fasting plasma glucose; OR, odds ratio; CI, confidence interval. * $p$ values were tested using univariate [a] and multivariate [b] logistic regression analyses. * Statistically significant. $p < 0.05$.

## 4. Discussion

This cross-sectional study involving a large population assessed the relationship between metabolic syndrome and hearing loss. This study is based on health examination data for relatively healthy patients. In this study, 12.1% or 11,413 subjects met the diagnostic criteria for metabolic disease. First, due to the nature of this study, we cannot rule out the possibility that the study population was biased toward people interested in health. In addition, it is possible that there were fewer subjects who met the criteria for metabolic syndrome because at the time of assessment subjects may have been taking medications to control blood pressure, blood sugar, and/or other blood levels. However, the results of this study are meaningful because sufficient number of subjects, 94,223 was included.

To compare the incidence of hearing loss in adults with and without metabolic syndrome after adjustment for age, the rates of hearing loss were analyzed in subjects with 3, 4, and 5 of the components of metabolic syndrome, and the factors most closely related to hearing loss were identified.

The result of this study demonstrated an association between hearing loss and metabolic syndrome. The threshold of PTA was significantly higher in the group with metabolic syndrome in Table 2, and the rate of hearing loss was also higher in the group with metabolic syndrome in Table 3. In addition, Table 5 shows that although statistical significance was not observed for 3 and 5 factors in the multivariable analysis, this can be attributed to a decrease in the number of relevant groups, and the odds ratio of hearing loss tends to increase according to the number of metabolic syndrome factors. In particular, after adjustment for other factors, four specific components of metabolic syndrome—waist circumference, blood pressure, and triglyceride and fasting blood glucose concentrations—were strongly associated with hearing loss.

Although the mechanism(s) underlying the correlation between metabolic syndrome and hearing impairment remain undetermined, peripheral vascular disorders may be associated with both of these conditions.

Analysis of data from the US National Nutrition Survey showed a link between hearing loss and high blood pressure [28]. Hypertension causes hemorrhage in the inner ear, leading to reductions in capillary blood flow and oxygen supply and resulting in progressive or sudden sensorineural hearing loss [29]. Hypertension also reduces blood flow by reducing the inner diameter of blood vessels in the inner ear through atherosclerosis [30].

Diabetes is associated with microvascular and neuropathy complications affecting the retina, kidneys, peripheral arteries, and peripheral nerves [31,32]. Pathological changes in diabetes can cause sensorineural hearing loss through damage to the blood vessels and nervous system of the inner ear. In autopsy studies of diabetic patients, changes in labyrinth artery, spiral ganglion, cochlear blood vessels, and cranial nerve 8 were observed [33]. Correlations have been observed between diabetes and hearing loss, [19,21,24] and high fasting blood glucose concentrations were found to be independently associated with hearing loss [7,34].

Recent studies have shown that increases in triglyceride concentrations are closely associated with reduced hearing function [35]. Vacuolar edema and degeneration of the vascular striatum were reported as pathological changes associated with dyslipidemia in guinea pigs fed a lipid-rich diet [36,37]. Decreased nitric oxide production and increased reactive oxygen levels due to dyslipidemia can lead to hearing damage [22,37–39]. Furthermore, HDL was shown to have anti-inflammatory, antioxidant, and anti-apoptotic effects that can attenuate the pathological changes caused by dyslipidemia [34,40] High TG/HDL ratio has been associated with hearing loss [23] as has low HDL [3].

Obesity has been associated with hearing loss in both humans and animals. Central obesity, increased waist circumference, and increased hearing threshold after BMI correction of the content of visceral adipose tissue were found to be related [20]. Obesity, as determined by BMI, has been associated with an increased risk of hearing loss [26]. Moreover, abdominal lipid-related factors were reported to be associated with hearing loss at specific frequency bands [25]. Abdominal adipose tissue has also been associated with hearing loss in women, [8] and weight-hip ratio (WHR) may be an indicator of the risk of hearing loss [18].

Seventeen previous studies have examined the relationship between metabolic diseases and hearing loss. Nine of these studies analyzed the correlation between the overall components of metabolic syndrome and hearing loss; four analyzed the correlations between indices such as BMI, WHR, and factors relevant to abdominal fats (FRA) and hearing loss; three analyzed the correlations of diabetes DM and HbA1c concentration with hearing loss, and one analyzed the correlation of TG/HDL ratio with hearing loss. Of these 17 studies, 12 were cross-sectional in design, two were prospective studies, two were retrospective studies, and one as a case-control study. Most of the study subjects were middle-aged.

One study reported that metabolic syndrome was related to high-frequency hearing loss in a noise-exposed population [27]. Two studies found that metabolic syndrome was related to hearing loss in elderly women [8,9]. Three studies reported the percentage of subjects with hearing loss increased as the number of diagnostic factors for metabolic syndrome increased, with the rate of hearing loss being high in patients with four or five factors [3,10,11]. A study in drivers from West Azerbaijan showed the importance of analyzing each component of metabolic syndrome, not metabolic syndrome itself, finding a correlation between each component of metabolic syndrome and hearing loss [12]. One study found that metabolic syndrome itself was not an independent risk factor for hearing loss; rather, increased fasting plasma glucose concentration was the only independent risk factor for hearing loss [22]. In comparison, another study found that metabolic syndrome itself and several of its specific components, such as central obesity, hyperglycemia, and low HDL, were positively associated with hearing loss [7].

Many studies have found a correlation between HDL and hearing loss. For example, one study in US adults found that low HDL correlated with hearing loss, with low HDL being most responsible for the correlation between hearing loss and metabolic syndrome. [3] Two studies in the Korean population reported that low HDL and high TG were highly correlated with hearing loss, [11,23] and one study in a Chinese population reported that hearing loss was positively correlated with low HDL, hyperglycemia, and central obesity [7].

Several studies also observed relationships between obesity-related anthropometric indices and hearing loss. For example, one study found that WHR may be a surrogate marker for predicting the risk of hearing loss, [18] whereas another study suggested that FRAs were associated with hearing loss at specific frequencies, as determined by sex and the presence of diabetes, and that visceral adipose tissue (VAT) is particularly important role for hearing [25]. Two studies found relationships between BMI and hearing loss, with one finding that underweight and severe obesity were associated with an increased prevalence of hearing loss in a Korean population, and the other reporting that overweight was associated with an increased risk of hearing loss in a Japanese population [26].

This study had several limitations. First, because it was a cross-sectional study, the causative relationships between hearing loss and components of metabolic syndrome could not be determined. Second, because these data were from health examinations, the correlation between the prevalence of metabolic syndrome and hearing loss could not be accurately determined. Third, this study did not evaluate subjects who received medical treatment for hearing loss, nor did it evaluate factors contributing to hearing loss, such as noise, ototoxic drugs, otitis media, and family history of hearing loss.

## 5. Conclusions

This cross-sectional study involving a large population analyzed the association between metabolic syndrome and hearing loss. Hearing loss showed a positive correlation with the number of diagnostic factors for metabolic syndrome, especially in subjects with four specific factors: high waist circumference, blood pressure, triglyceride concentration, and fasting blood glucose concentration.

This study highlights the importance of control of metabolic syndrome in management of hearing loss. Subjects with metabolic diseases should therefore undergo regular hearing tests and, if necessary, hearing rehabilitation along with the management and treatment of their metabolic diseases. In addition, patients and health professionals may not be aware of this information regarding association between metabolic syndrome and hearing loss; hence, this can be included in part of health education.

**Author Contributions:** Original draft preparation, writing—review and editing, and data curation, H.-S.R.; conceptualization, investigation, and data curation, M.-G.K. and D.-C.P.; methodology and resources, S.-H.K. and D.-W.K.; methodology and data curation, D.-C.P., S.-S.K., and D.-W.K.; conceptualization, writing—review and editing, and supervision, S.-G.Y. All authors have read and agreed to the published version of the manuscript.

**Funding:** This work was supported by the National Research Foundation of Korea (NRF) grant funded by the Korean government (NRF-2019R1A2C1086807).

**Institutional Review Board Statement:** The study was conducted according to the guidelines of the Declaration of Helsinki, and approved by the Institutional Review Board of Kyung Hee University Hospital (IRB No. 2019-07-065).

**Informed Consent Statement:** Patient consent was waived due to Cross-sectional design of this study.

**Data Availability Statement:** The data presented in this study are available on request from the corresponding author. The data are not publicly available because the health examination data of a private hospital was used.

**Conflicts of Interest:** The authors declare no conflict of interest.

## References

1. Cunningham, L.L.; Tucci, D.L. Hearing loss in adults. *N. Engl. J. Med.* **2017**, *377*, 2465–2473. [CrossRef] [PubMed]
2. Vos, T.; Flaxman, A.D.; Naghavi, M.; Lozano, R.; Michaud, C.; Ezzati, M.; Shibuya, K.; Salomon, J.A.; Abdalla, S.; Aboyans, V.; et al. Global, regional, and national incidence, prevalence, and years lived with disability for 301 acute and chronic diseases and injuries in 188 countries, 1990–2013: A systematic analysis for the Global Burden of Disease Study 2013. *Lancet* **2015**, *386*, 743–800. [CrossRef]
3. Sun, Y.-S.; Fang, W.-H.; Kao, T.-W.; Yang, H.-F.; Peng, T.-C.; Wu, L.-W.; Chang, Y.-W.; Chou, C.-Y.; Chen, W.-L. Components of metabolic syndrome as risk factors for hearing threshold shifts. *PLoS ONE* **2015**, *10*, e0134388. [CrossRef] [PubMed]
4. Alberti, K.; Zimmet, P.; Shaw, J. The metabolic syndrome—A new worldwide definition. *Lancet* **2005**, *366*, 1059–1062. [CrossRef]
5. Alberti, K.; Eckel, R.; Grundy, S.; Zimmet, P.; Cleeman, J.; Donato, K.; Fruchart, J.; James, W.; Loria, C.; Smith, S.C., Jr. Harmonizing the metabolic syndrome: A joint interim statement of the international diabetes federation task force on epidemiology and prevention; national heart, lung, and blood institute; American heart association; world heart federation; international atherosclerosis society; and international association for the study of obesity. *Circulation* **2009**, *120*, 1640–1645. [PubMed]
6. Malik, S.; Wong, N.; Franklin, S.; Kamath, T.; L'ltalien, G.; Pio, J.; Williams, G. Impact of the metabolic syndrome on mortality from coronary heart disease, cardiovascular disease, and all causes in United States adults. *Circulation* **2004**, *110*, 1245–1250. [CrossRef]
7. Han, X.; Wang, Z.; Wang, J.; Li, Y.; Hu, H.; Hu, Y.; Hu, Y.; Zhao, X.; Zhan, Y.; Yuan, J.; et al. Metabolic syndrome is associated with hearing loss among a middle-aged and older Chinese population: A cross-sectional study. *Ann. Med.* **2018**, *50*, 587–595. [CrossRef]
8. Kim, T.S.; Kim, E.H.; Chung, J.W. The association between age-related hearing impairment and metabolic syndrome in Korean women: 5-year follow-up observational study. *Metab. Syndr. Relat. Disord.* **2017**, *15*, 240–245. [CrossRef]

9. Kang, S.H.; Jung, D.J.; Cho, K.H.; Park, J.W.; Yoon, K.W.; Do, J.Y. The association between metabolic syndrome or chronic kidney disease and hearing thresholds in Koreans: The Korean National Health and Nutrition Examination Survey 2009-2012. *PLoS ONE* **2015**, *10*, e0120372. [CrossRef]
10. Shim, H.S.; Shin, H.J.; Kim, M.G.; Kim, J.S.; Jung, S.Y.; Kim, S.H.; Yeo, S.G. Metabolic syndrome is associated with hearing disturbance. *Acta Otolaryngol.* **2019**, *139*, 42–47. [CrossRef]
11. Jung, D.J.; Shin, H.J.; Kim, M.G.; Kim, J.S.; Jung, S.Y.; Kim, S.H.; Yeo, S.G. Association of metabolic syndrome with the incidence of hearing loss: A national population-based study. *PLoS ONE* **2019**, *14*, e0220370. [CrossRef]
12. Aghazadeh-Attari, J.; Mansorian, B.; Mirza-Aghazadeh-Attari, M.; Ahmadzadeh, J.; Mohebbi, I. Association between metabolic syndrome and sensorineural hearing loss: A cross-sectional study of 11,114 participants. *Diabetes Metab. Syndr. Obes.* **2017**, *10*, 459. [CrossRef]
13. National Cholesterol Education Program (US); Expert Panel on Detection & Treatment of High Blood Cholesterol in Adults. *Third Report of the National Cholesterol Education Program (NCEP) Expert Panel on Detection, Evaluation, and Treatment of High Blood Cholesterol in Adults (Adult Treatment Panel III)*; National Cholesterol Education Program (US): Washington, DC, USA, 2002.
14. Kim, K.S. A Review of Occupational Disease Certification Criteria for Noise-Induced Hearing Impairment. *Audiol. Speech Res.* **2017**, *13*, 265–271. [CrossRef]
15. Lee, Y.; Park, S.; Lee, S.J. Exploring Factors Related to Self-perceived Hearing Handicap in the Elderly with Moderate to Moderately-severe Hearing Loss. *Commun. Sci. Disord.* **2020**, *25*, 142–155. [CrossRef]
16. Shin, J.W.; Kim, S.W.; Kim, Y.W.; Jang, W.; Kim, B.H.; Lim, Y.S.; Park, S.W.; Cho, C.G. The Value of Posterior Semicircular Canal Function in Predicting Hearing Recovery of Sudden Sensorineural Hearing Loss. *Res. Vestib. Sci.* **2019**, *18*, 103–110. [CrossRef]
17. Kim, S.L.; Oh, S.J.; Kong, S.K.; Goh, E.K. Sudden Sensorineural Hearing Loss after Granulocyte-Colony Stimulating Factor Administration. *J. Clin. Otolaryngol. Head Neck Surg.* **2018**, *29*, 87–90. [CrossRef]
18. Kang, S.H.; Jung, D.J.; Lee, K.Y.; Choi, E.W.; Do, J.Y. Comparison of various anthropometric indices as risk factors for hearing impairment in Asian women. *PLoS ONE* **2015**, *10*, e0143119. [CrossRef]
19. Bener, A.; Al-Hamaq, A.; Abdulhadi, K.; Salahaldin, A.; Gansan, L. Interaction between diabetes mellitus and hypertension on risk of hearing loss in highly endogamous population. *Diabetes Metab. Synd.* **2017**, *11*, S45–S51. [CrossRef]
20. Kim, S.H.; Won, Y.S.; Kim, M.G.; Baek, Y.J.; Oh, I.H.; Yeo, S.G. Relationship between obesity and hearing loss. *Acta Otolaryngol.* **2016**, *136*, 1046–1050. [CrossRef]
21. Kang, S.H.; Jung, D.J.; Choi, E.W.; Park, J.W.; Cho, K.H.; Yoon, K.W.; Do, J.Y. Association between HbA1c level and hearing impairment in a nondiabetic adult population. *Metb. Synd. Relat. Disord.* **2016**, *14*, 129–134. [CrossRef]
22. Heinrich, U.-R.; Helling, K. Nitric oxide–a versatile key player in cochlear function and hearing disorders. *Nitric Oxide* **2012**, *27*, 106–116. [CrossRef] [PubMed]
23. Jung, D.J.; Do, J.Y.; Cho, K.H.; Kim, A.Y.; Kang, S.H. Association between triglyceride/high-density lipoprotein ratio and hearing impairment in a Korean population. *Postgrad. Med.* **2017**, *129*, 943–948. [CrossRef] [PubMed]
24. Nwosu, J.N.; Chime, E.N. Hearing thresholds in adult Nigerians with diabetes mellitus: A case–control study. *Diabetes Metab. Syndr. Obes. Targets Ther.* **2017**, *10*, 155. [CrossRef] [PubMed]
25. Lee, Y.; Park, M. Relationships among factors relevant to abdominal fat and age-related hearing loss. *Clin. Exp. Otorhinolaryngol.* **2017**, *10*, 309. [CrossRef]
26. Hu, H.; Tomita, K.; Kuwahara, K.; Yamamoto, M.; Uehara, A.; Kochi, T.; Eguchi, M.; Okazaki, H.; Hori, A.; Sasaki, N. Obesity and risk of hearing loss: A prospective cohort study. *Clin. Nutr.* **2020**, *39*, 870–875. [CrossRef]
27. Kim, J.; Cho, I.Y.; Yeo, Y.H.; Song, Y.M. Relationship between Metabolic Syndrome and Hearing Loss: Korea National Health and Nutritional Survey. *Korean J. Fam. Pract.* **2021**, *42*, 53. [CrossRef]
28. Agrawal, Y.; Platz, E.A.; Niparko, J.K. Prevalence of hearing loss and differences by demographic characteristics among US adults: Data from the National Health and Nutrition Examination Survey, 1999–2004. *Arch. Intern. Med.* **2008**, *168*, 1522–1530. [CrossRef]
29. Siegelaub, A.B.; Friedman, G.D.; Seltzer, C.C. Hearing loss in adults: Relation to age, sex, exposure to loud noise, and cigarette smoking. *Arch. Environ. Occup. Health* **1974**, *29*, 107–109. [CrossRef]
30. Bachor, E.; Selig, Y.K.; Jahnke, K.; Rettinger, G.; Karmody, C.S. Vascular variations of the inner ear. *Acta Otolaryngol.* **2001**, *121*, 35–41.
31. Centers for Disease Control and Prevention. *National Diabetes Statistics Report: Estimates of Diabetes and Its Burden in the United States 2014*; U.S. Department of Health and Human Services: Atlanta, GA, USA, 2014.
32. Cowie, C.C.; Rust, K.F.; Byrd-Holt, D.D.; Eberhardt, M.S.; Flegal, K.M.; Engelgau, M.M.; Saydah, S.H.; Williams, D.E.; Geiss, L.S.; Gregg, E.W. Prevalence of diabetes and impaired fasting glucose in adults in the US population: National Health And Nutrition Examination Survey 1999–2002. *Diabetes Care* **2006**, *29*, 1263–1268. [CrossRef]
33. Makishima, K.; Tanaka, K. Pathological changes of the inner ear and central auditory pathway in diabetics. *Ann. Otol. Rhinol. Laryngol.* **1971**, *80*, 218–228. [CrossRef]
34. Lee, H.Y.; Choi, Y.J.; Choi, H.J.; Choi, M.S.; Chang, D.S.; Kim, A.Y.; Cho, C.S. Metabolic syndrome is not an independent risk factor for hearing impairment. *J. Nutr. Health Aging* **2016**, *20*, 816–824. [CrossRef]
35. Saito, T.; Sato, K.; Saito, H. An experimental study of auditory dysfunction associated with hyperlipoproteinemia. *Arch. Otorhinolaryngol.* **1986**, *243*, 242–245. [CrossRef]

36. Lüscher, T.F.; Landmesser, U.; von Eckardstein, A.; Fogelman, A. High-density lipoprotein: Vascular protective effects, dysfunction, and potential as therapeutic target. *Circ. Res.* **2014**, *114*, 171–182. [CrossRef]
37. Satar, B.; Ozkaptan, Y.; Surucu, H.; Ozturk, H. Ultrastructural effects of hypercholesterolemia on the cochlea. *Otol. Neurotol.* **2001**, *22*, 786–789. [CrossRef]
38. Brechtelsbauer, P.; Nuttall, A.; Miller, J. Basal nitric oxide production in regulation of cochlear blood flow. *Hear. Res.* **1994**, *77*, 38–42. [CrossRef]
39. Henderson, D.; Bielefeld, E.; Harris, K.; Hu, B. The role of oxidative stress in noise-induced hearing loss. *Ear Hear.* **2006**, *27*, 1–19. [CrossRef]
40. Rosenson, R.S.; Brewer, H., Jr.; Ansell, B.; Barter, P.; Chapman, M.; Heinecke, J.; Kontush, A.; Tall, A.; Webb, N. Translation of high-density lipoprotein function into clinical practice: Current prospects and future challenges. *Circulation* **2013**, *128*, 1256–1267. [CrossRef]

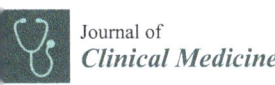 

*Article*

# Clinical and Genetic Characteristics of Finnish Patients with Autosomal Recessive and Dominant Non-Syndromic Hearing Loss Due to Pathogenic *TMC1* Variants

Minna Kraatari-Tiri [1,2], Maria K. Haanpää [3,4], Tytti Willberg [5], Pia Pohjola [4], Riikka Keski-Filppula [1,2], Outi Kuismin [1,2], Jukka S. Moilanen [1,2], Sanna Häkli [2,6] and Elisa Rahikkala [1,2,*]

1. Department of Clinical Genetics, Oulu University Hospital, 90029 Oulu, Finland; minna.kraatari@oulu.fi (M.K.-T.); riikka.keski-filppula@ppshp.fi (R.K.-F.); outi.kuismin@ppshp.fi (O.K.); jukka.moilanen@oulu.fi (J.S.M.)
2. PEDEGO Research Unit, Medical Research Center Oulu, Oulu University Hospital, and University of Oulu, 90014 Oulu, Finland; sanna.hakli@ppshp.fi
3. Department of Clinical Genetics, Turku University Hospital, 20521 Turku, Finland; maria.haanpaa@tyks.fi
4. Department of Genomics, Turku University Hospital, 20521 Turku, Finland; pia.pohjola@tyks.fi
5. Department of Otorhinolaryngology, Turku University Hospital, 20521 Turku, Finland; tytti.willberg@tyks.fi
6. Department of Otorhinolaryngology, Oulu University Hospital, 90029 Oulu, Finland
* Correspondence: elisa.rahikkala@ppshp.fi; Tel.: +358-8-315-3218; Fax: +358-8-315-3105

**Abstract:** Sensorineural hearing loss (SNHL) is one of the most common sensory deficits worldwide, and genetic factors contribute to at least 50–60% of the congenital hearing loss cases. The transmembrane channel-like protein 1 (*TMC1*) gene has been linked to autosomal recessive (DFNB7/11) and autosomal dominant (DFNA36) non-syndromic hearing loss, and it is a relatively common genetic cause of SNHL. Here, we report eight Finnish families with 11 affected family members with either recessively inherited homozygous or compound heterozygous *TMC1* variants associated with congenital moderate-to-profound hearing loss, or a dominantly inherited heterozygous *TMC1* variant associated with postlingual progressive hearing loss. We show that the *TMC1* c.1534C>T, p.(Arg512*) variant is likely a founder variant that is enriched in the Finnish population. We describe a novel recessive disease-causing *TMC1* c.968A>G, p.(Tyr323Cys) variant. We also show that individuals in this cohort who were diagnosed early and received timely hearing rehabilitation with hearing aids and cochlear implants (CI) have reached good speech perception in noise. Comparison of the genetic data with the outcome of CI rehabilitation increases our understanding of the extent to which underlying pathogenic gene variants explain the differences in CI rehabilitation outcomes.

**Keywords:** *TMC1*; hearing loss; cochlear implant; hearing rehabilitation; congenital

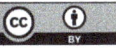

## 1. Introduction

Congenital moderate-to-profound bilateral sensorineural hearing loss (SNHL) affects at least 1 in 1000 infants [1], making SNHL is one of the most common sensory deficits worldwide. In developed countries, genetic hearing loss accounts for at least 50–60% of childhood hearing loss cases [2]. Inherited SNHL is often an isolated physical finding (non-syndromic SNHL) [3]. To date, more than 120 genes have been identified in association with monogenic non-syndromic hearing loss (https://hereditaryhearingloss.org/, accessed on 20 February 2022). In addition, hearing loss is associated with at least 400 different syndromes [4].

The transmembrane channel-like protein 1 (*TMC1*) gene encodes a transmembrane protein that acts as a component of the mechanotransduction channel in the auditory and vestibular hair cells of the inner ear [5]. *TMC1/2* mutant mice have no mechanosensitive current [6]. TMC1 is located at the tips of stereocilia of hair cells, where transduction occurs [7]. Pathogenic variants in *TMC1* alter the biophysical properties of hair cell mechanosensory transduction [8]. *TMC1* has been linked to autosomal recessive non-syndromic severe-to-profound hearing loss (DFNB7/11, OMIM #600974) and autosomal dominant late-onset progressive hearing loss (DFNA36, OMIM #606705) [9]. *TMC1* is a relatively common genetic cause of SNHL and accounts for 0.5–8.1% of patients with autosomal recessive SNHL (ARSNHL) in different ethnic populations [10–12].

In this study, we report eight Finnish families with 11 affected family members with recessively inherited homozygous, recessively inherited compound heterozygous, or dominantly inherited heterozygous *TMC1* variants.

## 2. Materials and Methods

### 2.1. Patient Recruitment

All individuals and their family members with pathogenic or likely pathogenic *TMC1* variants were contacted about the study, and all patients or their guardians gave their written informed consent for the research. The study was approved by the ethical review committee of Oulu University Hospital (EETTMK: 186/2020).

The patients were recruited from the departments of clinical genetics in Oulu University Hospital (Patients 1–8) and Turku University Hospital (Patients 9–11). In both clinics, genetic testing is offered to all children receiving a diagnosis of hearing loss, and to adults with hearing loss of unknown cause as a part of diagnostics.

### 2.2. Familial and Clinical Examination

The available medical records, as well as familial and clinical history, were evaluated. Eight (N = 8/11) affected individuals underwent an audiometry at 125–8000 Hz. Otoacoustic emission (OAE) testing (N = 6/11), transient evoked OAE (TEOAE) (N = 2/11), auditory brainstem response (ABR) (N = 6/11), and automated auditory brainstem response (AABR) (N = 2/11) were performed for the young individuals. These were not performed for the older individuals due to availability of the screening and different practices. Seven (N = 7/11) affected individuals underwent a speech-in-noise test. Speech perception was evaluated using spoken language; the adults conducted the Finnish matrix sentence test (FMST) and the children conducted the simplified Finnish matrix sentence test (FINSIMAT). Computed tomography (CT) scans and magnetic resonance imaging (MRI) were performed on those patients who had cochlear implants (CIs). The patients were subsequently referred to the Department of Clinical Genetics for pedigree construction and genetic evaluations.

### 2.3. Genetic Testing and Data Analysis

Peripheral blood samples were collected from available and consenting individuals, and genomic DNA was extracted using automated QIAsymphony device and Qiagen Qiasymphony DSP DNA Midi kit (Qiagen, Hilden, Germany). Traditionally, *GJB2* testing is performed before large gene panels. Six affected individuals were screened for pathogenic variants of *GJB2* by Sanger sequencing, with negative results.

Exome based hearing loss gene panels have been conducted over a period of last six years as part of clinical diagnostics. The gene panels performed vary depending on the laboratory where the test is conducted and the year the test is ordered. An exome-based next generation sequencing (NGS) hearing loss gene panels were performed in the Laboratory of Genome Diagnostics in Nijmegen, the Netherlands (gene panel versions DG-2.5 and DG-2.8) for two patients; Blueprint Genetics, Espoo, Finland (Comprehensive Hearing Loss and Deafness gene panel, version 6, 22 February 2020) for two patients; Tyks Genomics, Laboratory medicine, Turku, Finland for two patients, and Nordlab Oulu, Finland for two patients. In three families (Families 3, 5, and 8) with multiple participating affected individuals, targeted variant testing by Sanger sequencing was performed after the pathogenic variant was identified in the proband. In families with compound heterozygous *TMC1* variants, Sanger sequencing of parental samples was performed to confirm that the variants are in trans in patients. No other clinically relevant variants were found in the genetic testing.

## 3. Results

### 3.1. Clinical Characteristics of the Patients

The clinical characteristics of the affected cases for each family included in this study are summarized in Table 1, and the pedigrees are shown in Figure 1. Eleven affected individuals from eight different Finnish families were recruited for the study. Four were males, and seven were females, and their ages ranged between 0 and 57 years.

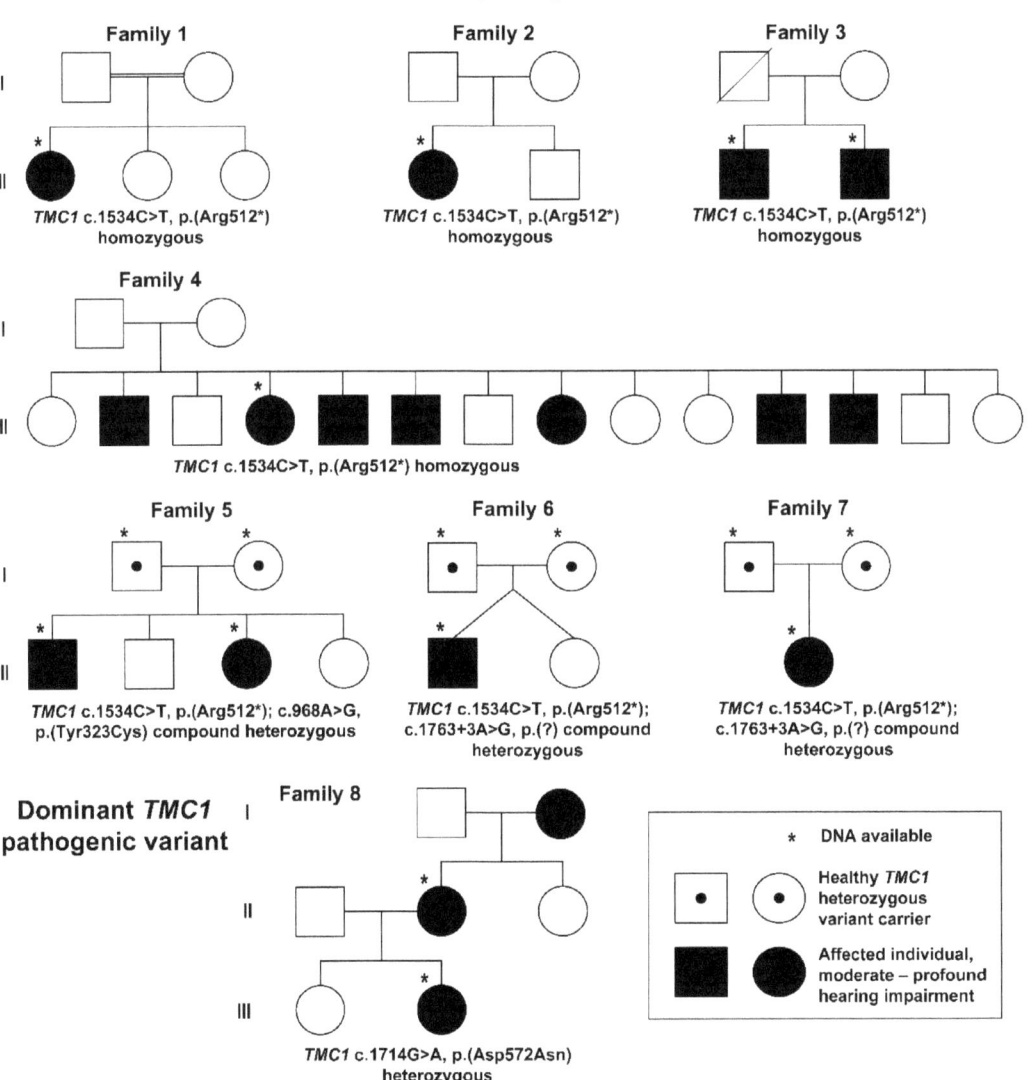

**Figure 1.** Pedigrees of the families in two (I–II) or three (I–III) generations. In six families, the *TMC1* c.1534C>T, p.(Arg512*); c.968A>G, p.(Tyr323Cys), and c.1763+3A>G, p.(?) variants segregated recessively. All the affected individuals showed profound congenital deafness. In one family, a dominantly inherited *TMC1* c.1714G>A, p.(Asp572Asn) segregated with the phenotype.

**Table 1.** Clinical characteristics of patients. Patients 1–9 had recessively inherited sensorineural hearing loss associated with biallelic pathogenic recessive *TMC1* variants. Patients 10 and 11 had a dominantly inherited hearing loss associated with a heterozygous pathogenic *TMC1* variant.

| | Patient 1 | Patient 2 | Patient 3 | Patient 4 | Patient 5 | Patient 6 | Patient 7 | Patient 8 | Patient 9 | Patient 10 | Patient 11 |
|---|---|---|---|---|---|---|---|---|---|---|---|
| Family | 1 | 2 | 3 | 3 | 4 | 5 | 5 | 6 | 7 | 8 | 8 |
| Current age | 21 | 5 | 42 | 46 | 53 | 23 | 18 | 7 | 0 | 57 | 21 |
| Sex | F | F | M | M | F | M | F | M | F | F | F |
| Genotype | c.1534C>T, p.(Arg512*), homozygous | c.1534C>T, p.(Arg512*), homozygous | c.1534C>T, p.(Arg512*), homozygous | c.1534C>T, p.(Arg512*), homozygous | c.1534C>T, p.(Arg512*), homozygous | c.1534C>T, p.(Arg512*) and c.968A>G, p.(Tyr323Cys) | c.1534C>T, p.(Arg512*) and c.968A>G, p.(Tyr323Cys) | c.1534C>T, p.(Arg512*) and c.1763+3A>G | c.1534C>T, p.(Arg512*) and c.1763+3A>G | c.1714G>A, p.(Asp572Asn) heterozygous | c.1714G>A, p.(Asp572Asn) heterozygous |
| Newborn screening | Abnormal | Abnormal | NA | NA | NA | NA | Abnormal | Abnormal | Abnormal | NA | NA |
| OAE | No response | No response | NA | NA | NA | No response | No response | No response | No response | NA | NA |
| TEOAE | NA | NA | NA | NA | NA | NA | NA | NA | No response | NA | NA |
| AABR | NA | No response | NA | NA | NA | NA | NA | NA | No response | NA | NA |
| ABR (dB) | No response | l.dx: no response/l.sin: 90 (4 kHz) and click 85 | NA | NA | NA | No response | No response | No response | Cochlear microphonics at 85, no neural responses at 85 | NA | NA |
| Speech-in-noise test | SRS +10 dB SNR l.a. 99%, SRT l.dx. −8.0 dB SNR, SRT l.sin −8.6 dB SNR | SRT l.dx. −5,9 dB SNR, SRT l.sin −4.9 dB SNR, SRT l.a. −6.6 dB SNR | NA | NA | NA | SRS +10 dB SNR l.a. 75%, SRT l.dx −2.3 dB SNR, SRT l.a. −3.4 dB SNR | SRS +10 dB SNR l.a. 100%, SRT l.dx −7.6 dB SNR, SRT l.a. −6.6 / −7.6 dB SNR | SRT l.dx −6.3 dB SNR, SRT l.sin −4.9 dB SNR, SRT l.a. −6.2 dB SNR | NA | SRS +10 dB SNR l.a. 94%, SRT l.sin. −1.3 dB SNR, SRT l.dx. −2.0 dB SNR, SRT l.a. −2.8 dB SNR | SRS +10 dB SNR l.a. 88%, SRT l.a. +0.4 dB SNR |
| Age at diagnosis | 7 m | 2 m | From birth | 1 y 8 m | From birth | From birth | 1 m | 8 m | From birth | 7 y | 7 y |
| Severity | Profound | Profound | Profound | Profound | Profound | Profound | Profound | Profound | Profound | Profound | Severe |
| Progression | No | No | No | No | No | No | No | No | No | Yes | Yes |
| Hearing aids (from the age) | Yes (7 m) | Yes (4 m) | No | No | Yes (1.5 y) | Yes (1 y 4 m) | Yes (3 m) | Yes (9 m) | Yes (4 m) | No | Yes |
| Cochlear implant (from the age) | Yes (1 y 5 m (right) and 13 y (left)) | Yes (1 y) | No | No | No | Yes (2 y 1 m (right) and 20 y 9 m (left)) | Yes (1 y (right) and 15 y 5 m (left)) | Yes (1 y 5 m (right) and 1y6m (left)) | Planned (8–9 m) | Yes (41 y (left) and 51 y (right)) | No |
| Balance problems | No | No | No | No | No | Yes | No | No | NA | No | No |
| Language perception | Good progress with CI use | Good progress with CI use | Sign language | Sign language | Sign language | Good progress with CI use | Good progress with CI use | Good progress with CI use | NA | Normal spoken language | Normal spoken language |

Abbreviations: OAE, otoacoustic emission; TEOAE, transient evoked OAE; ABR, auditory brainstem response; AABR, automated ABR; SRS, speech recognition score; SNR, signal-to-noise ratio; SRT, speech reception threshold; CI, cochlear implant; l.a., both sides; l.dx, right side; l.sin, left side.

In the families with a recessive pattern of inheritance (Families 1–7), the hearing loss was congenital. Three individuals (Patients 3–5 from Families 3 and 4) were born before the start of the newborn hearing screening program, and before CIs were available. Their hearing aid benefit was limited, and they all use sign language as their primary mode of communication. The newborn screenings were abnormal in all tested cases (N = 5/5, 100%), the OAE and TEOAE showed no responses (N = 6/6, 100% and N = 2/2, 100%, respectively), and the ABR was abnormal in all tested cases (N = 6/6, 100%). An audiogram revealed a bilateral profound SNHL in all the affected individuals (Figure 2A–F). One individual reported a balance problem, but his motor development was normal. The ophthalmological examination revealed one individual with deuteranopia and one individual with esophoria and hyperopia. Imaging studies were unremarkable. Seven individuals were fitted with hearing aids (between 3 months to 1.5 years of age) but obtained limited benefits. Bilateral simultaneous or consecutive CIs were later implanted in five individuals at the ages of 12 months to 2 years, and bilateral simultaneous CIs are planned for the youngest individual at the age of 8–9 months. All implanted patients showed good progress in language acquisition. In the best-aided condition (bilateral CIs), in quiet, the speech recognition scores ranged from 75% to 100%. The two youngest patients, who were tested with the FINSIMAT, had speech reception thresholds (SRTs) of −6.6 dB signal-to-noise ratio (SNR) and −6.2 dB SNR. The best-aided SRTs for the adults, determined with the FMST, ranged from −3.4 dB SNR to −8.6 dB SNR.

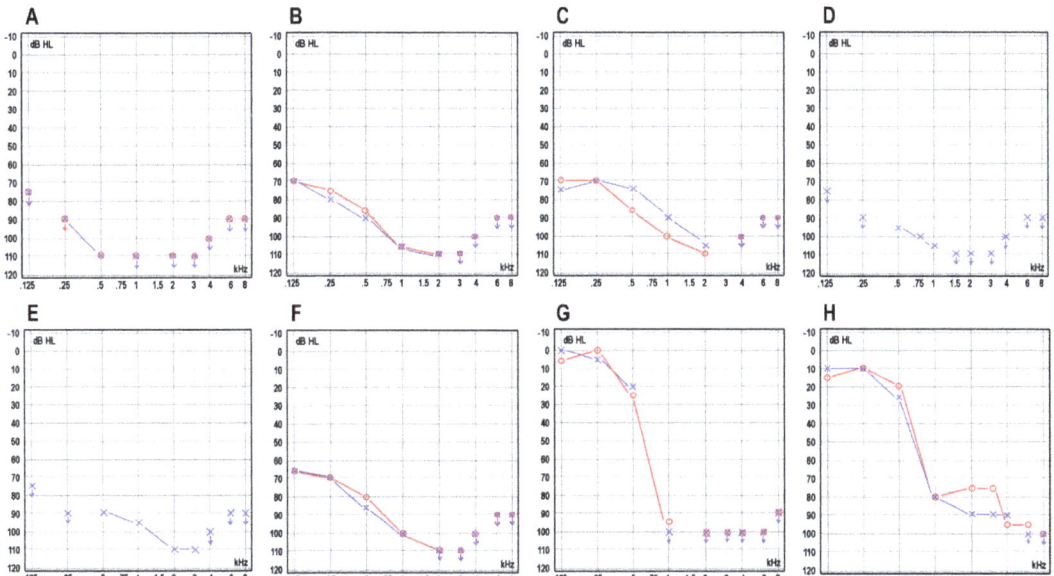

**Figure 2.** Pure tone audiograms (PTA) of the affected individuals. (**A**) Patient 1, (**B**) Patient 3, (**C**) Patient 5, (**D**) Patient 6, (**E**) Patient 7, and (**F**) Patient 8. All six of these patients showed severe-to-profound sensorineural hearing loss and mildly down-sloping curves associated with recessive pathogenic *TMC1* variants. (**G**) Patient 10 and (**H**) Patient 11 had deeply down-sloping curves, demonstrating predominant deterioration of higher frequencies associated with a dominant pathogenic *TMC1* variant. In all patients, the last available audiograms are shown. Patients 3, 5, and 11 have not received CIs. In Patients 1, 6, and 7, the audiograms shown are after the first, but before the second CI operation. In Patient 8 the audiogram shown is after bilateral CI operations. In Patient 10, the audiogram shown is before the CI operation. The red circles indicate the right ear and the blue X's indicate the left ear.

In family 8, with dominant inheritance, the onset of hearing loss was postlingual and was diagnosed at the age of 7 years. The hearing loss was progressive, and audiograms revealed down-sloping curves (Figure 2G,H). The older affected individual benefited from CIs, which she received in her left ear at the age of 41 and in her right ear at the age of 51. Her best-aided SRT with FMST was −2.8 dB SNR. The younger affected individual has been offered CIs but currently prefers to use hearing aids. Her best-aided SRT with the FMST was +0.4 dB SNR.

*3.2. Genetic Results*

Five individuals from families 1 to 4 were homozygous for the *TMC1* (NM_138691.3) c.1534C>T, p.(Arg512*) (hg38: chr9:72792320C>T, rs200171616) variant, which was classified as pathogenic according to the ACMG guidelines (PVS1, PM2, PP3, and PP5) [13]. This variant has previously been reported in the medical literature [9,14]. Two individuals from family 5 were compound heterozygous for the *TMC1* (NM_138691.3) variants c.1534C>T, p.(Arg512*) and c.968A>G, p.(Tyr323Cys) (hg38: chr9:72788422A>G, rs746724027). The latter is classified as likely pathogenic, according to the ACMG guidelines (PM2, PM3, PP1, and PP3), and, to the authors' knowledge, this variant has not yet been reported in the literature. Parental testing revealed that the variants were in different alleles. Two affected individuals from families 6 and 7 were compound heterozygous for the *TMC1* (NM_138691.3) variants c.1534C>T, p.(Arg512*) and c.1763+3A>G, p.(?) (hg38: chr9:72816213A>G, rs370898981). The latter is classified as pathogenic according to the ACMG guidelines (PS3, PM3, and PM2). *TMC1* c.1763+3A>G has previously been reported in the medical literature [15,16]. Parental testing revealed that the variants were in different alleles.

Two individuals from family 8 were heterozygous for the *TMC1* (NM_138691.3) c.1714G>A, p.(Asp572Asn), (hg38: chr9:72816161G>A, rs121908072). This heterozygous *TMC1* variant and severe hearing loss segregated dominantly in this family. *TMC1* c.1714G>A, p.(Asp572Asn) is classified as pathogenic according to the ACMG guidelines (PP5, PM1, PM2, and PM5).

## 4. Discussion

In this study, we reported nine individuals from seven Finnish families with congenital ARSNHL and biallelic TMC1 variants. We also reported two individuals from one Finnish family with autosomal dominant SNHL (ADSNHL) and a heterozygous TMC1 variant. All the affected individuals with recessively inherited TMC1 variants displayed severe-to-profound congenital hearing loss associated with down-sloping audiograms, where higher frequencies are the most severely affected. This is consistent with previous publications demonstrating that pathogenic recessive TMC1 variants cause moderate-to-profound hearing loss [17–20]. The individuals affected with ADSNHL displayed progressive postlingual sensorineural hearing loss that led to profound deafness and the need for CIs. In the previous publications, ADSNHL cases showed postlingual-onset progressive hearing loss, with predominant deterioration in the higher frequencies [18–21]. Only 1 of the 11 affected individuals in the present study had balance problems. This finding is in line with previous studies that found no vestibular symptoms associated with TMC1-associated HL cases [18,19].

Previous work has shown variable auditory outcome in patients with pathogenic biallelic *TMC1* variants [19,21–23]. Most reports are small case series with heterogeneous samples, which makes it difficult to assess the full effect of a particular genotype. Recent study reported three patients with pathogenic compound heterozygous *TMC1* variants demonstrating excellent functional outcome after CIs [22]. Interestingly, one of the patients in this study was compound heterozygous for the Finnish enriched *TMC1* c.1534C>T, p.(Arg512*) variant [22]. Another study reported 19 patients from 12 consanguineous Saudi families with pathogenic homozygous *TMC1* variants with variable auditory outcome after CIs [19]. In the latter study, both excellent and poor results were reported for individuals with the same variants emphasizing that a significant proportion of the variance in outcomes can be due to social and environmental factors, as well as other known explanatory factors such as the duration of the deafness before the CI operation.

In our study population, the individuals who had access to CIs in early childhood, and received timely hearing rehabilitation with hearing aids and CIs, have reached a good speech perception in quiet and in noise. No age-specific reference values have been established for children for the FINSIMAT, but the two youngest individuals in the present study had SRTs in a range similar to that of typically performing early implanted CI users of their age (Willberg, personal communication). The older, early implanted CI users also reached good speech perception. The average SRT for a bilateral CI user with the FMST was −5.4 dB SNR in a large, unselected group of Finnish CI users [24]. Two of the early implanted individuals in the present study reached an even better SRT, and another individual had a SRT of −3.4 dB, which can still be considered an adequate CI rehabilitation result. Similar to the outcomes from Gallo et al. [22], our outcomes are comparable to the outcomes of individuals with *GJB2*-associated DFNB1 [25]. Both individuals with ADSNHL had poorer speech perception in noise than the early implanted individuals with ARSNHL. For the younger individual, this was most likely due to insufficient amplification with hearing aids. For the older individual, the poor SRT may be a result of prolonged deafness in the high-frequency region before the CI rehabilitation.

Even though CIs have been highly successful in restoring hearing in severe and profound hearing loss, the rehabilitation results remain highly variable with a significant proportion of the variance still unexplained [26,27]. Implementation of large gene panels and exome sequencing in clinical practice has allowed frequent detection of causative pathogenic variants in patients with hearing loss. Comparing this etiological data systematically with the outcome of CI rehabilitation, especially with speech perception measures in noise, as they are sensitive to minor differences in functional hearing, we can increase our understanding of the extent to which the underlying pathogenic gene variants explain the differences in the CI rehabilitation outcomes.

The *TMC1* c.1534C>T, p.(Arg512*) is enriched in the Finnish population, with a minor allele frequency (MAF) 24 times higher in Finns (0.003344) than in non-Finnish Europeans (0.0001395) (gnomAD v.2.1.1, https://gnomad.broadinstitute.org/, accessed on 20 February 2022) [28]. The expected number of *TMC1* c.1534C>T, p.(Arg512*) homozygote patients in Finland is $(0.003344)^2 \times 5.5$ million or approximately 62, and the carrier frequency of this pathogenic variant is approximately 1/300 in the Finnish population. In this cohort, the *TMC1* c.1534C>T, p.(Arg512*) variant was identified in 14 of the 18 alleles (78%) of the ARSNHL patients, and was in either a homozygous or a compound heterozygous state in all patients. Based on the gnomAD and clinical data, we suggest that the *TMC1* p.(Arg512*) variant is likely a Finnish founder variant. As hearing loss is genetically highly heterogeneous, additional similar variants will possibly be identified as enriched in the Finnish population.

The *TMC1* c.1534C>T, p.(Arg512*) causes a premature stop codon. It is predicted to cause a loss of normal protein function either through protein truncation (512 out of 760 aa) or nonsense-mediated mRNA decay. *TMC1* c.1763+3A>G, p.(?) is predicted to cause a splice site defect leading also to a loss-of-function of normal TMC1. *TMC1* c.968A>G, p.(Tyr323Cys) was identified in two affected individuals in a compound heterozygote state with a known pathogenic *TMC1* c.1534C>T, p.(Arg512*). The mother of these two affected individuals was a healthy heterozygous carrier of this *TMC1* c.968A>G, p.(Tyr323Cys) variant suggesting that *TMC1* c.968A>G, p.(Tyr323Cys) is a recessive variant leading to a functional null allele.

In contrast, *TMC1* c.1714G>A, p.(Asp572Asn) is a well-known dominantly acting *TMC1* variant [9,20,29,30]. Amino acid 572 in *TMC1* is a critical functional residue for pathogenic dominant variants [9,20,29,30]. Nucleotide 1714 of *TMC1* is located within the hypermutable CpG context, thereby explaining its location as a mutational hot spot and its occurrence in different populations [9,29,30]. Dominant variants are likely to confer a specific dominant negative or gain-of-function effect, leading to dominant inheritance [20], whereas pathogenic recessive *TMC1* variants create a functional null allele and lead to recessive inheritance through a loss-of-function mechanism. It has been proposed that two mechanisms link pathogenic *TMC1* channel variants and deafness: decreased $Ca^{2+}$ permeability to all pathogenic variants, and decreased resting open probability in low $Ca^{2+}$ confined to pathogenic dominant variants [31].

## 5. Conclusions

We identified *TMC1* variants c.1534C>T, p.(Arg512*), c.968A>G, p.(Tyr323Cys), and c.1763+3A>G, p.(?) with profound congenital ARSNHL in seven Finnish families, and *TMC1* c.1714G>A, p.(Asp572Asn) with postlingual progressive ADSNHL in one Finnish family. To the authors' knowledge, the *TMC1* c.968A>G, p.(Tyr323Cys) variant is a novel variant expanding the knowledge of the genotypic spectrum of pathogenic *TMC1* variants. We also showed that the *TMC1* c.1534C>T, p.(Arg512*) variant is the most prevalent variant enriched in the Finnish population, suggesting a founder effect. To the authors' knowledge, these are the first reported cases of *TMC1*-related SNHL in Finland.

Our study demonstrates that the individuals who had access to CIs in early childhood, and received timely hearing rehabilitation with hearing aids and CIs, have reached a good speech perception in quiet and in noise. Comparison of the genetic data with the outcome of CI rehabilitation increases our understanding of the extent to which underlying pathogenic gene variants explain the differences in CI rehabilitation outcomes. It is even possible that in the future patients can be stratified based on the underlying gene defect into categories that can predict their rehabilitation outcomes.

**Author Contributions:** Conceptualization: M.K.-T. and E.R.; Formal Analysis: M.K.-T.; Funding acquisition: J.S.M. and E.R.; Investigation: M.K.-T. and S.H.; Resources: M.K.-T., M.K.H., T.W., P.P., R.K.-F., O.K., S.H. and E.R.; Supervision: E.R.; Visualization: S.H. and E.R. Writing—original draft: M.K.-T., M.K.H., T.W. and E.R.; Writing—review and editing: M.K.-T., M.K.H., T.W., P.P., R.K.-F., O.K., J.S.M., S.H. and E.R. All authors have read and agreed to the published version of the manuscript.

**Funding:** This study was funded by Academy of Finland (grant number 338446), Uolevi Mäki Foundation, and the Competitive State Research Financing of the Expert Responsibility Area of Oulu University Hospital (grant number VTR K36733).

**Institutional Review Board Statement:** The study was conducted in accordance with the Declaration of Helsinki, and approved by the Ethics Committee of the Northern Ostrobothnia Hospital District (Eettmk § 186, 17 August 2020).

**Informed Consent Statement:** Written informed consent was obtained from all patients or their guardians.

**Data Availability Statement:** The reported variants were submitted to the LOVD database hosted at Leiden University Medical Center, The Netherlands.

**Acknowledgments:** We would like to thank genetic nurse Sirpa Miettinen for recruiting patients and the families for participating in the study.

**Conflicts of Interest:** All authors declare no conflict of interest.

## References

1. Smith, R.J.H.; Bale, J.F.; White, K.R. Sensorineural Hearing Loss in Children. *Lancet* **2005**, *365*, 879–890. [CrossRef]
2. Koffler, T.; Ushakov, K.; Avraham, K.B. Genetics of Hearing Loss: Syndromic. *Otolaryngol. Clin. N. Am.* **2015**, *48*, 1041–1061. [CrossRef] [PubMed]
3. Parker, M.; Bitner-Glindzicz, M. Genetic Investigations in Childhood Deafness. *Arch. Dis Child.* **2015**, *100*, 271–278. [CrossRef]
4. Shearer, A.E.; Hildebrand, M.S.; Smith, R.J. Hereditary Hearing Loss and Deafness Overview. In *GeneReviews*®; Adam, M.P., Ardinger, H.H., Pagon, R.A., Wallace, S.E., Bean, L.J., Gripp, K.W., Mirzaa, G.M., Amemiya, A., Eds.; University of Washington, Seattle: Seattle, WA, USA, 1993.
5. Pan, B.; Géléoc, G.S.; Asai, Y.; Horwitz, G.C.; Kurima, K.; Ishikawa, K.; Kawashima, Y.; Griffith, A.J.; Holt, J.R. TMC1 and TMC2 Are Components of the Mechanotransduction Channel in Hair Cells of the Mammalian Inner Ear. *Neuron* **2013**, *79*, 504–515. [CrossRef]

6. Kawashima, Y.; Géléoc, G.S.G.; Kurima, K.; Labay, V.; Lelli, A.; Asai, Y.; Makishima, T.; Wu, D.K.; Della Santina, C.C.; Holt, J.R.; et al. Mechanotransduction in Mouse Inner Ear Hair Cells Requires Transmembrane Channel-like Genes. *J. Clin. Investig.* **2011**, *121*, 4796–4809. [CrossRef]
7. Kurima, K.; Ebrahim, S.; Pan, B.; Sedlacek, M.; Sengupta, P.; Millis, B.A.; Cui, R.; Nakanishi, H.; Fujikawa, T.; Kawashima, Y.; et al. TMC1 and TMC2 Localize at the Site of Mechanotransduction in Mammalian Inner Ear Hair Cell Stereocilia. *Cell Rep.* **2015**, *12*, 1606–1617. [CrossRef] [PubMed]
8. Pan, B.; Akyuz, N.; Liu, X.-P.; Asai, Y.; Nist-Lund, C.; Kurima, K.; Derfler, B.H.; György, B.; Limapichat, W.; Walujkar, S.; et al. TMC1 Forms the Pore of Mechanosensory Transduction Channels in Vertebrate Inner Ear Hair Cells. *Neuron* **2018**, *99*, 736–753. [CrossRef] [PubMed]
9. Kurima, K.; Peters, L.M.; Yang, Y.; Riazuddin, S.; Ahmed, Z.M.; Naz, S.; Arnaud, D.; Drury, S.; Mo, J.; Makishima, T.; et al. Dominant and Recessive Deafness Caused by Mutations of a Novel Gene, TMC1, Required for Cochlear Hair-Cell Function. *Nat. Genet.* **2002**, *30*, 277–284. [CrossRef] [PubMed]
10. Sirmaci, A.; Duman, D.; Oztürkmen-Akay, H.; Erbek, S.; Incesulu, A.; Oztürk-Hişmi, B.; Arici, Z.S.; Yüksel-Konuk, E.B.; Taşir-Yilmaz, S.; Tokgöz-Yilmaz, S.; et al. Mutations in TMC1 Contribute Significantly to Nonsyndromic Autosomal Recessive Sensorineural Hearing Loss: A Report of Five Novel Mutations. *Int. J. Pediatr. Otorhinolaryngol.* **2009**, *73*, 699–705. [CrossRef] [PubMed]
11. Sommen, M.; Schrauwen, I.; Vandeweyer, G.; Boeckx, N.; Corneveaux, J.J.; van den Ende, J.; Boudewyns, A.; De Leenheer, E.; Janssens, S.; Claes, K.; et al. DNA Diagnostics of Hereditary Hearing Loss: A Targeted Resequencing Approach Combined with a Mutation Classification System. *Hum. Mutat.* **2016**, *37*, 812–819. [CrossRef] [PubMed]
12. Zazo Seco, C.; Wesdorp, M.; Feenstra, I.; Pfundt, R.; Hehir-Kwa, J.Y.; Lelieveld, S.H.; Castelein, S.; Gilissen, C.; de Wijs, I.J.; Admiraal, R.J.; et al. The Diagnostic Yield of Whole-Exome Sequencing Targeting a Gene Panel for Hearing Impairment in The Netherlands. *Eur. J. Hum. Genet.* **2017**, *25*, 308–314. [CrossRef] [PubMed]
13. Richards, S.; Aziz, N.; Bale, S.; Bick, D.; Das, S.; Gastier-Foster, J.; Grody, W.W.; Hegde, M.; Lyon, E.; Spector, E.; et al. Standards and Guidelines for the Interpretation of Sequence Variants: A Joint Consensus Recommendation of the American College of Medical Genetics and Genomics and the Association for Molecular Pathology. *Genet. Med.* **2015**, *17*, 405–424. [CrossRef] [PubMed]
14. Bademci, G.; Foster, J.; Mahdieh, N.; Bonyadi, M.; Duman, D.; Cengiz, F.B.; Menendez, I.; Diaz-Horta, O.; Shirkavand, A.; Zeinali, S.; et al. Comprehensive Analysis via Exome Sequencing Uncovers Genetic Etiology in Autosomal Recessive Nonsyndromic Deafness in a Large Multiethnic Cohort. *Genet. Med.* **2016**, *18*, 364–371. [CrossRef] [PubMed]
15. de Heer, A.-M.R.; Collin, R.W.J.; Huygen, P.L.M.; Schraders, M.; Oostrik, J.; Rouwette, M.; Kunst, H.P.M.; Kremer, H.; Cremers, C.W.R.J. Progressive Sensorineural Hearing Loss and Normal Vestibular Function in a Dutch DFNB7/11 Family with a Novel Mutation in TMC1. *Audiol. Neurootol.* **2011**, *16*, 93–105. [CrossRef] [PubMed]
16. Schrauwen, I.; Sommen, M.; Corneveaux, J.J.; Reiman, R.A.; Hackett, N.J.; Claes, C.; Claes, K.; Bitner-Glindzicz, M.; Coucke, P.; Van Camp, G.; et al. A Sensitive and Specific Diagnostic Test for Hearing Loss Using a Microdroplet PCR-Based Approach and next Generation Sequencing. *Am. J. Med. Genet. A* **2013**, *161A*, 145–152. [CrossRef] [PubMed]
17. Imtiaz, A.; Maqsood, A.; Rehman, A.U.; Morell, R.J.; Holt, J.R.; Friedman, T.B.; Naz, S. Recessive Mutations of TMC1 Associated with Moderate to Severe Hearing Loss. *Neurogenetics* **2016**, *17*, 115–123. [CrossRef] [PubMed]
18. Nishio, S.-Y.; Usami, S.-I. Prevalence and Clinical Features of Autosomal Dominant and Recessive TMC1-Associated Hearing Loss. *Hum. Genet.* **2021**. [CrossRef]
19. Ramzan, K.; Al-Owain, M.; Al-Numair, N.S.; Afzal, S.; Al-Ageel, S.; Al-Amer, S.; Al-Baik, L.; Al-Otaibi, G.F.; Hashem, A.; Al-Mashharawi, E.; et al. Identification of TMC1 as a Relatively Common Cause for Nonsyndromic Hearing Loss in the Saudi Population. *Am. J. Med. Genet. B Neuropsychiatr. Genet.* **2020**, *183*, 172–180. [CrossRef]
20. Wang, H.; Wu, K.; Guan, J.; Yang, J.; Xie, L.; Xiong, F.; Lan, L.; Wang, D.; Wang, Q. Identification of Four TMC1 Variations in Different Chinese Families with Hereditary Hearing Loss. *Mol. Genet. Genom. Med.* **2018**, *6*, 504–513. [CrossRef]
21. Makishima, T.; Kurima, K.; Brewer, C.C.; Griffith, A.J. Early Onset and Rapid Progression of Dominant Nonsyndromic DFNA36 Hearing Loss. *Otol. Neurotol.* **2004**, *25*, 714–719. [CrossRef]
22. Gallo, S.; Trevisi, P.; Rigon, C.; Caserta, E.; Seif Ali, D.; Bovo, R.; Martini, A.; Cassina, M. Auditory Outcome after Cochlear Implantation in Children with DFNB7/11 Caused by Pathogenic Variants in TMC1 Gene. *Audiol. Neurootol.* **2021**, *26*, 157–163. [CrossRef] [PubMed]
23. Lee, S.-Y.; Oh, D.-Y.; Han, J.H.; Kim, M.Y.; Kim, B.; Kim, B.J.; Song, J.-J.; Koo, J.-W.; Lee, J.H.; Oh, S.H.; et al. Flexible Real-Time Polymerase Chain Reaction-Based Platforms for Detecting Deafness Mutations in Koreans: A Proposed Guideline for the Etiologic Diagnosis of Auditory Neuropathy Spectrum Disorder. *Diagnostics* **2020**, *10*, 672. [CrossRef]
24. Willberg, T.; Sivonen, V.; Linder, P.; Dietz, A. Comparing the Speech Perception of Cochlear Implant Users with Three Different Finnish Speech Intelligibility Tests in Noise. *J. Clin. Med.* **2021**, *10*, 3666. [CrossRef]
25. Black, J.; Hickson, L.; Black, B. Defining and Evaluating Success in Paediatric Cochlear Implantation—An Exploratory Study. *Int. J. Pediatr. Otorhinolaryngol.* **2012**, *76*, 1317–1326. [CrossRef] [PubMed]
26. Holden, L.K.; Finley, C.C.; Firszt, J.B.; Holden, T.A.; Brenner, C.; Potts, L.G.; Gotter, B.D.; Vanderhoof, S.S.; Mispagel, K.; Heydebrand, G.; et al. Factors Affecting Open-Set Word Recognition in Adults with Cochlear Implants. *Ear Hear.* **2013**, *34*, 342–360. [CrossRef] [PubMed]

27. Zhao, E.E.; Dornhoffer, J.R.; Loftus, C.; Nguyen, S.A.; Meyer, T.A.; Dubno, J.R.; McRackan, T.R. Association of Patient-Related Factors with Adult Cochlear Implant Speech Recognition Outcomes: A Meta-Analysis. *JAMA Otolaryngol. Head Neck Surg.* **2020**, *146*, 613–620. [CrossRef] [PubMed]
28. Karczewski, K.J.; Francioli, L.C.; Tiao, G.; Cummings, B.B.; Alföldi, J.; Wang, Q.; Collins, R.L.; Laricchia, K.M.; Ganna, A.; Birnbaum, D.P.; et al. The Mutational Constraint Spectrum Quantified from Variation in 141,456 Humans. *Nature* **2020**, *581*, 434–443. [CrossRef]
29. Hilgert, N.; Monahan, K.; Kurima, K.; Li, C.; Friedman, R.A.; Griffith, A.J.; Van Camp, G. Amino Acid 572 in TMC1: Hot Spot or Critical Functional Residue for Dominant Mutations Causing Hearing Impairment. *J. Hum. Genet.* **2009**, *54*, 188–190. [CrossRef]
30. Wei, Q.; Zhu, H.; Qian, X.; Chen, Z.; Yao, J.; Lu, Y.; Cao, X.; Xing, G. Targeted Genomic Capture and Massively Parallel Sequencing to Identify Novel Variants Causing Chinese Hereditary Hearing Loss. *J. Transl. Med.* **2014**, *12*, 311. [CrossRef]
31. Beurg, M.; Schimmenti, L.A.; Koleilat, A.; Amr, S.S.; Oza, A.; Barlow, A.J.; Ballesteros, A.; Fettiplace, R. New Tmc1 Deafness Mutations Impact Mechanotransduction in Auditory Hair Cells. *J. Neurosci.* **2021**, *41*, 4378–4391. [CrossRef]

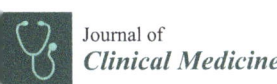 

Article

# A Prospective Study of Etiology and Auditory Profiles in Infants with Congenital Unilateral Sensorineural Hearing Loss

Marlin Johansson [1,2,*], Eva Karltorp [1,3], Kaijsa Edholm [1,4], Maria Drott [2,3] and Erik Berninger [1,2]

[1] Division of Ear, Nose and Throat Diseases, Department of Clinical Science, Intervention and Technology, Karolinska Institutet, 141 52 Stockholm, Sweden; eva.karltorp@regionstockholm.se (E.K.); kaijsa.edholm@regionstockholm.se (K.E.); erik.berninger@ki.se (E.B.)
[2] Department of Audiology and Neurotology, Karolinska University Hospital, 141 86 Stockholm, Sweden; maria.drott@regionstockholm.se
[3] Department of Hearing Implants, Karolinska University Hospital, 141 86 Stockholm, Sweden
[4] Department of Radiology, Karolinska University Hospital, 141 57 Stockholm, Sweden
* Correspondence: marlin.johansson@ki.se

**Abstract:** Congenital unilateral sensorineural hearing loss (uSNHL) is associated with speech-language delays and academic difficulties. Yet, controversy exists in the choice of diagnosis and intervention methods. A cross-sectional prospective design was used to study hearing loss cause in twenty infants with congenital uSNHL consecutively recruited from a universal neonatal hearing-screening program. All normal-hearing ears showed ≤20 dB nHL auditory brainstem response (ABR) thresholds (ABRthrs). The impaired ear median ABRthr was 55 dB nHL, where 40% had no recordable ABRthr. None of the subjects tested positive for congenital cytomegalovirus (CMV) infection. Fourteen subjects agreed to participate in magnetic resonance imaging (MRI). Malformations were common for all degrees of uSNHL and found in 64% of all scans. Half of the MRIs demonstrated cochlear nerve aplasia or severe hypoplasia and 29% showed inner ear malformations. Impaired ear and normal-hearing ear ABR input/output functions on a group level for subjects with ABRthrs < 90 dB nHL were parallel shifted. A significant difference in interaural acoustic reflex thresholds (ARTs) existed. In congenital uSNHL, MRI is powerful in finding a possible hearing loss cause, while congenital CMV infection may be relatively uncommon. ABRs and ARTs indicated an absence of loudness recruitment, with implications for further research on hearing devices.

**Keywords:** etiology; sensorineural hearing loss; unilateral hearing loss; imaging; cytomegalovirus; electrophysiology; pediatric; congenital; auditory dysfunction

## 1. Introduction

Congenital unilateral sensorineural hearing loss (uSNHL) is a chronic condition affecting approximately 1 in every 2000 newborns [1,2]. Children with uSNHL have a higher risk of speech-language delays, academic difficulties, and psychosocial challenges compared to children with normal hearing (e.g., [3–5]). They generally also have impaired binaural hearing, including sound source localization [6–9], and impaired speech recognition in noise [9–11].

Controversy exists in the choice of diagnostic methods for children with uSNHL. For example, some argue for using imaging [12–14], while a recent systematic review and meta-analysis argues that "imaging does not provide information that alters management or gives insight into prognosis or hereditary causes in most cases and therefore does not warrant strong recommendations" [15]. The prevalence of hearing loss causes may be different for congenital uSNHL, compared to uSNHL that emerges later in development. A systematic investigation should be of value for clinical routines, as congenital uSNHL represents one fourth of the sensorineural hearing losses found through the universal neonatal hearing-screening programs [2].

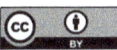

Malformations of the auditory system are more common in congenital uSNHL compared to bilateral SNHL [16,17]. The malformation prevalence depends on several factors, e.g., the use of magnetic resonance imaging (MRI) and/or computed tomography (CT). CT provides a good view of the bony labyrinth and middle ear, whereas soft-tissue resolution is higher with modern MRI and is therefore the preferred method for evaluating the vestibulocochlear nerve with its cochlear branch, the facial nerve, and the internal cochlear structures. The malformation prevalence with MRI is about 37–58% in children with uSNHL [12–14,18,19], and similarly around 36–67% for CT [13,20,21]. The prevalence may be somewhat higher, around 46–67%, when obviously acquired uSNHL has been excluded, e.g., meningitis or trauma [12,20,21]. However, more precise estimates of malformation prevalence for congenital uSNHL are lacking.

The congenital cytomegalovirus (cCMV) infection is believed to be the leading nongenetic cause for SNHL during the last few decades, with a prevalence of up to 20–30% in SNHL [22–24]. It is common that SNHL associated with cCMV infection is progressive and sometimes even fluctuating [24–26]. The debut of SNHL may even be more common after the neonatal period, so that many children with cCMV-associated SNHL will not be identified through universal neonatal hearing-screening (UNHS) programs [27,28]. Children with uSNHL (congenital and acquired) have previously been found to be cCMV positive in around 10% [14] to 20% of cases [29,30]. Still, the prevalence of uSNHL caused by cCMV infection needs more research, due to, e.g., small groups of children, the frequent uncertainty of uSNHL onset when not found through UNHS, and the variability in spread of cCMV infection over time and across countries [14,29,30].

Research of auditory profiles or hearing function in relation to etiology is lacking. Most research on etiology and auditory profiles in uSNHL focuses on cochlear implant (CI) candidates with profound uSNHL, i.e., single-sided deafness (SSD) (e.g., [30,31]), and is much less explored in mild-moderate uSNHL, i.e., potential hearing aid (HA) candidates. All patients with hearing loss experience elevated hearing thresholds in at least one ear, but other auditory functions may vary between patients. Loudness recruitment, i.e., an increased growth in perceived loudness as the intensity level of a signal increases, is an important amplification factor in a hearing aid, that most adult patients with cochlear hearing loss experience [32,33]. The prevalence of loudness recruitment in the pediatric population is sparsely explored, as young children are difficult to assess with psychoacoustic tests of loudness perception. The auditory brainstem response (ABR) may be used to estimate loudness perception by neural firing [34,35] and needs further study. Congenital uSNHL represents an excellent model for estimation due to the possibility of comparing the impaired ear (IE) with the normal-hearing ear (NE).

The aim was to describe congenital uSNHL (ranging from mild to profound) in infants, focusing on the causes, hearing function and the affected auditory mechanisms by using a prospective study design and a comprehensive test battery. Tests included MRI, cCMV infection testing, acoustic reflex threshold (ART) measurements to investigate middle ear, inner ear and neural function (e.g., [36,37]), and various otoacoustic emissions (OAEs) to investigate cochlear function [38,39]. The auditory brainstem response (ABR) was measured for site of lesion testing, hearing threshold estimation, and to study the function of the cochlea and auditory pathways (e.g., [40–42]). The ABR amplitude as a function of stimulus level, i.e., the input/output (I/O) function, was studied to estimate loudness recruitment.

## 2. Materials and Methods
### 2.1. Study Design

The subjects were recruited during the years 2019–2020 from the bedside UNHS program in Region Stockholm, which is based on multiple transient-evoked OAE (TEOAE) recordings and an automatic ABR (aABR). The UNHS program has been described previously (first TEOAE around postnatal day 3, 98% screened) [2,42–44], where the aABR screening before clinical ABR was first introduced in 2016 [45].

Eligible subjects were invited to participate in two research visits. ABRs, TEOAEs, distortion-product OAEs (DPOAEs), tympanograms, and ARTs were recorded at the first visit. The ABRs, TEOAEs and DPOAEs were recorded in an audiometric test room with low ambient sound levels, allowing determinations down to $-10$ dB HL (ISO8253-1 2010). The tympanograms and ARTs were measured in the audiometric test room or a quiet room. Otomicroscopy was performed by an experienced otologist to exclude middle ear disease. An oral case history was obtained from the infants' parents for additional information including parents' knowledge about relevant medical and development history, including prenatal and perinatal history. Testing for cCMV followed as soon as possible. The visit took approximately 2.5–3 h.

At a second research visit, all eligible subjects were invited to the MRI of the auditory system (inner ears and cochlear nerve).

This study was approved by the Swedish Ethical Review Authority (no: 2018/1500-31). Written informed consent was obtained from all parents with child custody.

*2.2. Subjects*

Several recruitment steps were undertaken with the aim of inviting all children born with uSNHL and excluding all children with temporary hearing loss, e.g., otitis media with effusion (OME). Inclusion criteria comprised: (1) One ear passing and one ear failing TEOAE UNHS; (2) An ABR threshold (ABRthr) > 30 dB nHL in the IE; and (3) An ABRthr of $\leq$20 dB nHL in the NE.

M.J. (first author) was notified when a neonate was suspected of having a unilateral hearing loss, i.e., failed several TEOAE tests in one ear and passed in the other ear, passed aABR screening in one ear ($\leq$30 dB nHL, i.e., the lowest sound level tested) and failed in the other ear (>30 dB nHL). TEOAE pass criteria included: $\geq$70% whole wave reproducibility, signal-to-noise ratio (SNR) $\geq$4 dB in at least three of the upper four wide-frequency bands provided by the ILO instrument, and $\geq$50 sweeps. The neonate's families were informed of the study and invited to the next step in the study recruitment process at the first audiologic test visit following UNHS if the ABR showed thresholds >30 dB nHL in the IE and a SNHL was alleged (based on the ABR, additional auditory steady-state response (ASSR), tympanograms, TEOAEs, and sometimes bone-conduction ABR), and $\leq$25 dB nHL in the NE.

In total, 48 out of 68 potential subjects based on the UNHS were excluded at the first audiologic test visit following screening or, in a few cases, at the first research visit as they did not fulfill the study inclusion criteria. This was typically due to OME that fully explained the elevated ABRthr in the IE, or an ABRthr $\leq$ 30 dB nHL in the IE, or bilateral hearing loss ($\geq$25 dB nHL in both ears).

Thus, 20 infants with congenital uSNHL were invited to the study, and the 20 families all consented to participate in the study (see Figure 1 for sample size compared to estimated sample).

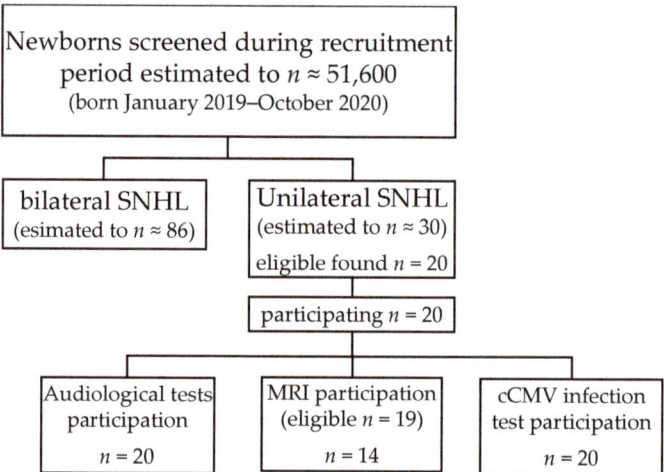

**Figure 1.** Estimated and included number of participants. Estimated numbers are based on previous universal neonatal hearing-screening results from Region Stockholm ([2], >30,000 screened, 98% coverage rate), and the documented number of newborns during 2019 and 2020 in Region Stockholm [46]. One subject was born with a heart anomaly, which is the reason for 19 subjects eligible for MRI. cCMV = congenital cytomegalovirus; MRI = magnetic resonance imaging; SNHL = sensorineural hearing loss.

*2.3. Auditory Brainstem Response (ABR)*

The ABR was recorded monaurally in both ears using 100 μs rarefaction clicks at a repetition rate of 39 Hz. Clicks were presented through insert earphones (EAR Tone; Etymotic Research Inc, Elk Grove Village, IL, USA) with Eclipse EP25 (program version 4.3.0.17, Interacoustics, Middelfart, Denmark).

The ABR was recorded in 10 dB steps whenever possible, from 70 dB nHL down to the threshold or 20 dB nHL minimum. The 70 dB nHL level was chosen as the main supra-threshold level for analysis of the ABR I–V interval. If the ABR waves I and V could not be discerned at 70 dB nHL, the input level was increased in 10 dB steps up to a maximum of 80 dB nHL for the NE, and 90 dB nHL for the IE.

The response quality was enhanced by the use of up to 10,000 sweeps at stimulus levels close to the ABRthr, and ≈2000 sweeps for the other stimulus levels. Calibration of 100 μsec clicks was performed according to ISO389-6 (2007) in an occluded ear simulator IEC60318-4 (2010) [47,48].

Ag/AgCl electrodes were placed on left and right mastoids (left, right), and the forehead (vertex, ground) for differential recording between ipsilateral mastoid (noninverting) and the forehead (inverting). The subject was placed in a supine position in the parent's arms or in a baby carrier. Lights in the audiometric test room were turned off during the ABR recordings in order to minimize electric interferences.

E.B. determined all the ABR waves, blinded to which subject and ear that was evaluated. The ABR latencies were determined using narrow-band filtering (digital filter, 300 to 1500 Hz), thereby obtaining a well-defined vertex-positive peak.

If no ABR-waves could be determined, the wave reproducibility ($\rho$) was objectively determined in the time domain (1–15 ms) for the entire ABR [42], and the lack of a response was confirmed if $\rho$ was <70% ($\rho$ = 70% corresponds to SNR = 3.7 dB [42]). The wave I of each ABR recording was objectively confirmed by a $\rho \geq 70\%$ within a time window of 1–1.5 ms encompassing the wave. The ABR wave V at the threshold was confirmed with a $\rho \geq 70\%$ within a time window of 1–1.5 ms encompassing the wave. The amplitudes for the ABR waves were quantified based on the difference between the vertex positive peak maximum and succeeding minimum [42].

Contralateral masking was applied when needed [49].

### 2.4. Transient-Evoked Otoacoustic Emission (TEOAE)

The TEOAEs were recorded in the non-linear quickscreen neonate diagnostic mode with Echoport ILO288 USB-II (Otodynamics Ltd., Hatfield, UK, program version 6, time window: 3.0–12.8 ms, click rate 78 Hz). For details on the non-linear stimulus paradigm see [50]. The Echoport interface was placed in the audiometric test room during the measurement together with the subject and accompanying parent, whereas the tester and computer were outside in the surrounding quiet room. All the TEOAE stimulus and response levels were recorded at the probe-tip in the outer ear canal using an electrically constant stimulus, corresponding to a typical stimulus level of 81.5–82 dB SPL peak [43,44]. The NE was tested first in 65% of subjects, and the right ear first in 60% of subjects, which may be important, as TEOAEs have been demonstrated to be larger in the ear tested first [51]. A sweep consisted of two sets of non-linear responses in response to four 80-μs click stimulations. Whole-wave reproducibility was calculated as the correlation coefficient of interleaved non-linear responses.

### 2.5. Distortion Product Otoacoustic Emission (DPOAE)

The DPOAEs were recorded using the same test setup as the TEOAEs with Echoport ILO288 USB-II (Otodynamics Ltd., Hatfield, UK, program version 6). The $2f_1$-$f_2$ cubic distortion product component was measured with a frequency ratio of the primaries of 1.22 ($f_2/f_1$). The stimulus consisted of two equal-level sinusoids with an expected sound pressure level of 75 dB SPL at the tympanic membrane (as used by, e.g., [52]). The DPOAEs were recorded with $f_2$ at 1, 1.5, 2, 3, 4, 6 and 8 kHz. The SNR was defined as the DPOAE level–(Noise + 2 SD) in dB. The NE was tested first in 63% of subjects, and the right ear first in 53% of subjects.

### 2.6. Tympanometry and Acoustic Stapedius Reflex Threshold (ART)

Tympanograms and ARTs were recorded in both ears with GSI Tympstar (Grason-Stadler, Eden Prairie, MN, USA) to primarily study the middle ear system and the function of the reflex arc. The ART was elicited ipsilaterally at tympanic peak pressure and at the stimulus frequency of 1000 Hz, using an ascending method in steps of 5 dB with a maximum of 105 dB HL (as recorded in a 2-cc coupler). The criterion for a reflex response was a repeatable compliance change corresponding to 0.02 mL or greater, supported with an impedance growth at a higher stimulus level.

### 2.7. Magnetic Resonance Imaging (MRI)

Subjects were excluded from MRI if they were too ill for sedation with dexmedetomidine, which was determined in two steps, first by the responsible otologist (E.K.), then by the MRI team physician. One subject was excluded from MRI due to a congenital heart abnormality. Another 5 out of 19 subjects declined MRI participation (Figure 1).

All but one of the 14 MRI scans were assessed with 3T scanners (Siemens Skyra, Erlangen, Germany, $n = 8$, or Siemens Prisma, Erlangen, Germany, $n = 5$), the exception being for S3, where a 1.5T scanner was used (GE Optima, GE Healthcare, Fairfield, CT, USA), as a back and spine MRI was prioritized additional to the auditory system MRI.

For all 3T scans, a protocol designed for pre-cochlear implantation was used. For assessment of the inner ear, a transversal high resolution T2 3D SPACE sequence with 0.5 mm slice thickness was used. The cochlear nerve was assessed using a T2 3D SPACE sequence acquired in an oblique sagittal plane perpendicular to the inner auditory canal. The protocol also included T1-weighted images (T1WI) and T2-weighted images (T2WI) of the temporal bone, as well as sagittal T1WI, transversal T2-weighted Fluid Attenuated Inversion Recovery images (T2 FLAIR), diffusion-weighted imaging (DWI) and susceptibility-weighted imaging (SWI) of the brain.

The 1.5T scan was performed using a protocol designed for the temporal bone. The inner ear was assessed using a transversal T2 3D FIESTA sequence with 0.6 mm thickness, and the cochlear nerve by making oblique sagittal reconstructions from this sequence. The scan also included sagittal and coronal T2WI as well as transversal T1WI, T2 FLAIR and DWI of the brain.

The MRI results were reviewed by one or two experienced neuroradiologists or head-neck radiologists, and later all results were double checked by K.E., an experienced head-neck radiologist.

*2.8. Congenital Cytomegalovirus (cCMV) Infection*

A blood sample was taken from the mother for CMV testing as soon as possible after the study inclusion. If the mother had a positive CMV-test (IgG and/or IgM antibodies) the child's newborn dried blood spot (DBS) card was then analyzed for CMV DNA with the polymerase chain reaction (PCR) technique. Exceptions were made from the study protocol for two subjects where the DBS cards were analyzed directly, as the mothers had not yet taken the blood sample after several months, despite repeated reminders, and one subject had already been CMV tested with a blood sample the same day as birth.

*2.9. Statistical Analysis*

All the statistical analyses were performed with Statistica version 13.5 (TIBCO software Inc., Palo Alto, CA, USA), except linear mixed modelling, which was performed with R version 3.4.2 (R Foundation for Statistical Computing, Vienna, Austria).

Mean and SD are primarily presented in this study for easy comparison with previous studies, although medians and interquartile ranges (IQRs) are presented when Kurtosis and Skewness were clearly different from zero, e.g., for ARTs and ABRthrs.

Nonparametric tests were used for statistical testing, due to small sample sizes.

Due to the parallel-shifted IE and NE ABR I/O functions on the group level, a post hoc analysis with linear mixed modelling of ABR amplitude was performed (waves I, III, and V, respectively), with the ear (NE/IE) and stimulus level as fixed effects and the subject as the random variable (Satterwaite's method for *t*-tests).

## 3. Results

*3.1. Subjects*

Twenty subjects with mild to profound congenital uSNHL participated in the study (50% males, 65% left IEs, 55% first-borns) (Table 1). Subjects 15 and 17 (S15 and S17) were born as dizygotic twins (not co-twins). Six subjects spent several days in the neonatal intensive care unit (NICU) after birth due to asphyxia, anal atresia, corpus callosum agenesis, jaundice, mild respiratory distress syndrome or heart abnormality (S1, S3, S10, S12, S14 and S19). S12 was born preterm before 37 weeks of gestation (36 weeks + 1 day). All other 19 subjects were born full-term (weeks 37 to 42).

The median chronological age at the first research visit, and the diagnosis of congenital uSNHL, was 2.2 months (Table 1). The otomicroscopic examinations were normal. However, S8 showed signs of OME when first scheduled for the visit (supported by a flat tympanogram and lack of TEOAEs in the NE) so the visit was rescheduled, hence the comparably late diagnosis (Table 1). S13 was also diagnosed with congenital uSNHL comparably late, due to COVID-19 outbreak during spring 2020 and disease risk groups in the family (Table 1).

**Table 1.** Characteristics of the 20 infants' impaired ears (IEs), with normal ear (NE) characteristics in parentheses when applicable (all NEs showed ABR thresholds of ≤20 dB nHL and are therefore not in parentheses).

| ID | IE | Sex | Age at Diagnosis (mos) | ABR Threshold IE (dB nHL) | ABR Wave I–V (ms) | ART (dB HL) | DPOAE (3 Frequencies or More) | MRI Result |
|---|---|---|---|---|---|---|---|---|
| 1 | L | M | 1.8 | 45 | 5.07 (4.90) | | | |
| 2 | L | F | 2.5 | 35 | 4.53 (3.93) | | X | N.A.D. |
| 3 | L | F | 2.1 | >90 | | 95 (90) | | Hypoplasia cochlea, aplasia/severe hypoplasia auditory nerve, semicircular canal dysplasia and EVA |
| 4 | R | F | 2.2 | 40 | | 80 (NT) | X | |
| 5 | L | M | 2.1 | 40 | 4.87 (4.70) | 95 (90) | X | N.A.D. |
| 6 | L | M | 2.0 | >90 | | >105 (75) | | Aplasia cochlea, aplasia/severe hypoplasia auditory nerve, labyrinth dysplasia and semicircular canal dysplasia |
| 7 | R | F | 2.0 | 45 | 4.73 (4.73) | 80 (75) | X | Bilateral EVA with probable IP II |
| 8 | R | F | 5.3 | >90 | | 95 (85) | | Aplasia/severe hypoplasia auditory nerve and hypoplasia inner ear canal |
| 9 | L | M | 2.2 | >90 | | >105 (85) | | |
| 10 | L | M | 2.7 | 40 | 4.94 (5.13) | 95 (85) | X | |
| 11 | R | M | 3.3 | >90 | | >105 (90) | | Aplasia/severe hypoplasia auditory nerve and hypoplasia inner ear canal |
| 12 | R | F | 1.8 | >90 | | >105 (85) | | Aplasia/severe hypoplasia auditory nerve and hypoplasia inner ear canal |
| 13 | L | F | 5.6 | >90 | | | | N.A.D. |
| 14 | L | M | 1.7 | >90 | | 95 (80) | | Aplasia/severe hypoplasia auditory nerve |
| 15 | L | M | 2.0 | 40 | 4.84 (4.80) | | | N.A.D. |
| 16 | L | F | 2.3 | 45 | 4.90 (4.57) | | | N.A.D. |
| 17 | L | M | 2.9 | 60 | | 100 (75) | | Aplasia/severe hypoplasia auditory nerve |
| 18 | R | F | 3.0 | 60 | | 100 (80) | | Unilateral EVA with probable IP II |
| 19 | L | M | 4.3 | 40 | 4.40 (4.87) | | | |
| 20 | R | F | 2.4 | 50 | 5.60 (4.83) | 85 (75) | | |

ABR = auditory brainstem response; ART = acoustic reflex threshold, ipsilateral, 1000 Hz; DPOAE = distortion-product otoacoustic emission with SNR > 0 dB; EVA = enlarged vestibular aqueduct; IE = impaired ear; IP II = cochlear incomplete partition type II; L = left; MRI = magnetic resonance imaging; N.A.D. = no anomaly detected; NT = no test; R = right.

### 3.2. Auditory Brainstem Response (ABR)

All subjects slept during the ABR recording. The maximum electrode impedances (33 Hz square wave) were low with a median of 1.5 kΩ (IQR = 1–2 kΩ, n = 20 subjects).

#### 3.2.1. ABR Thresholds (ABRthrs)

ABRthrs of 20 dB nHL were recorded in all NEs (n = 20), with a wave-V reproducibility of >73% within a time window of 1–1.5 ms encompassing the wave (median $\rho$ = 97%).

The median ABRthr was 55 dB nHL in the IE (IQR = 40 dB nHL-no response, n = 20). In 8 subjects (40%), no ABR waves could be discerned in the IE at 90 dB nHL (Table 1), indicating SSD (objectively supported by $\rho$ < 70%, i.e., SNR < 3.7 dB, for an analysis window of 1–15 ms [42]). For the subjects with discernible ABR waves, the median ABRthr was 43 dB nHL (IQR = 40–48 dB nHL, n = 12).

### 3.2.2. ABR I–V Intervals

The ABR interpeak I–V interval was used to determine the neural transmission time between the cochlea and upper brainstem. No statistically significant interaural difference existed in the ABR I–V wave interval (Wilcoxon matched pairs; $p = 0.26$, $n = 9$). However, the interaural between-subject variability was large (Table 1). At 70 dB nHL, the mean ± SD I–V interval was 4.80 ± 0.34 ms in the NE ($n = 17$) and 4.92 ± 0.34 ms in the IE ($n = 8$). At 80 dB nHL, it was 4.82 ± 0.31 ms in the NE ($n = 8$) and 4.81 ± 0.19 ms in the IE ($n = 7$).

### 3.2.3. ABR Latencies

Not surprisingly, the latency as a function of the stimulus level for waves I, III and V was similar when comparing the NE and IE for all the subjects (Figure 2) (Mann–Whitney U test: $ps > 0.05$). A slight, albeit significant, interaural wave-V latency difference existed for paired comparisons at 70 dB nHL (median difference 0.25 ms, $p = 0.03$, $n = 12$), and at 80 dB nHL (median difference 0.13 ms, $p = 0.04$, $n = 5$), but not at 40, 50 or 60 dB nHL (Wilcoxon's matched pairs test, see Table S1, Supplementary Materials). No statistically significant interaural difference existed in ABR latency for wave I and III at any stimulus level, neither paired nor unpaired (see Table S1, Supplementary Materials, $ps > 0.05$).

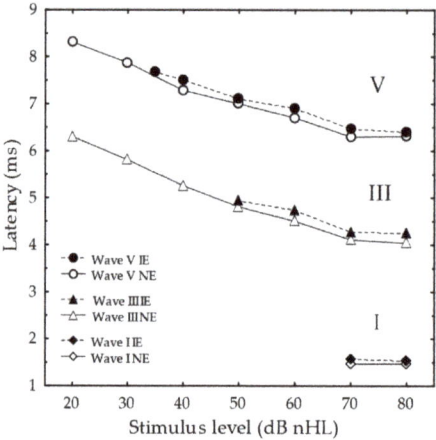

**Figure 2.** Mean Auditory brainstem response latency as a function of stimulus level (dB nHL) for wave V (circles), wave III (triangles) and wave I (rhombi) for the IE (filled) and the NE (open). The mboxemphns = 1, 6, 10, 9, 12, and 11 for wave I in the IE for 35, 40, 50, 60, 70, and 80 dB nHL, respectively, whereas the $ns$ = 20, 16, 16, 13, 9, 20, and 9 in the NE for 20, 30, 40, 50, 60, 70, and 80 dB nHL, respectively. For wave III the $ns$ = 7, 5, 11 and 10 in the IE for 50, 60, 70, and 80 dB nHL, respectively, whereas the $ns$ = 11, 13, 14, 11, 9, 20, and 9 in the NE for 20, 30, 40, 50, 60, 70, and 80 dB nHL, respectively. The wave I $ns$ = 8 and 7 for the IE and $ns$ = 17 and 8 for the NE at 70 and 80 dB nHL, respectively.

### 3.2.4. ABR Wave Amplitudes

The NE vs. IE I/O functions for waves I, III and V were parallel shifted (Figure 3).

Likewise, linear mixed modelling revealed a significant effect of ear (NE vs. IE) on wave V ($r_{totalmodel} = 0.78$, $p < 0.001$), wave-III ($r_{total\ model} = 0.76$, $p < 0.001$) and wave I ($r_{total\ model} = 0.64$, $p < 0.001$) amplitudes. The effect of the stimulus level was also significant ($p < 0.001$, $p < 0.001$, $p = 0.004$) for wave V, III, and I, respectively. Subject was a significant contributor to the model for wave III ($p < 0.001$) and I ($p < 0.001$).

For detailed ABR mean and median amplitude NE vs. IE difference by stimulus level with statistical significance (paired and unpaired) for wave I, III and V see Table S2, Supplementary Materials.

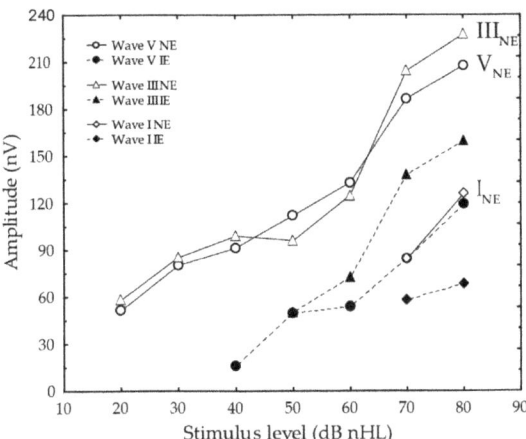

**Figure 3.** Mean auditory brainstem response amplitude as a function of stimulus level (dB nHL) for wave V (circles), wave III (triangles) and wave I (rhombi) demonstrates parallel shifted I/O functions, when comparing the NE (open) with the IE (filled). The $n$s = 20, 15, 16, 13, 9, 10, and 9 for Wave V in the NE for 20, 30, 40, 50, 60, 70, and 80 dB nHL, respectively, whereas $n$s = 6, 10, 9, 12, and 11 in the IE for 40, 50, 60, 70, and 80 dB nHL, respectively. For wave III the $n$s = 11, 12, 14, 11, 9, 20, and 9 in the NE for 20, 30, 40, 50, 60, 70, and 80 dB nHL, respectively, whereas $n$s = 7, 5, 11, and 10 in the IE for 50, 60, 70, and 80 dB nHL, respectively. The wave I $n$s = 8 and 7 for the IE and $n$s = 17 and 8 for the NE at 70 and 80 dB nHL, respectively.

### 3.3. Magnetic Resonance Imaging (MRI)

Seventy percent (14/20) of the subjects underwent MRI of the auditory systems (Table 1). One subject was excluded due to congenital heart abnormality, and another 5 subjects declined MRI participation for personal reasons. The median age for MRI was 8 months (IQR = 7–10 months).

Malformations of the auditory system were identified in 64% (9/14) of the subjects. The prevalence of malformations was higher in children with profound uSNHL, as 86% (6/7) of the children with an ABRthr >90 dB nHL showed malformations, whereas children with mild to profound uSNHL demonstrated a malformation prevalence of 43% (3/7; Table 1).

Half of the MRIs revealed no visible cochlear nerve (Figure 4) ($n$ = 7/14; S3, S6, S8, S11–12, S14 and S17), henceforth referred to as cochlear nerve aplasia, although severe hypoplasia cannot be excluded. All cochlear nerve aplasia was combined with hypoplasia of the vestibulocochlear nerve. Six of these seven subjects demonstrated no ABR response (or threshold > 90 dB nHL, i.e., SSD), while the ABRthr for S17 was 60 dB nHL (Table 1). Moreover, no visible cochlear nerve was combined with hypoplasia of the inner ear canal in three of the subjects (S8, S11–12; i.e., inner ear canal being evidently smaller on IE side compared to NE side).

Cochlear nerve aplasia in combination with an inner ear malformation was observed in two subjects: S6 with cochlear aplasia, labyrinth dysplasia and semicircular canal dysplasia, and S3 with cochlear hypoplasia, semicircular canal dysplasia and enlarged vestibular aqueduct (EVA). The total percentage of inner ear malformations was 29% (S3, S6–7, S18; Table 1). S3, S7 and S18 revealed EVA, bilateral for S7 (ABRthr of 45 dB nHL in the IE) and unilateral for S3 (SSD), as well as for S18 (ABRthr of 60 dB nHL in the IE). S7 progressed to a bilateral hearing loss at a hearing follow-up at 8 months of age, despite having an ABRthr of 20 dB nHL, as well as TEOAEs and DPOAEs, in the NE at 2 months of age.

Nothing abnormal was identified in the auditory pathway for S2, S5, S13, S15 and S16.

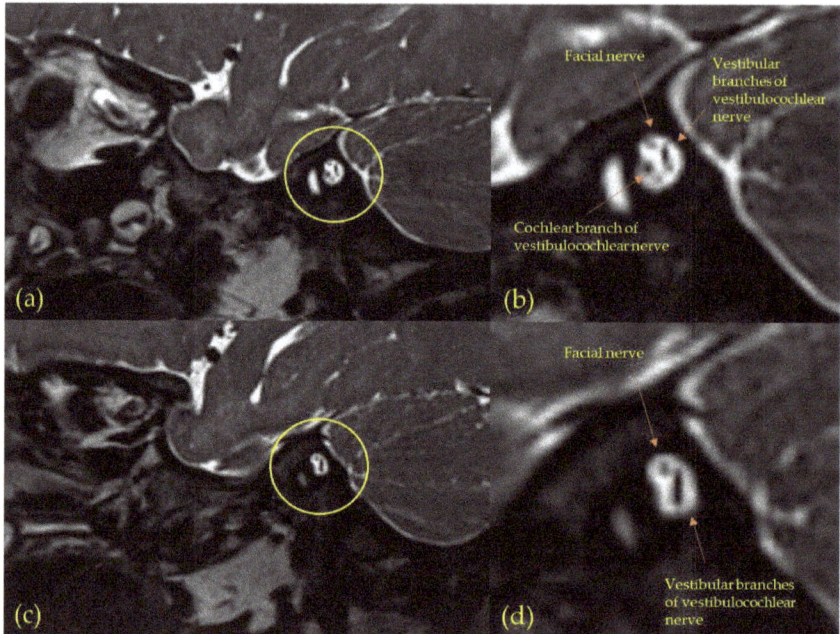

**Figure 4.** Typical MRI images of the inner auditory canal for subjects with cochlear nerve aplasia (oblique-sagittal view); (**a,b**) The normal-hearing ear (NE) of subject 11 (S11) showing a normal cochlear branch of the vestibucochlear nerve; (**c,d**) The impaired ear (IE) of S11 showing no visible cochlear nerve branch, indicating aplasia or severe hypoplasia.

*3.4. Congenital Cytomegalovirus (cCMV) Infection*

All subjects were CMV negative according to the PCR analysis on the DSP cards typically taken 48 h after birth ($n = 16$), plasma test on the same day as birth ($n = 1$), or the mother's IgG and IgM negative CMV blood test shortly after birth ($n = 3$). The mothers who were CMV IgG and IgM negative left the blood sample for the analysis within 3 months after childbirth (51–88 days).

*3.5. Tympanometry and Acoustic Stapedius Reflex Threshold (ART)*

The change in absolute compliance, measured in equivalent volume of air at tympanic peak pressure was almost identical in the two ears, with medians of 1 mL in the NE (IQR: 0.5–1.5 mL, $n = 19$) and 1 mL in the IE (IQR: 0.7–1.4 mL, $n = 16$). Similarly, the median tympanic peak pressure was 10 daPa in the NE (IQR: −5–40 daPa, $n = 19$) and 10 daPa and IE (IQR: −10–30 daPa, $n = 16$). The ears that could not be tested at the research visit (the IEs of S1, S2, S16 and S19, and the NE of S2) showed normal tympanograms at follow-up visits ($\geq 0.2$ mL compliance, −100 daPa to 100 daPa) in combination with no significant changes in hearing (ABRthrs, ARTs and/or TEOAEs).

An ipsilateral acoustic reflex test was completed in 70% of the infants in the NEs and 70% in the IEs. The median ART was 85 dB HL in the NEs (IQR: 75–90 dB HL, $n = 14$), and 95 dB HL in the IEs (IQR: 95 dB HL-no response, $n = 14$; Table 1 for the ART of the IEs for each subject). A statistically significant median interaural ART difference of 15 dB was found for the subjects with recordable ARTs in both ears (Wilcoxons matched pairs: $p = 0.008$, $n = 9$).

*3.6. Transient-Evoked Otoacoustic Emission (TEOAE)*

All TEOAE recordings in NEs showed a SNR > 4 dB in at least three of the upper four wide-frequency bands ($n$ = 18, no reliable/no recording for S2 and S10 at test, though all NEs had passed TEOAE screening previously). The mean ± SD response level was 19.8 ± 7.2 dB SPL ($n$ = 18) for NEs, similar to the 19–20 dB SPL in previous research of neonatal NEs with a similar test setup [43,44]. In Nes, the median stimulus level was 81.9 dB SPL peak (IQR: 81.6–83.1, $n$ = 18), the stimulus stability was high (median = 98%, IQR: 92–99, $n$ = 18), and a median of 233 sweeps were used (IQR: 160–260 sweeps; $n$ = 18). The whole-wave reproducibility was high with a median of 90% (IQR: 83–97%; $n$ = 18), and the median entire SNR was 6.4 dB (IQR: 3.8–12.8 dB, $n$ = 18). The IEs did not pass UNHS and likewise no TEOAEs could be recorded at the research visit ($n$ = 18, no reliable/no recording for S10 and S19 at test, though all IEs had not passed TEOAE screening previously).

*3.7. Distortion-Product Otoacoustic Emission (DPOAE)*

A DPOAE response, classified as a positive SNR, was recorded at three frequencies or more (1–8 kHz) in 16/17 NEs (only two NE frequency responses for S19, that held the noisiest recording) and at two frequencies or more for 17/17 NEs (no reliable/no DPOAE recording for S2, S10 and S15).

In comparison, a DPOAE response was recorded at three frequencies or more (1–8 kHz) in 5/18 IEs (S2, S4, S5, S7 and S10), all with corresponding IE ABRthrs of 35–45 dB nHL (no reliable/no DPOAE recording for S13 and S15) (Table 1). DPOAE responses at two frequencies or more were recorded in 7/18 IEs (for S2–5, S7, S10 and S17) and at one frequency or more in 13/18 IEs (S1–5, S7, S9–11, S16–19).

Although DPOAEs were recorded in some IEs, the DPOAE response levels (dB SPL) were generally weaker in the IEs compared to the NEs, as expected. For the frequencies with DPOAEs in the IEs (27 frequency recordings; DPOAE level−(Noise + 2 SD) > 0 dB), the median response level was −0.2 dB SPL (IQR: −3.8 to 6.3 dB SPL), in comparison to 17.7 dB SPL (IQR: 12.5–21.7 dB SPL, 94 frequency recordings) in the NEs.

## 4. Discussion

*4.1. Magnetic Resonance Imaging (MRI)*

Infants with mild to profound congenital uSNHL, consecutively recruited from the newborn hearing-screening program, were diagnosed with malformations of the auditory system in 64% of cases (9/14); 86% for congenital SSD (6/7) and 43% for mild to severe congenital uSNHL (3/7). Thus, the diagnostic yield of 64% was numerically somewhat higher than other studies of uSNHL and MRI of 37–58% [12–14,18,19]. However, compared to studies where apparently acquired uSNHL had been excluded (CT and/or MRI), the 64% was very similar to the previous 46–67% malformations [12,20,21]. A strength with this study design of congenital uSNHL was that the median diagnostic age was 2 months (Table 1), in comparison to the mean/median diagnostic age of around 4 years in previous studies, where apparently acquired uSNHL had been excluded [12,20,21]. A thorough audiologic examination was also performed in addition to the MRI. In agreement with previous studies of uSNHL, malformations were common for all degrees of uSNHL [13,16], and malformations were about twice as common for children with SSD compared to children with mild to severe uSNHL [16]. For mild to severe uSNHL the 43% malformation prevalence was similar to the 44–48% [13,16]. The 86% malformation prevalence for SSD was numerically higher than the 52–71% [13,16] found previously for SSD, probably due to the high prevalence of cochlear nerve aplasia found here.

The most common malformation was cochlear nerve aplasia in 50% of scans (7/14, Figure 4), which was numerically higher than what has been found in previous studies of children with uSNHL at 17–36% [12–14,18,19]. Not surprisingly, cochlear nerve aplasia was much more common for SSD (6/7, 86%) than for mild-to-severe uSNHL (1/7, 14%). The proportion of subjects with SSD compared to other degrees of uSNHL does not fully explain the high prevalence of cochlear nerve aplasia in this study, as 50% of the subjects who underwent MRI had SSD, which was similar to the 28–74% SSD in previous uSNHL studies [12–14,18,19]. The high prevalence of cochlear nerve aplasia may be due to our aim of only including infants with congenital uSNHL, by recruiting from the UNHS program, and diagnosing the uSNHL early (median age 2 months) and performing MRI as soon as possible (median age 8 months). For instance, one study found a prevalence of cochlear nerve aplasia or hypoplasia in 100% of infants with SSD ($n$ = 10) and 75% in preschool children with SSD ($n$ = 20), compared to 48% in children with SSD in general ($n$ = 50) [18], indicating that the diagnosis age matters. Furthermore, the MRI resolution needs to be sufficient to resolve individual nerves in the inner auditory canal and diagnose cochlear nerve aplasia or hypoplasia. A 3T MRI scanner was used in 93% of scans, the exception being for S3 where a 1.5 T scanner was used, as a back and spine MRI was prioritized additional to the auditory system MRI. Thus, the 3T scans may also contribute to the high prevalence of malformations, e.g., some studies included in a recent meta-analysis [15] found no cases of nerve aplasia or severe hypoplasia [53,54], and the MRI resolution was not described/specified, or found only a few percent cochlear nerve aplasia or severe hypoplasia [55] with MRI resolution at 1–2 Tesla.

The 29% inner ear malformations (4/14) were similar in prevalence to the 28–46% in previous studies [12–14,18], and so was the 21% EVA (3/14) compared to the 8–25% in previous studies [12–14,18]. The bilateral EVA quickly deteriorated to a bilateral SNHL, so the early MRI (at 7 months of age) contributed to a CI-fitting shortly after hearing loss onset.

*4.2. Congenital Cytomegalovirus (cCMV) Infection*

All subjects were cCMV negative. Children with uSNHL has previously been found to be cCMV positive in around 10% [14] to 20% of cases [29,30], so we expected some positive cases. The CMV PCR technique, used for the majority of subjects, has demonstrated a high negative predictive value (NPV) of 0.991 (95% CI = 0.972–0.997), as found by a meta-analysis based on 15 studies [56]. One contributing factor to the absence of cCMV infection could be that only congenital uSNHL was studied, compared to both acquired and congenital uSNHL [14,29,30]. About 30–50% children with cCMV that develop SNHL or uSNHL specifically do this during the neonatal period [27,28]. The first TEOAE measurement is also routinely performed very early, around postnatal day 3, in the UNHS program in Region Stockholm (98% screened) [2,43,44], compared to the neonatal period up to 2 months of age in previous studies [27,28]. Moreover, the spread of infections generally changes over time. The COVID-19 pandemic in 2020 to 2021 might have contributed to a lower prevalence of cCMV infection in infants, due to adjustments in hand hygiene and close contact with other people, as has been suggested from changes in cCMV prevalence in populations affected by strict lockdowns due to the pandemic [57,58].

Detecting cCMV-associated progressive uSNHL during the first years of life without universal neonatal cCMV screening is a challenge. Clinical protocols for finding these patients needs careful consideration, as they are potential CI candidates [30,59–61].

*4.3. Affected Mechanisms and Auditory Profiles*

The aim of this study included describing affected mechanisms in congenital uSNHL. We found that the ABR I/O function for the NE and IE were parallel shifted (Figure 3) and interaural amplitudes were significantly different at higher input levels, in contrast to the pattern previously observed in adults with cochlear hearing losses with recruitment [34,35]. Additionally, no significant interaural difference was found in ABR I-V intervals, indicating no reflection of auditory deprivation or retrocochlear influence on the IEs. The interaural difference in TEOAEs primarily supported the diagnosis of congenital uSNHL, with a NE and an IE from birth. The recordings of DPOAEs confirmed that the TEOAEs recorded here are more sensitive than DPOAEs evoked at 75/75 dB SPL in identifying minor cochlear hearing losses [52]. Not surprisingly, the subjects with DPOAEs at three frequencies or more demonstrated the lowest IE ABRthrs (i.e., 35–40 dB nHL). Similarly, the subjects that lacked DPOAEs also showed some of the highest IE ABRthrs (i.e., ≥60 dB nHL), which adds to research indicating that DPOAE I/O functions in children may be related to their behavior audiometric thresholds [62], although the relationship needs more study.

The parallel shift in ABR I/O functions was supported by the statistically significant effect of ear and stimulus level on waves I, III and V in the linear mixed model. From studies of adults with cochlear hearing loss and loudness recruitment, ABR amplitudes are expected to be significantly lower near the ABRthr in the IE than at the corresponding stimulus level in the NE, with similar amplitudes in the IE and NE at higher ABR stimulus levels of about 70–80 dB HL [34] and 60–80 dB nHL [35]. Thus, the parallel shifted functions suggest a reflection of a lack of recruitment on the group level, and/or a different type of hearing loss than cochlear hearing loss, predominantly affecting outer hair cells [34,35].

The absence of loudness recruitment was also reflected in the ARTs, as a significant interaural difference existed on the group level (Table 1). This agrees with previous study results, e.g., it was found that with higher stimulus levels, where equal loudness was judged between the ears, ARTs did not differ between the ears in adults with mild to moderate unilateral or asymmetrical SNHL and recruitment [63]. Additionally, this finding has been supported in human quinine experiments (induced hearing loss by affecting outer hair cells), where recruitment was reflected in changes in both in the TEOAE I/O function [64], and in ABR I/O function [35], with no change in ARTs, even up to a 46 dB hearing threshold shift [35,64]. It should be noted that parallel shifted NE and IE ABR I/O functions are typical for conductive hearing loss too. However, the interaural ABR latency difference for wave I, III and V was typical for SNHL, i.e., within the level of reproducibility (of about 0.2–0.3 ms) for NEs and IEs with cochlear hearing loss [65,66] (Figure 2 and Table S1, Supplementary Materials). Further support of no conductive component to the congenital uSNHL can be found in the indistinguishable tympanograms in the NE and IE, and the 10–15 dB interaural difference in ARTs.

ABR I/O functions in combination with ARTs may be useful clinical tools, especially the ABR, as it is already measured as a first or second step by many UNHS programs, and ABR I/O functions have shown to be similar for wave I and V from birth to adulthood [67,68]. The lack of loudness recruitment based on ABR I/O functions and ARTs on group level in children with congenital uSNHL presumably reflect the etiology behind the hearing loss, where, e.g., malformations of the auditory system are more common in unilateral compared to bilateral SNHL [16,17].

The ABR I/O function may add important information to be used in the choice of amplification and compression settings for pediatric patients. Most amplification guidelines for pediatric SNHL recommend the use of validated pediatric-focused prescriptive formulas, i.e., the desired sensation level (DSL) v.5 [69,70] or the national acoustic laboratory non-linear 2 (NAL NL2) [71] that focus on ensuring there is enough compression in the dynamic range to make sounds audible near thresholds and encourage that a wide range of input levels be compressed sufficiently [72,73]. These prescriptive formulas use the hearing thresholds as a function of frequency as a basis and take into account some additional auditory parameters. For loudness, the possibility of choosing between linear gain or wide dynamic range compression (WDRC) exists, and adjustments of the compression threshold can be made, and loudness discomfort levels (LDL) are taken into account for DSL v.5 [69,70]. The LDL is, to our knowledge, the only supra-threshold clinical data that can be applied to modify the prescriptive formulas of amplification. LDLs are not possible to measure in small children, and variability across subjects of all ages is large [74]. Thus, more research is needed into how supra-threshold data that reflect the individual's reduced dynamic range of hearing could be used in prescriptions to infants and children, e.g., the ABR I/O function studied here, as our groups' IE vs. NE I/O functions were different than those of adult listeners with cochlear hearing loss [34,35].

### 4.4. Strengths and Limitations

A strength of this diagnostic study is the prospective design of consecutively recruiting all children with congenital uSNHL in Region Stockholm during a two-year period, reducing sample bias. The median 55 dB nHL ABRthr, the 50% males and 65% left IEs ($n = 20$) were similar to the median 50 dB nHL ABRthr, the 56% males and 61% left IEs ($n = 18$) with congenital uSNHL previously screened in the UNHS program in Region Stockholm (>30,000 consecutively screened newborns, 98% coverage rate) [2], indicating a representative sample. Moreover, the median diagnostic age was much lower at 2 months of age, compared to about 4 years of age in etiology/imaging studies using similar subject groups [12,20,21]. Another strength is the detailed descriptions of auditory profiles and that all subjects revealed ABRthrs of $\leq$20 dB nHL in the NEs at the initial research visit, with healthy outer and middle ears bilaterally. The same audiological test instruments and audiologic test room was used for the measurements. ABRs, ARTs, TEOAEs, DPOAEs and tympanograms were recorded in an automatic and objective manner, and possible remaining between-subject variability due to, e.g., the inadequate placement of earphones or electrodes, was reduced by M.D., M.J. and E.B. performing and analyzing the audiologic measurements. The ABR wave analysis was performed in an objective and blinded manner. K.E. reviewed all MRI scans additional to the first review by one or two experienced neuroradiologists or head-neck radiologists.

Various recruitment steps were undertaken to invite all children born with uSNHL and excluding all children with temporary hearing loss. However, some children may have been missed in the recruitment process, despite our efforts to differentiate conductive from sensorineural components based on the tympanograms, ARTs, otomicroscopy by an experienced otologist, ABR amplitudes and latencies, and our attempts to reschedule follow-up visits to ensure normal hearing once OME was resolved. Based on earlier screening results in Region Stockholm, we expected about ten more participants (Figure 1), with 51,600 newborns screened in January 2019–October 2020 [46] and 0.058% congenital uSNHL prevalence [2], similar to other UNHS programs, e.g., 0.045% [1]. The COVID-19 pandemic may have contributed due to hospital anxiety in the beginning stages of the infection spread in Sweden, as we recruited 3 subjects born during the first 6 months of 2020 when the pandemic arrived in Sweden, compared to 6 subjects per 6 months in 2019. During the last 4 months of the recruitment of children born between July and October 2020 (recruitment stopped 31st of December 2020), after the first Swedish wave of COVID-19 infection, we recruited 5 infants, the expected number.

## 5. Conclusions

In this prospective etiology study of infants with congenital uSNHL, 64% of the MRIs revealed abnormal anatomical structures. In ears with a profound degree of uSNHL the malformation incidence was especially high at 86% ($n = 6/7$), though considerably high also in ears with mild to severe uSNHL at 43% ($n = 3/7$). The most common malformation was an absence of a cochlear nerve found in 50% of the MRI scans, followed by 29% inner ear malformations, of which 21% of all MRIs demonstrated EVA. Thus, MRI is powerful in finding possible causes for congenital uSNHL and may be used to find CI candidates with risks of unilateral to bilateral progression (e.g., ears with EVA). All 20 subjects tested negative for cCMV infection, indicating that it may be relatively uncommon with cCMV infection with very early uSNHL onset, although fluctuations in infection exposure over time should not be overlooked. The parallel shifted IE and NE ABR I/O functions and the interaural ART difference indicate that many children with mild-severe congenital uSNHL may not experience typical loudness recruitment associated with cochlear hearing loss. More research is needed on how supra-threshold measurements, such as the ABR I/O function and the ART, can be used to improve amplification and compression settings in pediatric hearing aids, as poor fittings may contribute to the large variability in hearing aid use and outcomes for children with uSNHL.

**Supplementary Materials:** The following supporting information can be downloaded at: https://www.mdpi.com/article/10.3390/jcm11143966/s1, Table S1: Auditory Brainstem Response (ABR) mean and median latency difference by stimulus level with statistical significance, Table S2: Auditory Brainstem Response (ABR) mean and median amplitude difference by stimulus level with statistical significance.

**Author Contributions:** Conceptualization, M.J. and E.B.; methodology, M.J. and E.B. with the assistance of E.K. and M.D.; validation, M.J., E.B. and K.E.; formal analysis, M.J., E.B., E.K. and K.E.; investigation, M.J, E.B. and M.D.; data curation, M.J. and E.B.; writing—original draft preparation, M.J. with assistance from E.B. and K.E.; writing—review and editing, all authors; project administration, M.J. with assistance from M.D.; funding acquisition, M.J. and E.B. All authors have read and agreed to the published version of the manuscript.

**Funding:** This research was funded by the Oticon Foundation (16-2108), the regional agreement on medical training and clinical research (ALF) between Region Stockholm and Karolinska Institutet, Hörselforskningsfonden (Swedish Hearing Research Foundation (2018-585)), Tysta Skolan Foundation (FB21-0009), Karolinska University Hospital, the Jerring foundation, Queen Silvia's Jubilee Fund and the Foundation of the Swedish Order of Freemasons.

**Institutional Review Board Statement:** The study was conducted in accordance with the Declaration of Helsinki and approved by the Swedish Ethical Review Authority (No: 2018/1500-31).

**Informed Consent Statement:** Informed consent was obtained from all subjects involved in the study through all parents with child custody.

**Data Availability Statement:** Data are sharable upon request.

**Acknowledgments:** The authors thank the participants and their parents. Additionally, Linda Nordin, Veronica Lilius (with team), and Andra Lazar at the Department of Audiology and Neurotology for helping with recruitment of subjects, Martin Eklöf for statistical assistance, Håkan Forsman and Magnus Vestin for technical assistance, and Sten Hellström for insightful comments on the manuscript.

**Conflicts of Interest:** Eva Karltorp is on the advisory board for MED-EL. The funders had no role in the design of the study; in the collection, analyses, or interpretation of data; in the writing of the manuscript, or in the decision to publish the results.

## References

1. Mehl, A.L.; Thomson, V. Newborn hearing screening: The great omission. *Pediatrics* **1998**, *101*, e4. [CrossRef] [PubMed]
2. Berninger, E.; Westling, B. Outcome of a universal newborn hearing-screening programme based on multiple transient-evoked otoacoustic emissions and clinical brainstem response audiometry. *Acta Otolaryngol.* **2011**, *131*, 728–739. [CrossRef] [PubMed]
3. McKay, S.; Gravel, J.S.; Tharpe, A.M. Amplification considerations for children with minimal or mild bilateral hearing loss and unilateral hearing loss. *Trends Amplif.* **2008**, *12*, 43–54. [CrossRef] [PubMed]
4. Kuppler, K.; Lewis, M.; Evans, A.K. A review of unilateral hearing loss and academic performance: Is it time to reassess traditional dogmata? *Int. J. Pediatr. Otorhinolaryngol.* **2013**, *77*, 617–622. [CrossRef] [PubMed]
5. Lieu, J.E.C.; Karzon, R.K.; Ead, B.; Tye-Murray, N. Do Audiologic Characteristics Predict Outcomes in Children With Unilateral Hearing Loss? *Otol. Neurotol.* **2013**, *34*, 1703–1710. [CrossRef] [PubMed]
6. Humes, L.E.; Allen, S.K.; Bess, F.H. Horizontal sound localization skills of unilaterally hearing-impaired children. *Audiology* **1980**, *19*, 508–518. [CrossRef]
7. Newton, V.E. Sound localisation in children with a severe unilateral hearing loss. *Audiology* **1983**, *22*, 189–198. [CrossRef]
8. Bess, F.H.; Tharpe, A.M. Unilateral hearing impairment in children. *Pediatrics* **1984**, *74*, 206–216. [CrossRef]
9. Bess, F.H.; Tharpe, A.M. Case history data on unilaterally hearing-impaired children. *Ear Hear.* **1986**, *7*, 14–19. [CrossRef]
10. Bovo, R.; Martini, A.; Agnoletto, M.; Beghi, A.; Carmignoto, D.; Milani, M.; Zangaglia, A.M. Auditory and academic performance of children with unilateral hearing loss. *Scand. Audiol. Suppl.* **1988**, *30*, 71–74.
11. Ruscetta, M.N.; Arjmand, E.M.; Pratt, S.R. Speech recognition abilities in noise for children with severe-to-profound unilateral hearing impairment. *Int. J. Pediatr. Otorhinolaryngol.* **2005**, *69*, 771–779. [CrossRef] [PubMed]
12. Orzan, E.; Pizzamiglio, G.; Gregori, M.; Marchi, R.; Torelli, L.; Muzzi, E. Correlation of cochlear aperture stenosis with cochlear nerve deficiency in congenital unilateral hearing loss and prognostic relevance for cochlear implantation. *Sci. Rep.* **2021**, *11*, 3338. [CrossRef] [PubMed]
13. van Beeck Calkoen, E.A.; Sanchez Aliaga, E.; Merkus, P.; Smit, C.F.; van de Kamp, J.M.; Mulder, M.F.; Goverts, S.T.; Hensen, E.F. High prevalence of abnormalities on CT and MR imaging in children with unilateral sensorineural hearing loss irrespective of age or degree of hearing loss. *Int. J. Pediatr. Otorhinolaryngol.* **2017**, *97*, 185–191. [CrossRef]

14. Paul, A.; Marlin, S.; Parodi, M.; Rouillon, I.; Guerlain, J.; Pingault, V.; Couloigner, V.; Garabedian, E.N.; Denoyelle, F.; Loundon, N. Unilateral Sensorineural Hearing Loss: Medical Context and Etiology. *Audiol. Neurootol.* **2017**, *22*, 83–88. [CrossRef]
15. Ropers, F.G.; Pham, E.N.B.; Kant, S.G.; Rotteveel, L.J.C.; Rings, E.; Verbist, B.M.; Dekkers, O.M. Assessment of the Clinical Benefit of Imaging in Children With Unilateral Sensorineural Hearing Loss: A Systematic Review and Meta-analysis. *JAMA Otolaryngol. Head Neck Surg.* **2019**, *145*, 431–443. [CrossRef]
16. McClay, J.E.; Booth, T.N.; Parry, D.A.; Johnson, R.; Roland, P. Evaluation of pediatric sensorineural hearing loss with magnetic resonance imaging. *Arch. Otolaryngol. Head Neck Surg.* **2008**, *134*, 945–952. [CrossRef] [PubMed]
17. Masuda, S.; Usui, S. Comparison of the prevalence and features of inner ear malformations in congenital unilateral and bilateral hearing loss. *Int. J. Pediatr. Otorhinolaryngol.* **2019**, *125*, 92–97. [CrossRef]
18. Clemmens, C.S.; Guidi, J.; Caroff, A.; Cohn, S.J.; Brant, J.A.; Laury, A.M.; Bilaniuk, L.T.; Germiller, J.A. Unilateral cochlear nerve deficiency in children. *Otolaryngol. Head Neck Surg.* **2013**, *149*, 318–325. [CrossRef]
19. Gruber, M.; Brown, C.; Mahadevan, M.; Neeff, M. Concomitant imaging and genetic findings in children with unilateral sensorineural hearing loss. *J. Laryngol. Otol.* **2017**, *131*, 688–695. [CrossRef]
20. Masuda, S.; Usui, S.; Matsunaga, T. High prevalence of inner-ear and/or internal auditory canal malformations in children with unilateral sensorineural hearing loss. *Int. J. Pediatr. Otorhinolaryngol.* **2013**, *77*, 228–232. [CrossRef]
21. Nakano, A.; Arimoto, Y.; Matsunaga, T. Cochlear nerve deficiency and associated clinical features in patients with bilateral and unilateral hearing loss. *Otol. Neurotol.* **2013**, *34*, 554–558. [CrossRef] [PubMed]
22. Barbi, M.; Binda, S.; Caroppo, S.; Ambrosetti, U.; Corbetta, C.; Sergi, P. A wider role for congenital cytomegalovirus infection in sensorineural hearing loss. *Pediatr. Infect. Dis. J.* **2003**, *22*, 39–42. [CrossRef] [PubMed]
23. Morton, C.C.; Nance, W.E. Newborn hearing screening—A silent revolution. *N. Engl. J. Med.* **2006**, *354*, 2151–2164. [CrossRef] [PubMed]
24. Vos, B.; Noll, D.; Whittingham, J.; Pigeon, M.; Bagatto, M.; Fitzpatrick, E.M. Cytomegalovirus-A Risk Factor for Childhood Hearing Loss: A Systematic Review. *Ear Hear.* **2021**, *42*, 1447–1461. [CrossRef]
25. Fowler, K.B.; McCollister, F.P.; Dahle, A.J.; Boppana, S.; Britt, W.J.; Pass, R.F. Progressive and fluctuating sensorineural hearing loss in children with asymptomatic congenital cytomegalovirus infection. *J. Pediatr.* **1997**, *130*, 624–630. [CrossRef]
26. Dahle, A.J.; Fowler, K.B.; Wright, J.D.; Boppana, S.B.; Britt, W.J.; Pass, R.F. Longitudinal investigation of hearing disorders in children with congenital cytomegalovirus. *J. Am. Acad. Audiol.* **2000**, *11*, 283–290. [CrossRef]
27. Fowler, K.B.; Dahle, A.J.; Boppana, S.B.; Pass, R.F. Newborn hearing screening: Will children with hearing loss caused by congenital cytomegalovirus infection be missed? *J. Pediatr.* **1999**, *135*, 60–64. [CrossRef]
28. Fowler, K.B.; McCollister, F.P.; Sabo, D.L.; Shoup, A.G.; Owen, K.E.; Woodruff, J.L.; Cox, E.; Mohamed, L.S.; Choo, D.I.; Boppana, S.B. A Targeted Approach for Congenital Cytomegalovirus Screening Within Newborn Hearing Screening. *Pediatrics* **2017**, *139*, e20162128. [CrossRef]
29. Karltorp, E.; Hellström, S.; Lewensohn-Fuchs, I.; Carlsson-Hansén, E.; Carlsson, P.I.; Engman, M.L. Congenital cytomegalovirus infection—A common cause of hearing loss of unknown aetiology. *Acta Paediatr.* **2012**, *101*, e357–e362. [CrossRef]
30. Arndt, S.; Prosse, S.; Laszig, R.; Wesarg, T.; Aschendorff, A.; Hassepass, F. Cochlear Implantation in Children with Single-Sided Deafness: Does Aetiology and Duration of Deafness Matter? *Audiol. Neurootol.* **2015**, *20*, 21–30. [CrossRef]
31. Gordon, K.A.; Henkin, Y.; Kral, A. Asymmetric Hearing During Development: The Aural Preference Syndrome and Treatment Options. *Pediatrics* **2015**, *136*, 141–153. [CrossRef]
32. Steinberg, J.C.; Gardner, M.B. The Dependence of Hearing Impairment on Sound Intensity. *J. Acoust. Soc. Am.* **1937**, *9*, 11–23. [CrossRef]
33. Moore, B.C. Perceptual consequences of cochlear hearing loss and their implications for the design of hearing aids. *Ear Hear.* **1996**, *17*, 133–161. [CrossRef] [PubMed]
34. Eggermont, J.J. Electrocochleography and Recruitment. *Ann. Otol. Rhinol. Laryngol.* **1977**, *86*, 138–149. [CrossRef] [PubMed]
35. Karlsson, K.K.; Berninger, E.; Gustafsson, L.L.; Alvan, G. Pronounced quinine-induced cochlear hearing loss. A mechanistic study in one volunteer at multiple stable plasma concentrations. *Audiol. Med.* **1995**, *4*, 12–24.
36. Jerger, J. Clinical Experience With Impedance Audiometry. *Arch. Otolaryngol.* **1970**, *92*, 311–324. [CrossRef]
37. Marchant, C.D.; McMillan, P.M.; Shurin, P.A.; Johnson, C.E.; Turczyk, V.A.; Feinstein, J.C.; Murdell Panek, D. Objective diagnosis of otitis media in early infancy by tympanometry and ipsilateral acoustic reflex thresholds. *J. Pediatr.* **1986**, *109*, 590–595. [CrossRef]
38. Shera, C.A.; Guinan, J.J., Jr. Evoked otoacoustic emissions arise by two fundamentally different mechanisms: A taxonomy for mammalian OAEs. *J. Acoust. Soc. Am.* **1999**, *105*, 782–798. [CrossRef]
39. Liberman, M.C.; Gao, J.; He, D.Z.Z.; Wu, X.; Jia, S.; Zuo, J. Prestin is required for electromotility of the outer hair cell and for the cochlear amplifier. *Nature* **2002**, *419*, 300–304. [CrossRef]
40. Gorga, M.P.; Worthington, D.W.; Reiland, J.K.; Beauchaine, K.A.; Goldgar, D.E. Some comparisons between auditory brain stem response thresholds, latencies, and the pure-tone audiogram. *Ear Hear.* **1985**, *6*, 105–112. [CrossRef]
41. Eggermont, J.J.; Don, M. Mechanisms of central conduction time prolongation in brain-stem auditory evoked potentials. *Arch. Neurol.* **1986**, *43*, 116–120. [CrossRef] [PubMed]
42. Berninger, E.; Olofsson, Å.; Leijon, A. Analysis of click-evoked auditory brainstem responses using time domain cross-correlations between interleaved responses. *Ear Hear.* **2014**, *35*, 318–329. [CrossRef] [PubMed]

43. Berninger, E. Characteristics of normal newborn transient-evoked otoacoustic emissions: Ear asymmetries and sex effects. *Int. J. Audiol.* **2007**, *46*, 661–669. [CrossRef] [PubMed]
44. Johansson, M.; Olofsson, Å.; Berninger, E. Twin study of neonatal transient-evoked otoacoustic emissions. *Hear. Res.* **2020**, *398*, 108108. [CrossRef] [PubMed]
45. Bussé, A.M.L.; Mackey, A.R.; Hoeve, H.L.J.; Goedegebure, A.; Carr, G.; Uhlén, I.M.; Simonsz, H.J. Assessment of hearing screening programmes across 47 countries or regions I: Provision of newborn hearing screening. *Int. J. Audiol.* **2021**, *60*, 821–830. [CrossRef]
46. Socialstyrelsen. Available online: https://sdb.socialstyrelsen.se/if_mfr_004/val.aspx (accessed on 2 June 2022).
47. *ISO389-6*; Acoustics—Reference Zero for the Calibration of Audiometric Equipment—Part 6: Reference Threshold of Hearing for Test Signals of Short Duration. International Organization for Standardization: Geneva, Switzerland, 2007.
48. *IEC60318-4*; Electroacoustics—Simulators of Human Head and Ear—Part 4: Occluded-Ear Simulator for the Measurement of Earphones Coupled to the Ear by Means of Ear Inserts. International Electrotechnical Commision: Geneva, Switzerland, 2010.
49. Sklare, D.A.; Denenberg, L.J. Interaural attenuation for tubephone insert earphones. *Ear Hear.* **1987**, *8*, 298–300. [CrossRef]
50. Kemp, D.T.; Ryan, S.; Bray, P. A guide to the effective use of otoacoustic emissions. *Ear Hear.* **1990**, *11*, 93–105. [CrossRef]
51. Thornton, A.R.; Marotta, N.; Kennedy, C.R. The order of testing effect in otoacoustic emissions and its consequences for sex and ear differences in neonates. *Hear. Res.* **2003**, *184*, 123–130. [CrossRef]
52. Berninger, E.; Karlsson, K.K.; Hellgren, U.; Eskilsson, G. Magnitude changes in transient evoked otoacoustic emissions and high-level 2f1-f2 distortion products in man during quinine administration. *Scand. Audiol.* **1995**, *24*, 27–32. [CrossRef]
53. Friedman, A.B.; Guillory, R.; Ramakrishnaiah, R.H.; Frank, R.; Gluth, M.B.; Richter, G.T.; Dornhoffer, J.L. Risk analysis of unilateral severe-to-profound sensorineural hearing loss in children. *Int. J. Pediatr. Otorhinolaryngol.* **2013**, *77*, 1128–1131. [CrossRef]
54. Haffey, T.; Fowler, N.; Anne, S. Evaluation of unilateral sensorineural hearing loss in the pediatric patient. *Int. J. Pediatr. Otorhinolaryngol.* **2013**, *77*, 955–958. [CrossRef] [PubMed]
55. Simons, J.P.; Mandell, D.L.; Arjmand, E.M. Computed Tomography and Magnetic Resonance Imaging in Pediatric Unilateral and Asymmetric Sensorineural Hearing Loss. *Arch Otolaryngol. Head Neck Surg.* **2006**, *132*, 186–192. [CrossRef] [PubMed]
56. Wang, L.; Xu, X.; Zhang, H.; Qian, J.; Zhu, J. Dried blood spots PCR assays to screen congenital cytomegalovirus infection: A meta-analysis. *Virol. J.* **2015**, *12*, 60. [CrossRef] [PubMed]
57. Fernandez, C.; Chasqueira, M.-J.; Marques, A.; Rodrigues, L.; Marçal, M.; Tuna, M.; Braz, M.C.; Neto, A.S.; Mendes, C.; Lito, D.; et al. Lower prevalence of congenital cytomegalovirus infection in Portugal: Possible impact of COVID-19 lockdown? *Eur. J. Pediatr.* **2022**, *181*, 1259–1262. [CrossRef]
58. Rios-Barnes, M.; Fontalvo, M.A.; Linan, N.; Plana, M.; Moreno, M.; Esteva, C.; Munoz-Almagro, C.; Noguera-Julian, A.; Alarcon, A.; Ríos-Barnés, M.; et al. Letter to the Editor on the original article: Lower prevalence of congenital cytomegalovirus infection in Portugal: Possible impact of COVID-19 lockdown? *Eur. J. Pediatr.* **2022**, *181*, 1293–1294. [CrossRef] [PubMed]
59. Polonenko, M.J.; Papsin, B.C.; Gordon, K.A. Children With Single-Sided Deafness Use Their Cochlear Implant. *Ear Hear.* **2017**, *38*, 681–689. [CrossRef]
60. Polonenko, M.J.; Gordon, K.A.; Cushing, S.L.; Papsin, B.C. Cortical organization restored by cochlear implantation in young children with single sided deafness. *Sci. Rep.* **2017**, *7*, 16900. [CrossRef]
61. Thomas, J.P.; Neumann, K.; Dazert, S.; Voelter, C. Cochlear Implantation in Children With Congenital Single-Sided Deafness. *Otol. Neurotol.* **2017**, *38*, 496–503. [CrossRef]
62. Janssen, T. A Review of the Effectiveness of Otoacoustic Emissions for Evaluating Hearing Status After Newborn Screening. *Otol. Neurotol.* **2013**, *34*, 1058–1063. [CrossRef]
63. Fitzzaland, R.E.; Borton, T.E. The acoustic reflex and loudness recruitment. *J. Otolaryngol.* **1977**, *6*, 460–465.
64. Berninger, E.; Karlsson, K.K.; Alvan, G. Quinine reduces the dynamic range of the human auditory system. *Acta Otolaryngol.* **1998**, *118*, 46–51. [PubMed]
65. Rosenhamer, H.J.; Lindström, B.; Lundborg, T. On the use of click-evoked electric brainstem responses in audiological diagnosis. I. The variability of the normal response. *Scand. Audiol.* **1978**, *7*, 193–205. [CrossRef] [PubMed]
66. Rosenhamer, H.J.; Lindström, B.; Lundborg, T. On the use of click-evoked electric brainstem responses in audiological diagnosis. IV. Interaural latency differences (wave V) in cochlear hearing loss. *Scand. Audiol.* **1981**, *10*, 67–73. [CrossRef] [PubMed]
67. Jiang, Z.D.; Zhang, L.; Wu, Y.Y.; Liu, X.Y. Brainstem auditory evoked responses from birth to adulthood: Development of wave amplitude. *Hear. Res.* **1993**, *68*, 35–41. [CrossRef]
68. Jiang, Z.D. Intensity Effect on Amplitude of Auditory Brainstem Responses in Human. *Scand Audiol.* **1991**, *20*, 41–47. [CrossRef]
69. Bagatto, M.P.; Moodie, S.; Scollie, S.; Seewald, R.; Moodie, S.; Pumford, J.; Liu, K.P. Clinical protocols for hearing instrument fitting in the Desired Sensation Level method. *Trends Amplif.* **2005**, *9*, 199–226. [CrossRef]
70. Scollie, S.; Seewald, R.; Cornelisse, L.; Moodie, S.; Bagatto, M.; Laurnagaray, D.; Beaulac, S.; Pumford, J. The Desired Sensation Level multistage input/output algorithm. *Trends Amplif.* **2005**, *9*, 159–197. [CrossRef]
71. Keidser, G.; Dillon, H.; Carter, L.; O'Brien, A. NAL-NL2 Empirical Adjustments. *Trends Amplif.* **2012**, *16*, 211–223. [CrossRef]
72. McCreery, R.W.; Bentler, R.A.; Roush, P.A. Characteristics of hearing aid fittings in infants and young children. *Ear Hear.* **2013**, *34*, 701–710. [CrossRef]
73. American Academy of Audiology. *American Academy of Audiology Clinical Practice Guidelines: Pediatric Amplification*; American Academy of Audiology: Reston, VA, USA, 2013; pp. 5–20.
74. Kawell, M.E.; Kopun, J.G.; Stelmachowicz, P.G. Loudness discomfort levels in children. *Ear Hear.* **1988**, *9*, 133–136. [CrossRef]

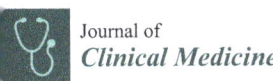

Article

# Analysis of the Results of Cytomegalovirus Testing Combined with Genetic Testing in Children with Congenital Hearing Loss

Yuan Jin [1], Xiaozhou Liu [1], Sen Chen [1], Jiale Xiang [2], Zhiyu Peng [2] and Yu Sun [1,*]

1 Department of Otorhinolaryngology, Union Hospital, Tongji Medical College, Huazhong University of Science and Technology, Wuhan 430022, China
2 College of Life Sciences, University of Chinese Academy of Sciences, Beijing 100049, China
* Correspondence: sunyu@hust.edu.cn

**Abstract:** To improve the etiological diagnosis of congenital hearing loss by combining whole-exome sequencing (WES) with cytomegalovirus (CMV) testing and to explore the potential benefits of adding CMV screening to newborn hearing screening, 80 children under 2 years of age with bilateral sensorineural hearing loss were recruited. Peripheral venous blood was extracted from the children for WES analysis. Saliva after mouthwash and the first urine in the morning were collected and used as samples to quantify CMV DNA copy number in urine and saliva by qPCR; among the 80 children with congenital deafness, 59 (74%) were found to have genetic variants that may cause congenital deafness, including 44 with *GJB2* or *SLC26A4* gene variant, 1 with *STRC* gene variant, and 14 with other genetic variants. A total of 12 children carried deafness gene variants associated with a syndrome; CMV test results showed that in two children, the CMV DNA copy number in saliva was >1000/mL, which indicates that they were CMV-positive, and their genetic test results were negative. A neonatal CMV test combined with genetic screening can improve the etiological diagnosis rate of congenital deafness, and the direct evidence of neonatal CMV infection deserves further verification.

**Keywords:** cytomegalovirus; congenital hearing loss; screening; genetic testing

## 1. Introduction

Congenital hearing loss is the most common sensory deficit in children. It has been reported that 1–2 per 1000 newborns have sensorineural hearing impairment [1]. More than 50% of cases of congenital hearing loss in children are attributed to genetic aetiologies [2]. To date, 218 genes causing deafness have been identified [3]. Among the non-genetic factors associated with congenital hearing loss, cytomegalovirus (CMV) infection is one of the most common, accounting for 10–20% of cases of sensorineural hearing impairment reported in children [4]. Countries and regions with different economic conditions have different rates of neonatal CMV infection. In general, the infection rate of human CMV in live newborns is 0.3–2.4% [5]. In developing countries, the incidence can reach 1–5% of all live births [6].

CMV mainly invades the liver, followed by the brain, bone marrow, lung, heart, and other organs, which can lead to neonatal birth defects and developmental disorders [7]. Approximately 85–90% of infected newborns have no symptoms at birth, and 10–15% of infected newborns have obvious symptoms of clinical infection [8]. Clinical manifestations of CMV include foetal growth restriction, low birth weight, central nervous system and multiple organ involvement with petechiae, hepatomegaly, splenomegaly, jaundice, pneumonia, and encephalitis [9]. These manifestations are severe and can cause a high perinatal mortality rate and major neurological sequelae in approximately 90% of surviving infants with symptomatic CMV [10]. In addition, 10–15% of infants with asymptomatic CMV develop long-term sequelae, including progressive sensorineural hearing difficulty and mental retardation [11]. These sequelae add to the complexity of the diagnosis of CMV infection.

If children with sensorineural hearing loss do not receive timely intervention, the development of their speaking ability, intelligence, and learning ability is seriously affected, which substantially impacts their individual development and future. Although newborn hearing screening is universal in most developed countries, screening for CMV in newborns is not widespread [12]. Determining whether congenital CMV infection or genetic factors are the cause of hearing loss in these newborns is important for early diagnosis and intervention. To improve the aetiological diagnosis rate of congenital deafness, we recruited children with congenital sensorineural disease and performed deafness genetic testing and CMV testing. Due to the high cost of whole-genome sequencing, we adopted a low-cost comprehensive genetic testing protocol. In this study, we identified several children who were CMV-positive via CMV screening and did not carry genetic variants that cause deafness. Although the CMV test results did not diagnose congenital CMV infection in these children, we considered their congenital hearing loss to be linked to congenital CMV infection based on their clinical symptoms. To more accurately diagnose the aetiology of congenital deafness, provide a more optimized diagnosis and treatment strategy, and improve the quality of life of children with congenital CMV, we propose adding high-sensitivity and high-specificity CMV screening to newborn hearing screening.

## 2. Materials and Methods

### 2.1. Clinical Examination

We recruited 80 children with bilateral hearing loss to this study. All participating children failed newborn hearing screening. Based on newborn hearing screening results, auditory steady-state response results, and medical history, these participants were diagnosed with congenital hearing loss. The children were 24 months of age or younger at the time of the testing. All children were physically examined, and their medical history was collected to identify other systemic disorders or abnormalities.

### 2.2. Variant Detection and Analysis

The *GJB2* and *SLC26A4* genes were first analysed by a multiplex polymerase chain reaction (PCR) amplicon sequencing assay. Low-pass genome sequencing was then used to analyse *GJB6* gene deletion. After excluding the aforementioned genes, *STRC/OTOA* analysis was performed using a kit (SALSA® MLPA® P461 DIS probe mix kit, MRC-Holland, Amsterdam, the Netherlands). Patients suffering from severe or profound hearing loss or who had negative results from *STRC/OTOA* analysis were further referred for exome sequencing. Exome sequencing was performed using KAPA HyperExome Probes (Roche, Pleasanton, CA, USA) accompanied by 100 bp paired-end sequencing on an MGISEQ-2000 platform (BGI-Wuhan, Wuhan, China). All detected sequence variants were confirmed via Sanger sequencing (single nucleotide variants), quantitative PCR (qPCR; exon-level copy number variations (CNVs)), or low-pass genome sequencing (subchromosomal CNVs). The sequencing results were all aligned to the reference human genome (hg19) using the Burrows–Wheeler Aligner (BWA) Multi-Vision software package. According to the sequencing results of two probands, Sanger sequencing was performed to confirm whether their parents had the same mutations. All SNVs and indels were referenced and compared with multiple databases, including the National Centre for Biotechnology Information (NCBI) GenBank database (https://www.ncbi.nlm.nih.gov/nuccore, accessed on 6 January 2021), the Database of Single Nucleotide Polymorphisms (dbSNP) (http://www.ncbi.nlm.nih.gov/projects/SNP, accessed on 6 January 2021), and the 1000 Genomes Database (https://www.internationalgenome.org, accessed on 6 January 2021).

### 2.3. Test for CMV Infection

Quantitative detection of CMV DNA content was performed by BGI Genomics (Wuhan, China). A total of 0.2 mL saliva and 2 mL urine was collected from each patient participating in the study for the detection of CMV infection. Specimens were stored at 4 °C until they were processed in the virology laboratory. We used 0.2 mL of urine or saliva to prepare DNA for quantitative detection of CMV DNA content by real-time fluorescence qPCR. A CMV test was considered positive when the saliva or urine samples were confirmed to be positive for CMV DNA (CMV DNA $\geq 1 \times 10^3$ copies/mL). Term infants with serum total bilirubin >220 µmol/L and preterm infants with serum total bilirubin >256 µmol/L were diagnosed with pathological neonatal jaundice.

## 3. Results
### 3.1. Rate of CMV Infection

Of the 80 children with congenital bilateral hearing loss in the study, 59 (74%) were found to have genetic variants that may cause congenital deafness, including 44 with *GJB2* or *SLC26A4* gene variant, 1 with *STRC* gene variant, and 14 with other genetic variants that may cause deafness. No genetic variants that can cause deafness were detected in the remaining 21 children. Among the 59 cases of children carrying a gene variant that may cause deafness, 12 children carried deafness gene variants associated with a syndrome; however, symptoms in addition to hearing loss were found in only five children upon further examination, and no signs or symptoms associated with a syndrome were observed upon subsequent clinical examination of the remaining seven children. CMV test results revealed that in two children, the CMV DNA copy number in saliva was >1000/mL, indicating that they were CMV-positive, and their genetic test results were negative, with no variants identified in genes that are known to cause deafness. The medical history of these two children included symptoms of congenital CMV infection, such as hyperbilirubinemia, ventricular defects, and patent ductus arteriosus. We summarise the information of all children with CMV-positive or CMV-false positive results in Table 1.

**Table 1.** Information on all children with CMV-positive or CMV-false positive results.

| Subject | Age at the Time of Sample Collection (Months) | CMV DNA Quantification in Saliva Sample | CMV DNA Quantification in Urine Sample | Variants in Congenital Hearing Loss–Related Genes |
|---|---|---|---|---|
| 1 | 4 | 413,976.2 | 48,028.8 | *GJB2* c. 560_605dup/c. 235del C |
| 2 | 7 | 114,985.0 | negative | - |
| 3 | 6 | 93,588.6 | negative | *SLC26A4* c. 919-2 A > G/c. 589 G > A |
| 4 | 7 | 90,400.3 | 60,704.0 | *GJB2* c. 263 C > T |
| 5 | 8 | 48,376.9 | 6928.1 | *KCNQ1* c. 1684 A > GT/EXON 8-9 DEL |
| 6 | 7 | 37,786.3 | negative | - |
| 7 | 3 | 14,382.9 | negative | *GJB2* c. 299_300 del AT/c. 235del C |
| 8 | 21 | negative | negative | - |
| 9 | 18 | negative | negative | - |
| 10 | 22 | negative | negative | *GJB2* c. 235del C/c. 235del C |
| 11 | 12 | negative | negative | *MYO7A* c. 6320 G > A/c. 612 C > G |
| 12 | 22 | negative | negative | - |
| 13 | 20 | negative | negative | *GJB2* c. 235del C/c. 176_191del |

### 3.2. Clinical Data

Auditory Brainstem Response (ABR) was used to detect the hearing thresholds of the subjects. For Subject 2, the hearing threshold of the left ear was 55 dB, and the hearing threshold of the right ear was 60 dB; for Subject 6, the hearing threshold of the left ear was 100 dB, and the hearing threshold of the right ear was 90 dB. The pure-tone average was categorised as normal, mild (26–40 dB), moderate (41–55 dB), moderately severe (56–70 dB), severe (71–90 dB), or profound (>90 dB).

Subject 2 suffered from bilateral congenital deafness. The parents of Subject 2 stated that Subject 2 was born with neonatal hyperbilirubinemia, neonatal pneumonia, and hypoalbuminemia. These were verified in Subject 2's medical history and examination. Subject 6 was born with congenital heart disease (congenital patent ductus arteriosus). These are symptoms that may be observed in children with congenital CMV infection (Figure 1).

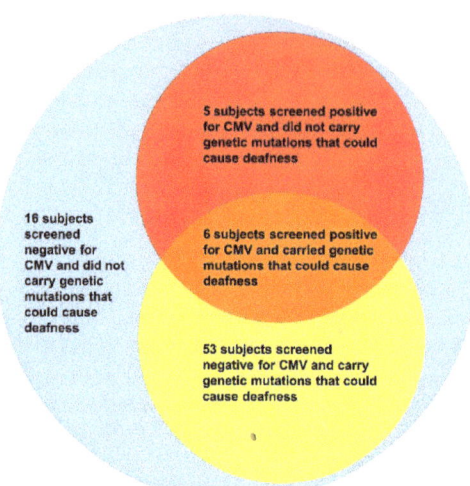

**Figure 1.** Graph of CMV screening and next-generation sequencing results.

## 4. Discussion

Numerous studies have reported that CMV infection can cause congenital SNHL in children [13]; however, newborn CMV screening has not yet been established in routine practice in most countries. TORCH tests are performed on women of childbearing age in countries such as China [14]. Notably, many women around the world of reproductive age are seropositive for CMV [15]. In addition, it has been reported that women who are seropositive for CMV antibodies and may be immune may carry CMV-infected infants who are also at significant risk of congenital SNHL [16].

In our study, we collected blood, saliva, and urine samples and clinical data from 80 children who failed newborn hearing screening and attempted to diagnose these children with congenital deafness via next-generation sequencing and CMV screening. All 80 children were under 2 years of age at the time of the study. According to previous reports, the detection rate of CMV in newborns' serum samples is lower than in saliva and urine samples. Serum samples were found to be positive in less than 40% of CMV-infected neonates. This suggests that saliva and urine samples are more suitable for newborn CMV screening. Saliva has a high detection rate but is prone to false-positive results; therefore, further testing on urine samples must be conducted in patients with CMV-positive saliva. In this study, CMV was detected in the saliva samples of 13 children and urine samples of 11 children. However, we considered children to be positive for CMV infection only when the CMV copy number detected in saliva or urine samples was >1000/mL. As shown in Table 1, there were two CMV-positive cases. Whole-exome sequencing revealed that they did not carry genetic variants that could cause hearing loss. In addition, the two children had a history of other clinical symptoms similar to those caused by congenital CMV infection. We believe that their congenital hearing loss may have been caused by congenital CMV infection.

In our study, genetic factors were found to account for 59/80 (74%) cases of congenital deafness. The proportion of children who are CMV-positive and do not carry the gene variant site is 0.025%. This value is much lower than the infection rate of CMV in children with SNHL [4,5]. This may be because the children we selected were all born with SNHL and were younger than 2 years of age. However, a considerable proportion of the hearing loss caused by congenital CMV infection is delayed hearing loss. Children who tested positive for CMV may have had a congenital infection, perinatal infection, or postnatal infection. However, we were not able to pinpoint the timing of CMV infection in the children. Moreover, we can only determine that these children had CMV infection; we cannot conclude whether their congenital hearing loss is related to CMV infection. As a result, diagnosis and treatment of these children is difficult. Notably, no association between urine or saliva CMV viral content and hearing loss severity was observed in our study. Of course, CMV virus levels in urine or saliva do not reflect the situation in the cochlea.

Early diagnosis and provision of antiviral therapy can help children with CMV infection lead normal lives. The efficacy of antiviral therapy in neonates with isolated SNHL due to CMV remains controversial. Because the replication of CMV in patients rebounds immediately after cessation of antiviral therapy, and SNHL in infants with CMV is often delayed; researchers question whether short-term antiviral therapy would have long-term benefit in the progression of SNHL [17]. However, it is worth noting that some studies have shown that infants born with isolated SNHL due to CMV were found to benefit from prolonged antiviral treatment. Marian G Michaels et al. treated nine symptomatic CMV-infected children with chronic intravenous or oral ganciclovir, seven had no progression of hearing loss, and two had improved hearing thresholds [18]. The placebo-controlled trial of valganciclovir therapy in neonates with symptomatic congenital CMV disease by David W Kimberlin et al. found that total-ear hearing (i.e., hearing in one or both ears that can be evaluated) was more likely to be improved or to remain normal at 12 months in the 6-month valganciclovir therapy group than in the 6-week valganciclovir therapy group [19]. The improvement in total-ear hearing was maintained at 24 months. In a retrospective study, Yehonatan Pasternak et al. found that infants born with isolated SNHL due to CMV showed significant improvement in hearing status and no deterioration of unaffected ears at baseline after receiving long-term antiviral therapy (intravenous ganciclovir 5 mg/kg/d for 6 weeks followed by oral valganciclovir or oral valganciclovir 17 mg/kg/dose in two daily doses for 12 weeks, then one daily dose until completion of 12 months of treatment) [20]. Although these antiviral treatments increase the risk of neutropenia, the benefit of long-term antiviral therapy on hearing in congenital CMV-infected patients deserves attention [19,20]. Antivirals should be started in the first month of life, and therapy must be based on a definitive diagnosis of CMV infection [21]. Therefore, screening for CMV in neonates is valuable.

Numerous studies have reported CMV screening combined with genetic testing for deafness in newborns who did not pass newborn hearing screening tests [22]. However, newborn CMV screening is not yet routinely performed in most countries. Foreign studies have shown that 68.3% of pregnant women have positive serum CMV IgG, of whom approximately 0.8% have active CMV infection [23]. In the United States, approximately 20,000 to 30,000 newborns are born with congenital CMV infection each year, of whom approximately 10–15% will suffer hearing impairment in childhood [24]. In China, approximately 95.3% of pregnant women are serum CMV-IgG positive [25]; among them, 3.5% were found to have acute or active CMV infection. Most newborns with congenital CMV infection are asymptomatic. We emphasise that newborn CMV screening is essential to identifying the aetiology of congenital deafness in newborns. The lack of newborn screening for CMV makes the diagnosis of congenital deafness difficult. Furthermore, we also propose including CMV screening in newborn hearing screening. However, there are problems in neonatal CMV screening that should be taken into consideration.

At present, there are no technical difficulties in the general screening for CMV in newborns, and a variety of samples and methods have been used to detect CMV. CMV screening of neonatal saliva samples by CMV PCR assay and collection of neonatal urine samples for further confirmation by PCR is an efficient and convenient method. However, widespread investigations have substantial economic costs. We can further reduce the risk of neonatal congenital CMV infection by developing CMV vaccines and reducing the exposure risk of women of childbearing age; however, ambiguity in diagnosis can lead to untimely interventions and antiretroviral treatment, causing children with SNHL to miss the optimal period of treatment and seriously hinder their healthy growth and development. We should calculate and balance the economic costs and social benefits of universal neonatal CMV screening. Studies have reported the potential cost-effectiveness and health benefits of universal screening among Chinese newborns [12]. Given that congenital CMV infection can cause progressive hearing loss, follow-up medical services such as hearing tests, examinations for other systemic diseases, and mental health counselling should also be provided, which increases the burden on the medical system. In any case, we need to set goals and create detailed plans to act as soon as possible.

## 5. Conclusions

Neonatal CMV testing combined with genetic screening can improve the aetiological diagnosis rate of congenital deafness, and direct evidence of neonatal CMV infection warrants further verification.

**Author Contributions:** Z.P. and Y.S. designed the study, Y.J. and X.L. wrote and edited the manuscript in equal parts, and Y.J., X.L., S.C., J.X., Z.P. and Y.S. contributed to the data analysis. All authors have read and agreed to the published version of the manuscript.

**Funding:** Study funded by the National Natural Science Foundation of China (grant numbers 82071058) and the National Key Research and Development Program of China No.2021YFF0702303.

**Institutional Review Board Statement:** The study was conducted by the Declaration of Helsinki, and approved by the Ethics Committee of Tongji Medical College, Huazhong University of Science and Technology (S193, 28 July 2021).

**Informed Consent Statement:** Informed consent was obtained from all subjects involved in the study. Written informed consent has been obtained from the patients to publish this paper.

**Data Availability Statement:** The data used and analysed during the current study are available from the corresponding author on reasonable request. The data are not publicly available due to privacy or ethical restrictions.

**Acknowledgments:** We acknowledge support from the National Natural Science Foundation of China.

**Conflicts of Interest:** The authors declare no conflict of interest.

## References

1. Hilgert, N.; Smith, R.J.H.; van Camp, G. Forty-six genes causing nonsyndromic hearing impairment: Which ones should be analyzed in DNA diagnostics? *Mutat. Res.* **2009**, *681*, 189–196. [CrossRef] [PubMed]
2. Smith, R.J.; Bale, J.F., Jr.; White, K.R. Sensorineural hearing loss in children. *Lancet* **2005**, *365*, 879–890. [CrossRef]
3. Available online: https://hereditaryhearingloss.org/ (accessed on 5 May 2022).
4. Goderis, J.; De Leenheer, E.; Smets, K.; Van Hoecke, H.; Keymeulen, A.; Dhooge, I. Hearing loss and congenital CMV infection: A systematic review. *Pediatrics* **2014**, *134*, 972–982. [CrossRef] [PubMed]
5. Fowler, K.B.; Stagno, S.; Pass, R.F. Maternal age and congenital cytomegalovirus infection: Screening of two diverse newborn populations, 1980–1990. *J. Infect. Dis.* **1993**, *168*, 552–556. [CrossRef]
6. Dollard, S.C.; Grosse, S.D.; Ross, D.S. New estimates of the prevalence of neurological and sensory sequelae and mortality associated with congenital cytomegalovirus infection. *Rev. Med. Virol.* **2007**, *17*, 355–363. [CrossRef]
7. Dar, L.; Pati, S.K.; Patro, A.R.K.; Deorari, A.K.; Rai, S.; Kant, S.; Broor, S.; Fowler, K.B.; Britt, W.J.; Boppana, S.B. Congenital cytomegalovirus infection in a highly seropositive semi-urban population in India. *Pediatr. Infect. Dis. J.* **2008**, *27*, 841–843. [CrossRef]
8. Kaye, S.; Miles, D.; Antoine, P.; Burny, W.; Ojuola, B.; Kaye, P.; Rowland-Jones, S.; Whittle, H.; Van Der Sande, M.; Marchant, A. Virological and immunological correlates of mother-to-child transmission of cytomegalovirus in the Gambia. *J. Infect. Dis.* **2008**, *197*, 1307–1314. [CrossRef]
9. Van der Sande, M.A.B.; Kaye, S.; Miles, D.J.C.; Waight, P.; Jeffries, D.J.; Ojuola, O.O.; Palmero, M.; Pinder, M.; Ismaili, J.; Flanagan, K.L.; et al. Risk factors for and clinical outcome of congenital cytomegalovirus infection in a peri-urban West-African birth cohort. *PLoS ONE* **2007**, *2*, e492. [CrossRef]
10. Davis, N.L.; King, C.C.; Kourtis, A.P. Cytomegalovirus infection in pregnancy. *Birth Defects Res.* **2017**, *109*, 336–346. [CrossRef] [PubMed]
11. Stagno, S.; Whitley, R.J. Herpesvirus infections of pregnancy. Part II: Herpes simplex virus and varicella-zoster virus infections. *N. Engl. J. Med.* **1985**, *313*, 1327–1330. [CrossRef]
12. Schleiss, M.R. Antiviral Therapy and Its Long-Term Impact on Hearing Loss Caused by Congenital Cytomegalovirus: Much Remains to Be Learned! *J. Pediatric Infect. Dis. Soc.* **2022**, *11*, 186–189. [CrossRef]

13. Michaels, M.G.; Greenberg, D.P.; Sabo, D.L.; Wald, E.R. Treatment of children with congenital cytomegalovirus infection with ganciclovir. *Pediatr. Infect. Dis. J.* **2003**, *22*, 504–509. [CrossRef] [PubMed]
14. Harrison, G.J.D. Newborn Screening for Congenital Cytomegalovirus Infection… It Is Time. *Clin. Infect. Dis.* **2020**, *70*, 1385–1387.
15. Liu, Y.F.; Wu, Y.; Wang, F.; Wang, S.; Zhao, W.; Chen, L.; Tu, S.; Qian, Y.; Liao, Y.; Huang, Y.; et al. The Association Between Previous TORCH Infections and Pregnancy and Neonatal Outcomes in IVF/ICSI-ET: A Retrospective Cohort Study. *Front. Endocrinol.* **2020**, *11*, 466. [CrossRef] [PubMed]
16. Uchida, A.; Tanimura, K.; Morizane, M.; Fujioka, K.; Morioka, I.; Oohashi, M.; Minematsu, T.; Yamada, H. Clinical Factors Associated With Congenital Cytomegalovirus Infection: A Cohort Study of Pregnant Women and Newborns. *Clin. Infect. Dis.* **2020**, *71*, 2833–2839. [CrossRef] [PubMed]
17. Schleiss, M.R.; Permar, S.R.; Plotkin, S.A. Progress toward Development of a Vaccine against Congenital Cytomegalovirus Infection. *Clin. Vaccine Immunol.* **2017**, *24*, e00268-17. [CrossRef]
18. Britt, W.J. Maternal Immunity and the Natural History of Congenital Human Cytomegalovirus Infection. *Viruses* **2018**, *10*, 405. [CrossRef]
19. Lanzieri, T.M.; Chung, W.; Flores, M.; Blum, P.; Caviness, A.C.; Bialek, S.R.; Grosse, S.D.; Miller, J.A.; Demmler-Harrison, G. Hearing Loss in Children With Asymptomatic Congenital Cytomegalovirus Infection. *Pediatrics* **2017**, *139*, e20162610. [CrossRef]
20. Lu, C.-Y.; Tsao, P.-N.; Ke, Y.-Y.; Lin, Y.-H.; Lin, Y.-H.; Hung, C.-C.; Su, Y.-N.; Hsu, W.-C.; Hsieh, W.-S.; Huang, L.-M.; et al. Concurrent Hearing, Genetic, and Cytomegalovirus Screening in Newborns, Taiwan. *J. Pediatr.* **2018**, *199*, 144–150.e1. [CrossRef]
21. Vos, B.; Noll, D.; Whittingham, J.; Pigeon, M.; Bagatto, M.; Fitzpatrick, E.M. Cytomegalovirus-A Risk Factor for Childhood Hearing Loss: A Systematic Review. *Ear Hear.* **2021**, *42*, 1447–1461. [CrossRef]
22. De Paschale, M.; Agrappi, C.; Manco, M.T.; Paganini, A.; Clerici, P. Incidence and risk of cytomegalovirus infection during pregnancy in an urban area of Northern Italy. *Infect. Dis. Obstet. Gynecol.* **2009**, *2009*, 206505. [CrossRef]
23. Buxmann, H.; Hamprecht, K.; Meyer-Wittkopf, M.; Friese, K. Primary Human Cytomegalovirus (HCMV) Infection in Pregnancy. *Dtsch. Arztebl. Int.* **2017**, *114*, 45–52. [CrossRef] [PubMed]
24. Hilditch, C.; Keir, A.K. Cost-effectiveness of universal and targeted newborn screening for congenital cytomegalovirus infection. *Acta Paediatr.* **2018**, *107*, 906. [CrossRef] [PubMed]
25. Huang, Y.; Li, T.; Yu, H.; Tang, J.; Song, Q.; Guo, X.; Wang, H.; Li, C.; Wang, J.; Liang, C.; et al. Maternal CMV seroprevalence rate in early gestation and congenital cytomegalovirus infection in a Chinese population. *Emerg. Microbes Infect.* **2021**, *10*, 1824–1831. [CrossRef] [PubMed]

*Journal of*
*Clinical Medicine*

*Article*

# Candidacy for Cochlear Implantation in Prelingual Profoundly Deaf Adult Patients

Ghizlene Lahlou [1,2,*], Hannah Daoudi [1,2], Evelyne Ferrary [1,2], Huan Jia [3], Marion De Bergh [1], Yann Nguyen [1,2], Olivier Sterkers [1,2] and Isabelle Mosnier [1,2]

1. Unité Fonctionnelle Implants Auditifs, Département d'Oto-Rhino-Laryngologie, Groupe Hospitalo-Universitaire Pitié-Salpêtrière, APHP Sorbonne Université, 75013 Paris, France; hannahpaule.daoudi@aphp.fr (H.D.); evelyne.ferrary@inserm.fr (E.F.); marion.de-bergh@aphp.fr (M.D.B.); yann.nguyen@aphp.fr (Y.N.); o.sterkers@gmail.com (O.S.); isabelle.mosnier@aphp.fr (I.M.)
2. Technologie et Thérapie Génique de la Surdité, Inserm/Institut Pasteur, Institut de l'Audition, 75012 Paris, France
3. Shanghai Key Laboratory of Translational Medicine on Ear and Nose Diseases (14DZ2260300), Department of Otolaryngology-HNS, Shanghai Ninth People's Hospital, Shanghai Jiao-Tong University School of Medicine, Shanghai 200025, China; huan.jia.orl@shsmu.edu.cn
* Correspondence: ghizlene.lahlou@aphp.fr; Tel.: +33-1-8482-7847 (ext. 75013)

**Abstract:** Cochlear implantation is usually not recommended for prelingual profoundly deaf adults, although some of these patients might benefit from it. This study aims to define the candidates for cochlear implantation in this population. This retrospective study reviewed 34 prelingual profoundly deaf patients who had received a cochlear implant at $32 \pm 1.7$ years old (16–55), with at least 1 year of follow-up. Speech perception and quality of life were assessed before and 3, 6, and 12 months after cochlear implantation, then every year thereafter. According to the word speech intelligibility in quiet (WSI) 1 year after implantation, two groups were identified: good performer (GP) with WSI $\geq$ 50% ($n = 15$), and poor performer (PP) with WSI $\leq$ 40% ($n = 19$). At the 1 year mark, mean WSI improved by $28 \pm 4.6\%$ ($-20$–100) ($p < 0.0001$). In GP, the intelligibility for words and sentences, communication and quality of life scales improved. In PP, the communication scale improved, but not auditory performance or quality of life. GP and PP differed pre-operatively in speech production, communication abilities, and WSI in best-aided conditions. In prelingual profoundly deaf adults, a dramatic auditory performance benefit could be expected after cochlear implantation if the patients have some degree of speech intelligibility in aided conditions and have developed oral communication and speech production.

**Keywords:** cochlear implant; prelingual profound hearing loss; speech perception; quality of life

## 1. Introduction

Cochlear implantation is a well-established treatment to restore communication in patients with post-lingual severe-to-profound hearing loss regarding their age, and in prelingually deaf infants [1–3]. Because of the short sensitive period for language development in infants, the shorter the auditory deprivation, the better the auditory performance and oral language acquisition that would be achieved after cochlear implantation [4,5]. Indeed, late cochlear implantation (after 5 years of age) is usually not recommended for non-progressive congenital or prelingual profound hearing loss [6,7], as prelingual profoundly deaf patients implanted when adults achieved lower auditory performance with their cochlear implant than those of post-lingual cochlear implanted users [8,9], although several studies have emphasized some benefits in auditory scores [8,10–15], quality of life [16,17], or self-esteem [11] in these late-implanted prelingual profoundly deaf patients. However, some patients implanted when adult who achieved poor performance after cochlear implantation have been reported to abandon the device [13], raising the question of who would be the prelingual profoundly deaf adult candidates to achieve sufficient benefit for a daily use. In a recent systematic review of the literature, there were not enough data to predict the auditory performance and analyze the prognosis factors of cochlear implantation outcomes in this population [18,19]. Most of the studies were small and heterogenous, including late-implanted prelingually and/or perilingually deaf patients, presumably because of the few validated indications to date for cochlear implantation in these populations.

The aim of the present study is to analyze cochlear implantation outcomes in a population of prelingual profoundly deaf adults to define the putative candidates who would attain a real benefit in daily life.

## 2. Materials and Methods

### 2.1. Patients

A monocentric retrospective cohort study was conducted in a tertiary referral center and included patients with unilateral or bilateral cochlear implant for a prelingual bilateral profound hearing loss, which were implanted over 15 years old without an upper age limit, between 2004 and 2019. The decision for a cochlear implantation was made after a multidisciplinary evaluation that included clinical, audiometric, speech, psychological and radiological assessments, and in accordance with the national guidelines for cochlear implantation [6,7,20], i.e., a speech discrimination ≤50% at 60 dB for disyllabic words in silence in the best-aided conditions. Patients were selected among a cohort of all cochlear implant recipients operated on in our department and noted as "congenital hearing loss" (Figure 1). Selection criteria were: (1) prelingual hearing loss diagnosed before the age of 4 years old, reported as severe to profound at diagnosis according to the medical file; (2) postoperative follow-up of at least 1 year; and (3) preoperative audiometric data available. Unilateral or bilateral, either simultaneous or sequential, cochlear implantations were performed with 3 different cochlear implant brands from Cochlear™, Med-El™, and Oticon™. Decision making for a bilateral cochlear implantation was dependent on deafness history, patient's request and motivation. All surgeries and devices were covered by government funds. Sequential bilateral cochlear implantation was performed with the objective of achieving a better performance, especially in noisy conditions.

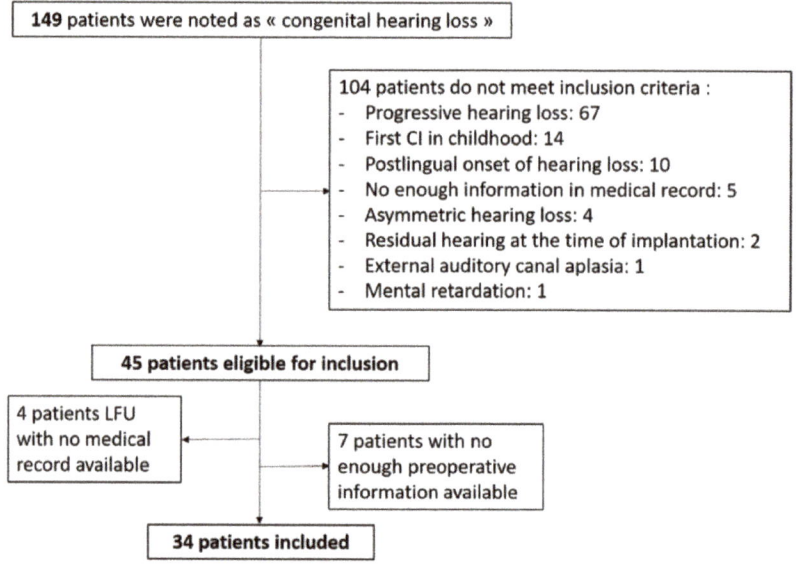

**Figure 1.** Flowchart of patient inclusion.

All patients or parents of teenagers provided written informed consent allowing the analysis of their data in accordance with the reference methodology of the National Commission for Data Protection and Liberties (CNIL-France, N°2040854). The study complies with the Declaration of Helsinki code ("World Medical Association Declaration of Helsinki. Recommendations Guiding Physicians in Biomedical Research Involving Human Subjects", 1997).

Data were collected on demographics, characteristics of hearing loss, pre-operative audiometric measurements, pre- and postoperative speech evaluation, and communication skills assessment. According to the medical charts, etiology, age and degree of hearing loss at diagnosis, age of first hearing aid fitting, and duration of hearing aid use were collected. A genetic cause of hearing loss was either proved by molecular analysis (Sanger), in the case of a bi-allelic mutation of *GJB2* (CONNEXIN 26 gene), or assumed to be a genetic-related hearing loss because of a familial history of similar hearing loss in a first-degree relative, or because of characteristic inner ear malformation (bilateral enlarged vestibular aqueduct). Socio-professional categories were classified into seven classes according to the main stages of French education (Poitrenaud's scale—Table S1) [21].

*2.2. Auditory Performance and Communication Evaluations*

Hearing was evaluated in a soundproof booth first with headphones and then in free field in quiet. Before implantation, pure tone average (PTA) and speech intelligibility without hearing aid using disyllabic words (Fournier lists) were measured with headphones. Speech intelligibility without and with lip-reading was evaluated in free field with a signal presented at 60 dB HL from the front, in best-aided conditions (with either uni- or bilateral hearing aids) before implant, and with cochlear implant alone after implantation. The following tests were systematically conducted in quiet: speech intelligibility using disyllabic words (Word Speech Intelligibility, WSI) and speech intelligibility for sentences (Marginal Benefit for Acoustic Amplification, MBAA). The results are expressed as the percentage of correct words for disyllabic lists, and as the percentage of correct words and sentences for the MBAA sentences.

The main outcome was WSI with cochlear implant alone 1 year after implantation. For simultaneous or sequential bilateral implantations, the evaluation was performed unilaterally on the best ear or first implanted ear, respectively. Patients were divided in two groups according to WSI with cochlear implant alone at 1 year: good performer (GP) when WSI ranged between 50% and 100%, and poor performer (PP) when WSI was less than 50%. A WSI below 50% was considered as a poor performance as it corresponds to the 25th percentile of all cochlear implant adult recipients in our center during the same period ($n$ = 612, unpublished data).

Before implantation, auditory tests in noisy conditions were not performed because of the severity of hearing loss. In some instances, speech intelligibility achieved sufficient level 1 year after implantation to be tested in noisy conditions, which was performed with a speech-to-noise ratio of 10 dB (SNR10), and subsequently each year. For patients with a sequential bilateral implantation, a complementary analysis compared the auditory performance in best-aided conditions before and 1 year after the second implantation.

Communication skills were assessed before and after implantation using the Category of Auditory Performance scale (CAP, Table S2) [22], scaled from 1 (no awareness of environmental sound) to 9 (can use the telephone with an unfamiliar talker). The usual mode of communication used before implantation was noted (code, sign language or oral). Moreover, the scores obtained with the APHAB (Abbreviated Profile of Hearing Aid Benefit) questionnaire were also studied, expressed from 0 (no difficulty) to 100% (maximal impact of hearing loss on communication) [23]. The language assessment was performed before implantation using the Speech Intelligibility Rating (SIR, Table S3), scaled from 1 (pre-recognizable words in spoken language) to 5 (connected speech intelligible to all listeners; the patient is easily understood in everyday contexts) [24]. After implantation, the follow-up protocol was standardized, and results were assessed using speech intelligibility for disyllabic words and MBAA scores at 3, 6, 12, and 24 months, APHAB and CAP at 1 year, and every year thereafter.

*2.3. Statistical Analysis*

Statistical analysis was performed using GraphPad Prism® (version 8.2.0, San Diego, CA, USA). Values were expressed as mean ± standard error of mean (SEM) (min–max). Two-way ANOVA, Wilcoxon, and Mann–Whitney tests were used to compare quantitative data, and Fisher's and chi-squared tests were used for qualitative data. A $p$ value < 0.05 was considered to be significant.

## 3. Results

*3.1. Population*

Thirty-four patients were included in the study (Table 1). Hearing loss was diagnosed at 21 ± 2.2 months (1–46), as severe and profound in 15 cases (44%) and 19 cases (56%), respectively. At the age of implantation (32 ± 1.7 years (16–55)), all patients were profoundly deaf (non-aided auditory thresholds >90 dB for both ears), and the mean preoperative WSI in best-aided conditions was 12 ± 2.4% (0–50). A confirmed or presumed genetic cause of hearing loss was found for 50% of patients ($n$ = 17), including 12 patients with a confirmed mutation of *GJB2* (CONNEXINE 26 gene). The other etiologies were unknown for 11 (32%), intra-uterine infection for 4 (12%), a neonatal meningitis for 1 (3%), and a prematurity for 1 (3%). Implantation was unilateral for 18 patients (53%), bilateral sequential for 9 (26%), and bilateral simultaneous for 7 (21%). All preoperative data are detailed in Table 1.

*3.2. Cochlear Implant Outcomes*

Post-implantation follow-up was 4 ± 0.5 years (1–10). The mean WSI at 1 year was 36 ± 5.1% (0–100), and the median was 35% (interquartile range (7.5–60)). Compared to the preoperative scores, the mean WSI improved by 28 ± 4.6% (−20–100) ($p$ < 0.0001, $n$ = 34, Wilcoxon test). At 1 year post-implantation, 15 patients (44%) achieved a WSI of at least 50%, and the 19 others (56%) inferior to 50%; they were considered as good (GP) and poor (PP) performers, respectively (Table 1).

As shown in Figure 2A, WSI increased as early as 3 months post-implantation for GP to reach 65 ± 4.1% (50–100) at 1 year ($p$ < 0.0001, two-way ANOVA, $n$ = 15, Table 2). Excellent WSI scores ranging from 70 to 100% were achieved in seven cases, four being unilaterally implanted and the other three being contra-laterally operated on later (Table 1). For PP, no significant improvement was observed with a difference of +10 ± 3.3% (0–20) 1 year after implantation compared to preoperative scores ($p$ = 0.052, two-way ANOVA, $n$ = 19) (Table 2). Moreover, no word recognition was obtained in eight cases, half of them having been bilaterally and simultaneously implanted (Table 1). Whatever the auditory performance achieved after 1 year, WSI remained stable up to 10 years (Figure 2B).

**Table 1.** Characteristics of implanted patients classified in function of speech intelligibility of disyllabic word score in quiet (WSI) with one cochlear implant 1 year after implantation (best or first implant outcomes are given for simultaneous or sequential bilateral implantation, respectively). Good and poor performers are patients 1 to 15 and 16 to 34, respectively.

| Patient | Sex | HL Etiology | HL Class at dg † | Age at dg (Months) | Age at First HA (Months) CI Ear | Age at First HA (Months) Non-CI Ear | Duration without HA (Years) | Social Category | CAP | SIR | Communication ‡ | Preoperative PTA (dB) CI Ear | Preoperative PTA (dB) Non-CI Ear | Type of Implantation | Age at CI (Years) | Year of First CI | CI Model | WSI at One Year (%) |
|---|---|---|---|---|---|---|---|---|---|---|---|---|---|---|---|---|---|---|
| 1 | F | Unknown | S | 12 | 12 | 12 | 1 | 7 | 5 | 5 | O | 115 | 114 | Unilateral | 29 | 2019 | CI522 | 100 |
| 2 | F | Unknown | P | 24 | 24 | 24 | 2 | 7 | 7 | 5 | O | 102.5 | 99 | Bilateral seq. | 22 | 2010 | Ci512 | 90 |
| 3 | M | Cnx 26 | P | 24 | 24 | 24 | 2 | 7 | NR | 5 | O | 120 | 111 | Bilateral seq. | 26 | 2015 | CI24RE | 80 |
| 4 | F | Unknown | S | 12 | 12 | 12 | 1 | 7 | 5 | 5 | O | 99 | 98 | Unilateral | 39 | 2014 | CI24RE | 70 |
| 5 | F | Cnx 26 | P | 12 | 12 | 12 | 1 | 6 | 6 | 5 | O | 99 | 99 | Unilateral | 16 | 2013 | CI24RE | 70 |
| 6 | M | Cnx 26 | S | 12 | 60 | 60 | 5 | 4 | 5 | 4 | O | 115 | 104 | Unilateral | 52 | 2018 | CI522 | 70 |
| 7 | F | IUI | P | 1 | 3 | 3 | 0 | 7 | 4 | 5 | O | 115 | 102.5 | Bilateral seq. | 45 | 2013 | CI522 | 70 |
| 8 | F | Unknown | S | 24 | 24 | 24 | 2 | 6 | 5 | 5 | O | 109 | 99 | Bilateral seq. | 30 | 2012 | Med-El Flex31 | 60 |
| 9 | M | Meningiti | S | 3 | 96 | 144 | 8 | 1 | 5 | 4 | O | 105 | 105 | Bilateral sim. | 47 | 2018 | Neuro ZTI Evo | 60 |
| 10 | F | Cnx 26 | P | 16 | 16 | 16 | 1 | 7 | 6 | 5 | O | 102 | 96 | Unilateral | 32 | 2012 | CI24RE | 50 |
| 11 | F | Genetic | S | 40 | 40 | 40 | 3 | 7 | 5 | 4 | O + S | 109 | 112 | Bilateral seq. | 27 | 2012 | CI422 | 50 |
| 12 | F | IUI | P | 9 | 9 | 9 | 5 | 2 | 2 | 2 | O + S | 117 | 111 | Bilateral sim. | 20 | 2007 | Med-El | 50 |
| 13 | M | Cnx 26 | S | 15 | 16 | 16 | 1 | 7 | 5 | 4 | O | 111 | 109 | Unilateral | 32 | 2018 | CI522 | 50 |
| 14 | F | Unknown | P | 24 | 24 | 24 | 2 | 7 | 5 | 5 | O | 109 | 99 | Unilateral | 27 | 2018 | CI522 | 50 |
| 15 | M | Unknown | S | 18 | 18 | 18 | 1.5 | 7 | 3 | 5 | O | 97.5 | 95 | Unilateral | 20 | 2013 | CI422 | 50 |
| 16 | M | Unknown | S | 9 | 9 | 9 | 1 | 7 | 3 | 5 | O | 111 | 99 | Unilateral | 31 | 2013 | Ci422 | 40 |
| 17 | F | Cnx 26 | S | 6 | 6 | 6 | 0 | 7 | 5 | 5 | O | 116 | 108 | Bilateral sim. | 39 | 2016 | Ci512 | 40 |
| 18 | F | Cnx 26 | P | 45 | 167 | 45 | 14 | 7 | NR | NR | O + S | 114 | 115 | Unilateral | 45 | 2004 | Ci24CA | 30 |
| 19 | M | Unknown | P | 18 | 18 | 18 | 1 | 6 | 5 | 4 | O | 99 | 91 | Unilateral | 21 | 2012 | Ci24RE | 30 |
| 20 | F | Cnx 26 | P | 9 | 9 | 9 | 1 | 7 | 5 | 3 | O + S | 112 | 108 | Bilateral seq. | 25 | 2012 | CI24RE | 30 |
| 21 | M | Cnx 26 | P | 12 | 12 | 12 | 6 | 6 | NR | NR | O + S | 110 | 106 | Unilateral | 33 | 2007 | Digisonic SP | 20 |
| 22 | M | Unknown | S | 36 | 36 | 36 | 3 | 6 | 5 | 3 | O + S | 115 | 116 | Unilateral | 32 | 2008 | CI24RE | 20 |
| 23 | F | Unknown | P | 3 | 3 | 3 | 0 | 7 | 4 | 2 | O + S | 110 | 104 | Unilateral | 18 | 2011 | CI24RE | 20 |
| 24 | F | Cnx 26 | P | 12 | 12 | 12 | 1 | 6 | 5 | 4 | O + S | 110 | 105 | Bilateral seq. | 30 | 2015 | Ci422 | 10 |
| 25 | M | Genetic | S | 36 | 36 | 36 | 3 | 6 | 5 | 4 | O + S | 99 | 115 | Unilateral | 21 | 2014 | Digisonic SP | 10 |
| 26 | F | Cnx 26 | P | 24 | 24 | 24 | 2 | 7 | 3 | 4 | O + S | 110 | 107 | Unilateral | 24 | 2016 | Ci422 | 10 |
| 27 | M | Genetic | S | 46 | 46 | 46 | 4 | 6 | 5 | 5 | O | 115 | 110 | Bilateral seq. | 41 | 2010 | CI24RE | 0 |
| 28 | M | Premature | S | 24 | 29 | 29 | 2 | 3 | 3 | 3 | O + C | 99 | 94 | Unilateral | 33 | 2011 | Med-El Ti100 | 0 |
| 29 | F | Genetic | P | 18 | 71 | 71 | 36 | 6 | 4 | 4 | O | 109 | 110 | Bilateral sim. | 43 | 2008 | CI24RE | 0 |

Table 1. Cont.

| Patient | Sex | HL Etiology | HL Class at dg [¥] | Age at dg (Months) | Age at First HA (Months) CI Ear | Age at First HA (Months) Non-CI Ear | Duration without HA (Years) | Social Category | CAP | SIR | Communication [†] | Preoperative PTA (dB) CI Ear | Preoperative PTA (dB) Non-CI Ear | Type of Implantation | Age at CI (Years) | Year of First CI | CI Model | WSI at One Year (%) |
|---|---|---|---|---|---|---|---|---|---|---|---|---|---|---|---|---|---|---|
| 30 | F | IUI | P | 46 | - | - | 30 | 1 | 1 | 1 | C | 111 | 100 | Bilateral sim. | 30 | 2013 | Digisonic SP | 0 |
| 31 | F | Unknown | P | 36 | 36 | 36 | 10 | 4 | 1 | 1 | S | 120 | 120 | Bilateral sim. | 23 | 2013 | Digisonic SP | 0 |
| 32 | F | Cnx 26 | S | 12 | 12 | 12 | 1 | 7 | 5 | 4 | O | 110 | 112 | Bilateral sim. | 41 | 2015 | Ci422 | 0 |
| 33 | M | Genetic | P | 36 | NR | NR | NR | 4 | 3 | 2 | O + S | 116 | 120 | Unilateral | 24 | 2019 | NeuroZTI Evo | 0 |
| 34 | F | IUI | P | 36 | 120 | 36 | 10 | 4 | 2 | 3 | O | 112 | 111 | Bilateral seq. | 55 | 2013 | Digisonic Evo | 0 |

HL.: Hearing loss; Cnx: connexin; IUI: intra-uterine infection; dg: diagnosis; HA: hearing aid; CI: cochlear implant; CAP: Category of Auditory Performance; SIR: Speech Intelligibility Rating; PTA (dB): pure tone audiometry (decibel); Bilateral seq: sequential; Bilateral sim: simultaneous; WSI: speech intelligibility for disyllabic words in quiet; NR: not-reported. [¥]: S is for severe and P for profound. [†]: O is for oral, S for sign, C for code. The grey color is for good performers group.

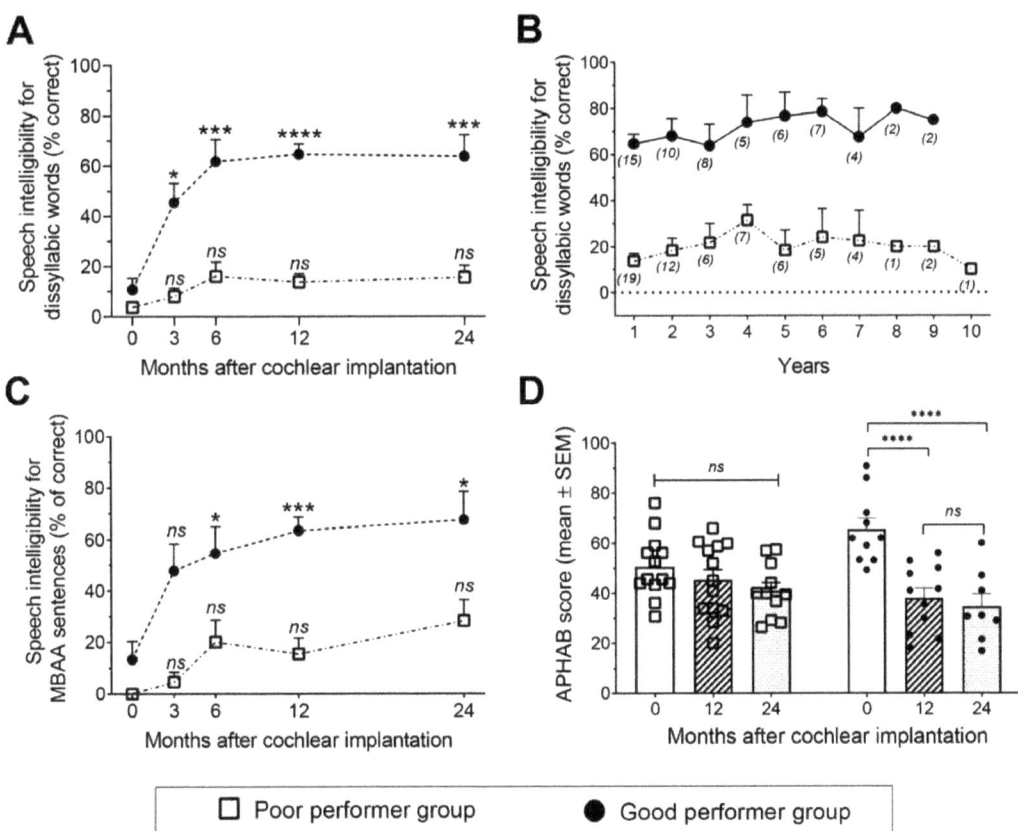

**Figure 2.** Post-operative evolution after cochlear implantation. (**A**) Speech intelligibility without lipreading for disyllabic words in silence in the 2 groups. Compared to the preoperative scores, an improvement was observed for the good performer group at 3 months ($p = 0.015$), 6 months ($p = 0.0002$), 1 year ($p < 0.0001$), and 2 years ($p = 0.0005$) post-implantation. For the poor performer group, no significant improvement was found. $n$ = 15, 11, 11, 15, 8 for the good performer group, and 19, 10, 10, 19, 11 for the poor performer group, respectively at 0, 3, 6, 12, and 24 months after cochlear implantation. (**B**) Evolution of speech intelligibility for disyllabic words over time in the 2 groups. ($n$) are the number of patients at each time point. (**C**) Speech intelligibility without lipreading for MBAA sentences in the 2 groups. Compared to the preoperative scores, an improvement was observed for the good performer group at 6 months ($p = 0.024$), 1 year ($p = 0.0007$), and 2 years ($p = 0.011$) post-implantation. For the poor performer group, no significant improvement was found. $n$ = 12, 11, 10, 14, 7 for the good performer group, and 9, 7, 8, 13, 10 for the poor performer group, respectively at 0, 3, 6, 12, and 24 months after cochlear implantation. (**D**) Mean ± SEM of APHAB scores before, 1 and 2 years after implantation in the 2 groups, showing an improvement only for the good performer group ($p < 0.0001$). APHAB, Abbreviated Profile of Hearing Aid Benefit. Data are mean ± SEM; a two-way ANOVA with a Tukey multiple comparisons test was performed for statistical analysis. * $p < 0.05$; *** $p < 0.0005$, **** $p < 0.0001$, $ns$: non significant.

**Table 2.** Auditory performance in quiet with cochlear implant alone (best or first implanted ear for bilateral simultaneous or sequential implantation, respectively) and communication performance before and 1 year post-implantation in the two groups.

|  | Poor Performers | | | Good Performers | | |
|---|---|---|---|---|---|---|
|  | Preoperative | 1 Year Post-CI | *p*-Value | Preoperative | 1 Year Post-CI | *p*-Value |
| Speech intelligibility |  |  |  |  |  |  |
| Disyllabic words | 4 ± 1.9 (0–30), *n* = 19 | 14 ± 3.4 (0–40), *n* = 19 | 0.052 ¥ | 11 ± 4.6 (0–50), *n* = 15 | 65 ± 4.1 (50–100), *n* = 15 | <0.0001 ¥ |
| Words in sentences | 2 ± 1.6 (0–14), *n* = 9 | 30 ± 8.6 (0–77), *n* = 12 | 0.13 ¥ | 20 ± 8.9 (0–92), *n* = 12 | 75 ± 6.7 (30–100), *n* = 14 | 0.001 ¥ |
| Sentences | 0 ± 0 (0–0), *n* = 9 | 15 ± 6.2 (0–60), *n* = 13 | 0.25 ¥ | 13 ± 7 (0–80), *n* = 12 | 64 ± 5.2 (33–100), *n* = 14 | 0.0007 ¥ |
| CAP |  |  |  |  |  |  |
| 1 | 2 | 0 |  | 0 | 0 |  |
| 2 | 1 | 1 |  | 1 | 0 |  |
| 3 | 4 | 0 |  | 1 | 0 |  |
| 4 | 2 | 6 |  | 1 | 0 |  |
| 5 | 8 | 4 | 0.015 ∞ | 8 | 2 | 0.0003 ∞ |
| 6 | 0 | 3 |  | 2 | 3 |  |
| 7 | 0 | 2 |  | 1 | 2 |  |
| 8 | 0 | 1 |  | 0 | 3 |  |
| 9 | 0 | 0 |  | 0 | 4 |  |

Good and poor performers had a speech intelligibility for disyllabic words in quiet ≥ and <50% at 1 year, respectively. CAP: Communication Auditory Performance; CI: cochlear implant. Data are given as mean ± SEM in % (range), and *n* for the intelligibility scores, and *n* for the CAP scores. ¥: two-way ANOVA; ∞: chi-squared test.

Speech intelligibility for sentences without lipreading increased as early as 6 months post-implantation for GP achieving 64 ± 5.2% (33–100) at 1 year ($p$ = 0.0007, two-way ANOVA, $n$ = 12), but not for PP (Figure 2C, Table 2).

The addition of lip-reading did not change the WSI in the two groups: 74 ± 9.3% (0–100) ($n$ = 14) vs. 98 ± 2.0% (90–100) ($n$ = 5) for GP ($p$ > 0.9, Wilcoxon test) and 58 ± 7.9% (0–90) ($n$ = 17) vs. 56 ± 10.9% (0–100) ($n$ = 13) for PP ($p$ = 0.8, Wilcoxon test) before and 1 year after implantation, respectively.

Communication evaluated using the CAP score improved at 1 year post-implantation in both PP and GP (respectively $p$ = 0.015 and $p$ = 0.0003, chi-squared test, Table 2). At 1 year post-implantation, all patients of the GP group improved the CAP score, and 86% of them ($n$ = 12/14 patients) reached a CAP ≥ 6, being able to understand common phrases without lip-reading. For PP, an improvement of the CAP score was achieved in 11/16 patients (69%), for whom CAP was available preoperatively and 1 year post-implantation, reaching a CAP ≥ 6 in only 35% of them.

Compared to the preoperative score, the APHAB score decreased 1 year after implantation for GP (−28 ± 3.6 (−38 to −18), $n$ = 10, $p$ < 0.0001), showing an improvement of their quality of life, and remained stable up to the second year of follow-up. No change on the APHAB score was observed for PP (Figure 2D).

Among the 34 implanted patients, 32 (94%) were all day long users, and time to time for the 2 others who were in the PP group. No patient has abandoned the device in the long term.

### 3.3. Analysis of Preoperative Factors

The 2 groups were similar in terms of age at diagnosis of hearing loss ($p$ = 0.5, Mann–Whitney test), etiology of hearing loss ($p$ = 0.2, chi-squared test), preoperative PTA ($p$ = 0.3 and $p$ = 0.08, respectively, for ipsi- and contralateral ear, Mann–Whitney test), age at first implantation ($p$ = 0.7, Mann–Whitney test), and socio-professional categories ($p$ = 0.2, chi-squared test) (Table 1). However, in best-aided conditions, preoperative speech intelligibility for disyllabic words without and with lip-reading was higher for GP compared to PP ($p = 0.022$ and $p = 0.012$, respectively, Mann–Whitney test, Figure 3A).

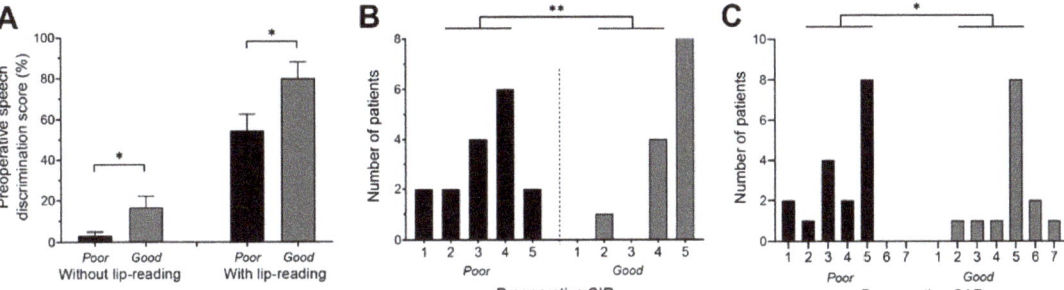

**Figure 3.** Preoperative assessments in the 2 groups. (**A**) Preoperative speech intelligibility for disyllabic words evaluated in optimal listening condition (i.e., with the 2 hearing aids if used) without and with lip-reading. Good performer group (GP) obtained better scores compared with to the poor performer group (PP) for the speech intelligibility without and with lip-reading (respectively $p = 0.022$, $n = 15$ for GP and 18 for PP, and $p = 0.012$, $n = 13$ for GP and 18 for PP, Mann–Whitney test). (**B**) Preoperative Speech Intelligibility Rating (SIR) scores. GP ($n = 15$) had better scores compared with PP ($n = 16$) ($p = 0.003$, chi-squared test, 3 missing values in PP). (**C**) Preoperative Category of Auditory Performance (CAP) scores. GP ($n = 14$) had better scores compared with PP ($n = 17$) ($p = 0.032$, chi-squared test, 1 missing for GP and 2 for PP). Data are mean ± SEM (**A**) and $n$ (**B**,**C**). * $p < 0.05$; ** $p < 0.005$.

All patients except eight were equipped with a bilateral hearing aid at the time of diagnosis of deafness, with no significant difference between the two groups for age of the first hearing aid ($p = 0.7$ and $p = 0.4$, respectively, for ipsi- and contralateral ear, Mann–Whitney test, Table 1). Among the eight remaining patients (24%), six were PP: one patient did not use any hearing aid before cochlear implantation, two were equipped in only one ear at the time of diagnosis, and three were equipped several years after diagnosis. The last two were GP: one patient had a bilateral hearing aid at the age of 5 years, and one was equipped in only one ear at the time of diagnosis (Table 1). At the time of implantation, 29 patients (85%) used their hearing aid in the implanted ear up to surgery, except for PP, a patient who never used a hearing aid, and 3 who had abandoned their hearing aid, and for GP, 1 patient had abandoned the hearing aid 5 years before implantation. There was no difference in the duration of hearing loss without hearing aid between the two groups ($p = 0.8$, Mann–Whitney test, Table 1).

All patients, apart from 2 in PP, used oral communication before implantation, alone (20/34 patients, 59%) or in combination with sign language in (12/34 patients, 35%) (Table 1). More patients used only oral communication in GP compared to PP (87% vs. 37%, $p = 0.005$, Fisher's test). Additionally, the preoperative SIR scores in GP were higher compared to PP ($p = 0.003$, chi-squared test, Figure 3B), 93% of GP patients having a connected speech intelligible to a listener who had no experience (score of 5) or little experience (score of 4) of a deaf person's speech. Finally, the preoperative CAP scores in GP were high compared to PP ($p = 0.03$, chi-squared test, Figure 3C).

### 3.4. Benefits of Bilateralisation in the Case of Sequential Cochlear Implantation

A total of 9 patients (26%) had a sequential implantation, 5/15 and 4/19 in GP and PP, respectively, with a mean delay between the 2 implantations of $3 \pm 0.9$ (0.5–7.8) years. All these patients were still using their hearing aid in the non-implanted ear until the contralateral implantation. When comparing the auditory performance in best-aided conditions, no difference was found for WSI or for sentences intelligibility in quiet and in noise before and 1 year after the second cochlear implantation (Table 3). Additionally, there was no difference for APHAB score, nor for CAP score (Table 3). Although no difference was objectified, all sequential bilaterally implanted patients whatever the performance group used both cochlear implant processor all day long, and speech intelligibility scores in noisy conditions for sentences and words in sentences improved by more than 20% in GP (not significant), but not in PP (Table 3).

**Table 3.** Evolution in good and poor performers groups before and 1 year after the second implantation in bilateral sequential implantation patients ($n = 9$). Good ($n = 5$) and poor ($n = 4$) performers had a speech intelligibility for disyllabic words in quiet $\geq$ and <50% at 1 year after the first implantation, respectively (see Table 1).

|  | Poor Performers ($n = 4$) | | | Good Performers ($n = 5$) | | |
|---|---|---|---|---|---|---|
|  | Before the 2nd | 1 Year Post-2nd | $p$-Value | Before the 2nd | 1 Year Post-2nd | $p$-Value |
| SI in quiet |  |  |  |  |  |  |
| Disyllabic words | 33 ± 16.5 (10–70), $n = 4$ | 50 ± 13.5 (30–90), $n = 4$ | 0.4 ¥ | 82 ± 11.1 (50–100), $n = 5$ | 88 ± 6.3 (70–100), $n = 4$ | 0.9 ¥ |
| Words in sentences | 48 ± 21.2 (0–94), $n = 4$ | 66 ± 13.0 (44–89), $n = 3$ | 0.9 ¥ | 83 ± 9.3 (51–100), $n = 5$ | 89 ± 10.5 (68–100), $n = 3$ | 0.7 ¥ |
| Sentences | 33 ± 17.7 (0–80), $n = 4$ | 49 ± 17.4 (20–80), $n = 3$ | 0.8 ¥ | 69 ± 13.6 (33–100), $n = 5$ | 80 ± 16.6 (47–100), $n = 3$ | 0.5 ¥ |
| SI in noise |  |  |  |  |  |  |
| Words in sentences | 25 ± 18.4 (0–78), $n = 4$ | 38 ± 14.4 (11–60), $n = 3$ | 0.9 ¥ | 55 ± 18.6 (3–91), $n = 5$ | 78 ± 11.7 (56–100), $n = 4$ | 0.1 ¥ |
| Sentences | 15 ± 15.0 (0–60), $n = 4$ | 20 ± 7.5 (7–33), $n = 3$ | 0.9 ¥ | 41 ± 17.4 (0–80), $n = 5$ | 62 ± 20.1 (27–100), $n = 4$ | 0.07 ¥ |
| APHAB | 45 ± 4.8 (33–57), $n = 4$ | 45 ± 4.7 (37–57), $n = 4$ | >0.9 ‡ | 48 ± 7.1 (33–67), $n = 5$ | 39 ± 8.6 (15–57), $n = 4$ | 0.6 ‡ |
| CAP |  |  |  |  |  |  |
| 5 | 1 | 1 |  | 1 | 0 |  |
| 6 | 0 | 0 |  | 1 | 0 |  |
| 7 | 0 | 1 | 0.8 ∞ | 1 | 0 | 0.09 ∞ |
| 8 | 2 | 1 |  | 1 | 2 |  |
| 9 | 1 | 1 |  | 1 | 2 |  |

SI: Speech intelligibility; CAP: Communication Auditory Performance. Data are mean ± SEM (range) in % for the intelligibility scores and the APHAB score, and $n$ for the CAP score. ¥: two-way ANOVA; ∞: chi-squared test; ‡: Wilcoxon test.

## 4. Discussion

In the present retrospective study, 34 adult patients with profound prelingual hearing loss were included and demonstrated a dramatic increase in auditory performance as evaluated 1 year after cochlear implantation with 1 cochlear implant alone using disyllabic words in quiet, regardless of whether patients were unilaterally or bilaterally implanted, although scores ranged from none to 100%. This is in line with other studies on series of patients demonstrating improvements for words [10,11,16], phonemes [10,13,25], and sentence recognition scores in quiet [10–13,16,17,26–28], although prelingual and perilingual hearing loss were in most cases mixed. This study reports among the largest cohorts of prelingually deaf adults cochlear implant recipients in the literature and analyzes the outcomes in terms of speech intelligibility for words and sentences, as well as in terms of quality of life and communication skills.

In this series, 44% of patients experienced a dramatic increase in auditory performance with a mean speech intelligibility in silence of 65 ± 4.1% (GP), similar to post-lingually implanted profoundly deaf adult scores (67% to 76% depending on the test used [1,29,30]). Accordingly, the speech intelligibility for disyllabic words in quiet of all the patients in the French cohort recently implanted at adult age reached 67% [30]. Having such good performance after a delayed cochlear implantation is a surprising fact, as it is commonly accepted that auditory performance after cochlear implantation in adults is significantly lower in patients with prelingual hearing loss compared to post-lingually acquired hearing loss, and that the duration of auditory deprivation is a major prognostic factor [8,9,31]. However, some prelingually deaf patients, who did not have a cochlear implant at an early stage, could really benefit from a cochlear implantation even if delayed, and obtain better speech intelligibility, as well as improved communication skills and quality of life.

For the other 56% of prelingually deaf patients with poor auditory performance (PP), a slight or no improvement was observed for disyllabic word intelligibility 1 year after the cochlear implantation with no further improvement, at variance with previously reported by others [32–34]. However, the everyday communication, as evaluated with the CAP score, was improved, and most of the recipients, except two, are all day long users. Moreover, some of them asked for a second cochlear implant on the other ear. Thus, judging the input of the cochlear implantation only on auditory performance does not give a complete picture of the individual benefit in this population.

Concerning subjective evaluation, the APHAB questionnaire, specific to hearing loss, quantifies the trouble experienced in communicating in everyday life situations, and is routinely used to evaluate post-lingual deaf adults. Prelingually deaf adults have a long history of coping with their hearing handicap and have developed communication strategies so that they are not as dramatically affected in their social communication as post-lingually deaf adults. In this study, they obtained better scores in the APHAB questionnaire compared to post-lingual hearing-impaired adults before implantation [30]. Therefore, this questionnaire is probably insufficient to highlight the benefit of cochlear implantation in the particular cases of prelingual poor performers. Other studies have shown that the main improvements for this deaf population were on primary sound processing, sense of safety, and self-confidence [11,16]. If the cochlear implant does not provide enough improvement for speech perception without lip-reading, it could be a real help in audiovisual conditions, processing environmental sounds, or at least as an alert device. The subjective benefit and preoperative expectations have to be taken into account to assess the real input of cochlear implantation in this population.

Based on this study, multiple preoperative factors could predict good auditory performance after cochlear implantation. First, preoperative speech perception in best-aided conditions, with or without lip-reading, appears to be a good preoperative prognostic factor, as already reported [10,15,28,35]. Second, preoperative communication, referring to the type of language used by the patient (code, sign language, or oral) and to the CAP score, appeared to be a major prognostic factor, as already mentioned in several studies [15,16,25,26,28]. In this study, most patients used oral communication, alone or in combination with signed language, showing probably some benefit of their hearing aid and a history of intensive speech therapy in childhood. Preoperative communication is probably an indicator of whether the auditory cortex has a quite normal organization or not, as it has been proved that visual processing causes a functional shift of the auditory cortex into the visual processing pathway [36]. In addition, the intelligibility of the patient's speech appears to be a prognostic factor in this study as in others [15,16,25,35], suggesting that the better the patient's speech was, the better their oral and auditory skills were developed in childhood. Third, hearing aid use until the day of cochlear implantation should also be taken into consideration before making the decision for cochlear implantation in an adult prelingually deaf patient, even though it does not appear to be a significant prognostic factor in this study, since the great majority of included patients wore their hearing aid until the cochlear implantation. However, most of the patients who did not wear hearing aids for a long period of several years did not achieve any word recognition. Finally, patient's motivation has to be deeply analyzed before cochlear implantation. In this study, patients came with a request for improved communication, often in the context of a change in their everyday life, such as starting higher education, new work, family, of after meeting cochlear implant recipients. Based on these results, we propose a decision algorithm for cochlear implantation in adulthood in the case of prelingual deafness (Figure 4). A bilateral simultaneous implantation should be discussed with great caution even in front of an express demand of the patient and/or his/her family. Alternatively, the benefit of a bilateral sequential implantation has to be made on a longer period of follow-up than 1 year after the contralateral procedure to evidence better performance in noisy conditions than with a unilateral cochlear implant [37]. Whether a contralateral implantation should be restricted to good performers or to all the patients is still a matter of debate.

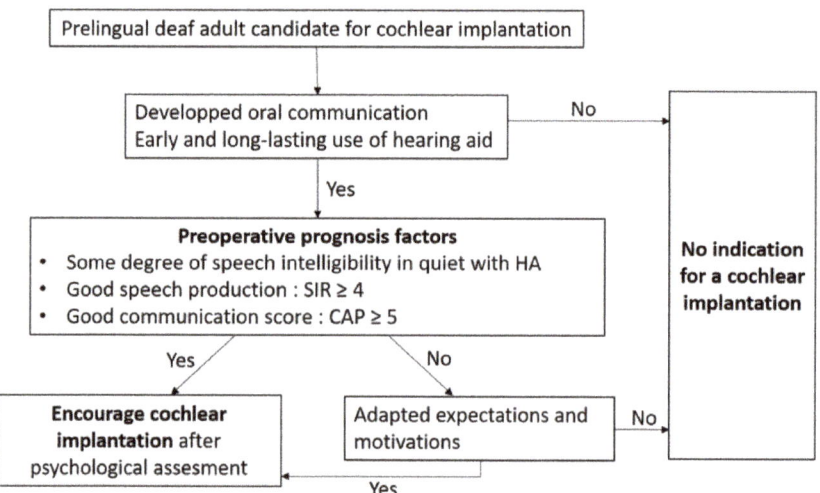

**Figure 4.** Decision algorithm for cochlear implantation in the case of an adult patient with prelingual severe-to-profound hearing loss. HA: hearing aid; SIR: Speech Intelligibility Response; CAP: Communication Auditory Performance.

This study has some limitations, as it was a retrospective analysis, with some missing data, making the power of the study weaker. Additionally, a selection bias is possible since the diagnosis of hearing loss was made many years ago. In addition, some patients who were operated on several years earlier, especially patients using sign language alone, were lost to follow-up, or were not evaluated properly before implantation, and were not included in this study (Figure 1). Finally, it would be interesting to evaluate the duration of post-operative speech therapy reeducation, which is probably longer for patients with prelingual hearing loss compared to post-lingual ones.

## 5. Conclusions

Cochlear implantation could be considered an adequate option for adults with prelingual onset profound hearing loss who request it, after an exhaustive evaluation of speech intelligibility, communication, speech production and expectations of the patient. For patients with developed oral communication, good speech production, and some degree of speech intelligibility with their hearing aid, a dramatic benefit should be expected, making these patients good candidates for cochlear implantation at the adult age. For those who experienced no measurable benefit on speech perception, the use of the cochlear implant processor might improve their communication skills. A proper assessment, adapted to these non-conventional cochlear implantation candidates, is thus needed pre- and post-operatively for this particular population of prelingual profoundly deaf adults.

**Supplementary Materials:** The following supporting information can be downloaded at: https://www.mdpi.com/article/10.3390/jcm11071874/s1, Table S1: Socio-professional levels according to Poitrenaud's scale. Table S2: The Category of Auditory Performance (CAP) scale. Table S3: The Speech Intelligibility Rating scale (SIR) scale.

**Author Contributions:** Conceptualization, G.L., E.F., O.S. and I.M.; methodology, G.L. and E.F.; software, G.L.; validation, O.S., Y.N. and I.M.; formal analysis, G.L. and H.J.; investigation, G.L., H.D. and M.D.B.; data curation, G.L., H.D. and M.D.B.; writing—original draft preparation, G.L.; writing—review and editing, O.S., E.F. and I.M. All authors have read and agreed to the published version of the manuscript.

**Funding:** This research received no external funding.

**Institutional Review Board Statement:** The study was conducted according to the guidelines of the Declaration of Helsinki. Ethical review and approval were waived for this study, due its retrospective nature with no intervention.

**Informed Consent Statement:** Informed consent was obtained from all subjects involved in the study.

**Data Availability Statement:** The data that support the findings of this study are available on re-quest from the corresponding author. The data are not publicly available due to privacy restriction.

**Acknowledgments:** We thank Fondation pour l'Audition and Institut Pasteur for their support (Starting Grant IDA 2020). We would like to acknowledge Emmanuelle Ambert-Dahan and Amélie Callies for their help in collecting data.

**Conflicts of Interest:** The authors declare no conflict of interest.

# References

1. Lenarz, M.; Sönmez, H.; Joseph, G.; Büchner, A.; Lenarz, T. Long-Term Performance of Cochlear Implants in Postlingually Deafened Adults. *Otolaryngol.-Head Neck Surg.* **2012**, *147*, 112–118. [CrossRef] [PubMed]
2. Gaylor, J.M.; Raman, G.; Chung, M.; Lee, J.; Rao, M.; Lau, J.; Poe, D.S. Cochlear implantation in adults: A systematic review and meta-analysis. *JAMA Otolaryngol.-Head Neck Surg.* **2013**, *139*, 265–272. [CrossRef]
3. McRackan, T.R.; Bauschard, M.; Hatch, J.L.; Franko-Tobin, E.; Droghini, H.R.; Nguyen, S.A.; Dubno, J.R. Meta-analysis of quality-of-life improvement after cochlear implantation and associations with speech recognition abilities. *Laryngoscope* **2018**, *128*, 982–990. [CrossRef] [PubMed]
4. Black, J.; Hickson, L.; Black, B.; Perry, C. Prognostic indicators in paediatric cochlear implant surgery: A systematic literature review. *Cochlear Implant. Int.* **2011**, *12*, 67–93. [CrossRef] [PubMed]
5. Moreno-Torres, I.; Madrid-Cánovas, S.; Blanco-Montañez, G. Sensitive periods and language in cochlear implant users. *J. Child Lang.* **2016**, *43*, 479–504. [CrossRef]
6. HAS. *Le Traitement de la Surdité par Implants Cochléaires ou du Tronc Cérébral*; HAS: Paris, France, 2012.
7. Simon, F.; Roman, S.; Truy, E.; Barone, P.; Belmin, J.; Blanchet, C.; Borel, S.; Charpiot, A.; Coez, A.; Deguine, O.; et al. Guidelines (short version) of the French society of otorhinolaryngology (SFORL) on pediatric cochlear implant indications. *Eur. Ann. Otorhinolaryngol. Head Neck Dis.* **2019**, *136*, 385–391. [CrossRef]
8. Kumar, R.S.; Mawman, D.; Sankaran, D.; Melling, C.; O'Driscoll, M.; Freeman, S.M.; Lloyd, S.K.W. Cochlear implantation in early deafened, late implanted adults: Do they benefit? *Cochlear Implant. Int.* **2016**, *17*, 22–25. [CrossRef]
9. Kraaijenga, V.J.C.; Smit, A.L.; Stegeman, I.; Smilde, J.J.M.; van Zanten, G.A.; Grolman, W. Factors that influence outcomes in cochlear implantation in adults, based on patient-related characteristics—A retrospective study. *Clin. Otolaryngol.* **2016**, *41*, 585–592. [CrossRef]
10. Arisi, E.; Forti, S.; Pagani, D.; Todini, L.; Torretta, S.; Ambrosetti, U.; Pignataro, L. Cochlear implantation in adolescents with prelinguistic deafness. *Otolaryngol. Head Neck Surg.* **2010**, *142*, 804–808. [CrossRef]
11. Bosco, E.; Nicastri, M.; Ballantyne, D.; Viccaro, M.; Ruoppolo, G.; Maddalena, A.I.; Mancini, P. Long term results in late implanted adolescent and adult CI recipients. *Eur. Arch. Oto-Rhino-Laryngol.* **2013**, *270*, 2611–2620. [CrossRef]
12. Heywood, R.L.; Vickers, D.A.; Pinto, F.; Fereos, G.; Shaida, A. Assessment and outcome in non-traditional cochlear implant candidates. *Audiol. Neurotol.* **2017**, *21*, 383–390. [CrossRef] [PubMed]
13. Lammers, M.J.W.; Versnel, H.; Topsakal, V.; Zanten, G.A.V.; Grolman, W. Predicting performance and non-use in prelingually deaf and late-implanted cochlear implant users. *Otol. Neurotol.* **2018**, *39*, e436–e442. [CrossRef] [PubMed]
14. Klop, W.M.C.; Briaire, J.J.; Stiggelbout, A.M.; Frijns, J.H.M. Cochlear implant outcomes and quality of life in adults with prelingual deafness. *Laryngoscope* **2007**, *117*, 1982–1987. [CrossRef] [PubMed]
15. O'Gara, S.J.; Cullington, H.E.; Grasmeder, M.L.; Adamou, M.; Matthews, E.S. factors affecting speech perception improvement post implantation in congenitally deaf adults. *Ear Hear.* **2016**, *37*, 671–679. [CrossRef]
16. Debruyne, J.; Janssen, M.; Brokx, J. Late cochlear implantation in early-deafened adults: A detailed analysis of auditory and self-perceived benefits. *Audiol. Neurotol.* **2018**, *22*, 364–376. [CrossRef] [PubMed]
17. Duchesne, L.; Millette, I.; Bhérer, M.; Gobeil, S. Auditory performance and subjective benefits in adults with congenital or prelinguistic deafness who receive cochlear implants during adulthood. *Cochlear Implant. Int.* **2017**, *18*, 143–152. [CrossRef]

18. Debruyne, J.; Janssen, A.; Brokx, J. Systematic review on late cochlear implantation in early-deafened adults and adolescents: Clinical effectiveness. *Ear Hear.* **2020**, *41*, 1417–1430. [CrossRef]
19. Debruyne, J.; Janssen, A.; Brokx, J. Systematic review on late cochlear implantation in early-deafened adults and adolescents: Predictors of performance. *Ear Hear.* **2020**, *41*, 1431–1441. [CrossRef]
20. Hermann, R.; Lescanne, E.; Loundon, N.; Barone, P.; Belmin, J.; Blanchet, C.; Borel, S.; Charpiot, A.; Coez, A.; Deguine, O.; et al. French society of ENT (SFORL) guidelines. Indications for cochlear implantation in adults. *Eur. Ann. Otorhinolaryngol. Head Neck Dis.* **2019**, *136*, 193–197. [CrossRef]
21. Kalafat, M.; Hugonot-Diener, L.; Poitrenaud, J. Standardisation et étalonnage français du "Mini-Mental State", version GRECO. *Rev. Neuropsychol.* **2003**, *13*, 209–236.
22. Archbold, S.; Lutman, M.; Marshall, D. Categories of auditory performance. *Ann. Otol Rhinol Laryngol. Suppl.* **1995**, *166*, 312–314. [PubMed]
23. Cox, R.; Alexander, G. The abbreviated profile of hearing aid benefit. *Ear Hear.* **1995**, *16*, 176–186. [CrossRef] [PubMed]
24. Allen, C.; Nikolopoulos, T.; Dyar, D.; O'Donoghue, G. Reliability of a rating scale for measuring speech intelligibility after pediatric cochlear implantation. *Otol. Neurotol.* **2001**, *22*, 631–633. [CrossRef] [PubMed]
25. Rousset, A.; Dowell, R.; Leigh, J. Receptive language as a predictor of cochlear implant outcome for prelingually deaf adults. *Int. J. Audiol.* **2016**, *55*, S24–S30. [CrossRef] [PubMed]
26. Caposecco, A.; Hickson, L.; Pedley, K. Cochlear implant outcomes in adults and adolescents with early-onset hearing loss. *Ear Hear.* **2012**, *33*, 209–220. [CrossRef]
27. Craddock, L.; Cooper, H.; Riley, A.; Wright, T. Cochlear implants for pre-lingually profoundly deaf adults. *Cochlear Implant. Int.* **2016**, *17*, 26–30. [CrossRef]
28. Yang, W.S.; Moon, I.S.; Kim, H.N.; Lee, W.S.; Lee, S.E.; Choi, J.Y. Delayed cochlear implantation in adults with prelingual severe-to-profound hearing loss. *Otol. Neurotol.* **2011**, *32*, 223–228. [CrossRef]
29. Holden, L.K.; Au, D.; Finley, C.C.; Ph, D.; Firszt, J.B.; Timothy, A.; Brenner, C.; Potts, L.G.; Gotter, B.D.; Vanderhoof, S.S.; et al. Factors affecting open-set word recognition in adults with cochlear implants. *Ear Hear.* **2013**, *34*, 342–360. [CrossRef]
30. Mosnier, I.; Ferrary, E.; Aubry, K.; Bordure, P.; Bozorg-Grayeli, A.; Deguine, O.; Eyermann, C.; Franco-Vidal, V.; Godey, B.; Guevara, N.; et al. The French national cochlear implant registry (EPIIC): Cochlear implantation in adults over 65 years old. *Eur. Ann. Otorhinolaryngol. Head Neck Dis.* **2020**, *137*, S19–S25. [CrossRef]
31. Lazard, D.S.; Giraud, A.L.; Gnansia, D.; Meyer, B.; Sterkers, O. Understanding the deafened brain: Implications for cochlear implant rehabilitation. *Eur. Ann. Otorhinolaryngol. Head Neck Dis.* **2012**, *129*, 98–103. [CrossRef]
32. Debruyne, J.A.; Francart, T.; Janssen, A.M.L.; Douma, K.; Brokx, J.P.L. Fitting prelingually deafened adult cochlear implant users based on electrode discrimination performance. *Int. J. Audiol.* **2017**, *56*, 174–185. [CrossRef] [PubMed]
33. Santarelli, R.; De Filippi, R.; Genovese, E.; Arslan, E. Cochlear implantation outcome in prelingually deafened young adults: A speech perception study. *Audiol. Neurotol.* **2008**, *13*, 257–265. [CrossRef] [PubMed]
34. Cusumano, C.; Friedmann, D.R.; Fang, Y.; Wang, B.; Roland, J.T.; Waltzman, S.B. Performance plateau in prelingually and postlingually deafened adult cochlear implant recipients. *Otol. Neurotol.* **2017**, *38*, 334–338. [CrossRef] [PubMed]
35. Van Dijkhuizen, J.N.; Boermans, P.P.B.M.; Briaire, J.J.; Frijns, J.H.M. Intelligibility of the patient's speech predicts the likelihood of cochlear implant success in prelingually deaf adults. *Ear Hear.* **2016**, *37*, e302–e310. [CrossRef] [PubMed]
36. Lyness, C.R.; Woll, B.; Campbell, R.; Cardin, V. How does visual language affect crossmodal plasticity and cochlear implant success? *Neurosci. Biobehav. Rev.* **2013**, *37*, 2621–2630. [CrossRef]
37. De Seta, D.; Nguyen, Y.; Vanier, A.; Ferrary, E.; Bebear, J.P.; Godey, B.; Robier, A.; Mondain, M.; Deguine, O.; Sterkers, O.; et al. Five-year hearing outcomes in bilateral simultaneously cochlear-implanted adult patients. *Audiol. Neurotol.* **2016**, *21*, 261–267. [CrossRef]

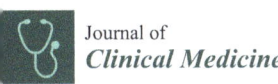

*Article*

# Functional Outcomes and Quality of Life after Cochlear Implantation in Patients with Long-Term Deafness

Attila Ovari [1,2,*], Lisa Hühnlein [2], David Nguyen-Dalinger [2,3,4], Daniel Fabian Strüder [5], Christoph Külkens [2,3,4], Oliver Niclaus [2,3,4] and Jens Eduard Meyer [1,2,3]

1 Department of Oto-Rhino-Laryngology, Head and Neck Surgery, Plastic Surgery, Asklepios Klinik St. Georg, 20099 Hamburg, Germany
2 Asklepios Medical School, Semmelweis University, 20099 Hamburg, Germany
3 Hanseatisches Cochlea Implantat Zentrum (HCIZ), 22417 Hamburg, Germany
4 Department of Oto-Rhino-Laryngology, Head and Neck Surgery, Facial Plastic Surgery, Asklepios Klinik Nord-Heidberg, 22417 Hamburg, Germany
5 Department of Oto-Rhino-Laryngology, Head and Neck Surgery "Otto Koerner", University Medical Center, 18057 Rostock, Germany
* Correspondence: atiova@gmail.com; Tel.: +49-40-1818852237; Fax: +49-1818853864

**Citation:** Ovari, A.; Hühnlein, L.; Nguyen-Dalinger, D.; Strüder, D.F.; Külkens, C.; Niclaus, O.; Meyer, J.E. Functional Outcomes and Quality of Life after Cochlear Implantation in Patients with Long-Term Deafness. *J. Clin. Med.* **2022**, *11*, 5156. https://doi.org/10.3390/jcm11175156

Academic Editor: George Psillas

Received: 21 July 2022
Accepted: 30 August 2022
Published: 31 August 2022

**Publisher's Note:** MDPI stays neutral with regard to jurisdictional claims in published maps and institutional affiliations.

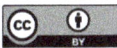

**Copyright:** © 2022 by the authors. Licensee MDPI, Basel, Switzerland. This article is an open access article distributed under the terms and conditions of the Creative Commons Attribution (CC BY) license (https://creativecommons.org/licenses/by/4.0/).

**Abstract:** Background: Hearing-related quality of life (QoL) after cochlear implantation (CI) is as important as audiological performance. We evaluated the functional results and QoL after CI in a heterogeneous patient cohort with emphasis on patients with long-term deafness (>10 years). Methods: Twenty-eight patients ($n$ = 32 implanted ears, within $n$ = 12 long-term deaf ears) implanted with a mid-scala electrode array were included in this retrospective mono-centric cohort study. Speech intelligibility for monosyllables (SIM), speech reception thresholds ($SRT_{50}$) and QoL with Nijmegen Cochlear Implant Questionnaire (NCIQ) were registered. Correlation of SIM and QoL was analyzed. Results: SIM and $SRT_{50}$ improved significantly 12 months postoperatively up to 54.8 ± 29.1% and 49.3 ± 9.6 dB SPL, respectively. SIM progressively improved up to 1 year, but some early-deafened, late implanted patients developed speech understanding several years after implantation. The global and all subdomain QoL scores increased significantly up to 12 months postoperatively and we found a correlation of SIM and global QoL score at 12 months postoperatively. Several patients of the "poor performer" (SIM < 40%) group reported high improvement of hearing-related QoL. Conclusions: Cochlear implantation provides a benefit in hearing-related QoL, even in some patients with low postoperative speech intelligibility results. Consequently, hearing-related QoL scores should be routinely used as outcome measure beside standard speech understanding tests, as well. Further studies with a prospective multi-centric design are needed to identify factors influencing post-implantation functional results and QoL in the patient group of long-term deafness.

**Keywords:** cochlear implants; long-term deafness; mid-scala electrode; Freiburger speech intelligibility test for monosyllables; Nijmegen Cochlear Implant Questionnaire; quality of life

## 1. Introduction

The standard outcome measure of cochlear implants (CIs) is the speech intelligibility test. However, quality of life (QoL) after cochlear implantation is as important as audiological performance. Several studies have evaluated the impact cochlear implantation on QoL and demonstrated significant postoperative improvements in hearing-related quality of life questionnaires [1–5], or in hearing-related domains of general health status questionnaires [2,5]. The Nijmegen Cochlear Implant Questionnaire (NCIQ) is a disease-specific questionnaire, which was adapted to different languages and is widely used to evaluate health-related QoL after cochlear implantation [2,6–14]. The NCIQ, developed 22 years ago, is still recommended as first-line measurement tool of QoL in patients after CI [15] and is used as a "legacy" patient-reported outcome measure for comparison of newer

QoL measurement tools; for example, the Cochlear Implant Quality of Life (CIQOL)-35 Profile instrument and CIQOL-10 Global measure [16]. At the same time, the majority of NCIQ subdomains and the global QoL score have a poor construct validity in confirmatory factor analysis, only the basic sound performance and activity limitation show strong psychometric properties [16].

*1.1. Hearing Outcome and QoL of Late Implanted Patients*

A high proportion of late implanted (after >10 years deafness) patients has poor functional results [17], but little is known about the hearing-related QoL in this patient group. High user satisfaction rates have consistently been reported in studies on early-deafened late implanted CI users, even in subjects with almost negligible gain in auditory performance [17–22]. Early-deafened, late implanted patients can show significant postoperative improvements measured with the NCIQ [2,5,17,23] despite minimal gain in speech understanding. In 2011, van Dijkhuizen et al. only found a significant correlation between speech perception outcomes and the subdomain "advanced sound perception" of the NCIQ [4], whereas both Peasgood et al. [20] and Straatman et al. [5] found no significant correlations between auditory outcome measures and scores on the Glasgow Benefit Inventory. Additionally, Straatman et al. found no significant correlations between phoneme benefit scores and the generic Health Utilities Index 3, or the postoperative changes on the NCIQ [5]. The authors hypothesized that prelingually deafened adults, in contrast to postlingually deafened adults, might be satisfied with just minimal improvements in hearing abilities. The hearing outcome with CI relates significantly in early-deafened and late implanted patients with preoperative speech intelligibility [23], communication mode as a child [17,24–26], and preoperative speech-understanding scores [17,24,26,27]. However, no correlation was found with duration of deafness [17,23,24,27] or with etiology [25,27] in this patient group. Whereas post-lingually deafened patients generally reach their maximum performance between 6 to 12 months [28], early-deafened patients may continue improving their hearing performance over 1 year postoperatively [29]. However, other studies found no further improvement after 1 year of follow-up [23]. One may argue that poor performers have no benefit of cochlear implantation as their speech understanding remains under 40%. However, patients with early-onset hearing loss and poor speech discrimination may be able to understand suprasegmental cues after implantation [17]. Moreover, the integration of visual speech information with auditory information provided by the CI allows higher scores in audio-visual condition [30]. Consequently, the evaluation of the real gain of CI in prelingually deafened patients should enclose suprasegmental and audio-visual cues [23]. The factors determining the large inter-individual differences in speech intelligibility postoperatively seen in this patient group are mainly unknown, but a recent study identified the preoperative consonant-nucleus-consonant (CNC) word recognition score and the preoperative pure tone averages of the implanted ear as the factors explaining 63.5% of the variation in postoperative speech understanding with CI [31]. Indeed, significant study results can be found about the influence of other preimplantation factors, such as patients' speech-understanding scores and preoperative hearing aid use [17,23,31].

*1.2. The HiFocus Mid-Scala Electrode Array*

The Cis HiRes 90K Advantage and the HiRes Ultra were commercially introduced 2012 and 2016, respectively. A new cochlear electrode array designed for the placement in the middle portion of the scala tympani, the HiFocus Mid-scala electrode (MSE) is the array used with these types of Cis since 2013 [32]. The MSE sits adjacent to the medial wall of the Scala tympani and is not in contact with the sensitive structures of the cochlea [33], minimizing the frictional forces on the lateral or medial wall during insertion [34]. The mean insertion force of MSE is less than 10 mN, corresponding to about 10% of the force expected for a normal straight electrode array with a similar insertion depth [34]. The MSE has a lower probability of dislocation into the scala vestibuli (scalar shift) than lateral or perimodiolar electrode arrays [35,36]. The functional advantages of the mid-scalar position are lower electrical thresholds, higher dynamic ranges and lower channel interaction compared to electrodes that are usually placed more peripherally in the Scala tympani [37]. The degree of hearing preservation is also higher with the MSE [38–40]. A comparison with the HiFocus 1J lateral wall electrode showed no difference in speech perception outcomes, despite the shallower insertion depth of MSE [41]. Additionally, MSE achieved a more consistent insertion depth than HiFocus 1J [39,41]. Battmer et al. compared the MSE with the Helix perimodiolar electrode array and they found that cochlear implantation with MSE led to significantly better postoperative SIM in quiet at each control interval from 3 to 12 months, at the same time, performance of both electrodes was in noise similar [42]. However, the biggest study to date with $n = 328$ participants comparing the outcome of MSE, lateral wall (LW) and perimodiolar (PM) electrodes showed no significant differences in hearing results [43]. However, studies dealing with quality of life (QoL) outcomes of MSE are lacking.

Taken together, the aim of this mono-centric retrospective cohort study was to evaluate the hearing performance and the QoL in a heterogenous patient group regarding duration and cause of deafness, but all implanted with the same CI electrode array (MSE). An emphasis was put on the performance and QoL of implantees with a long history (>10 years) of deafness, as controversial study results can be found on these subjects in the literature. The development of speech recognition and QoL scores should be analyzed over the follow-up period of one year and the relation of these two measures should be examined in this study, either.

## 2. Materials and methods

### 2.1. Patient Population

Epidemiological data are summarized in Table 1.

**Table 1.** Summary of the epidemiological data.

| Operated Patients | Operated Ears | Age at Implantation (Years) | Contralateral Ear | Cause of Deafness | Duration of Deafness (Years) |
|---|---|---|---|---|---|
| $n = 28$ Women $n = 18$ (64.3%) Men $n = 10$ (35.7%) Bilaterally implanted $n = 4$ (14.3%) | $n = 32$ left ears $n = 15$ (46.9%) right ears $n = 17$ (53.1%) | $54.2 \pm 15.85$ (range: 23–82) | normal hearing $n = 5$ (15.6%) moderate hearing loss $n = 5$ (15.6%) severe hearing loss $n = 4$ (12.5%) profound hearing loss $n = 16$ (50.0%) congenital deafness $n = 2$ (6.3%) bilateral implantation $n = 4$ (12.5%) | SIHL $n = 6$ (18.8%) SSD $n = 5$ (15.6%) PSHL $n = 11$ (34.4%) congenital $n = 4$ (12.5%) genetic $n = 1$ (3.13%) surgery $n = 1$ (3.13%) surgical removal of vestibular schwannoma $n = 1$ (3.13%) | <10 years: $n = 20$ (62.5%) >10 years: $n = 12$ (37.5%) |

The cochlear implantations were carried out from December 2013 to November 2017 using the Advanced Bionics HiRes 90K Advantage ($n = 27$, 84.4%) or HiRes Ultra ($n = 5$, 13.6%) with the HiFocus Mid-scala electrode. The Naída Q70 or 90 sound processor was used in every patient.

### 2.2. Surgical Technique

All patients were operated by using a minimal retroauricular incision, extended antrotomy and regular posterior tympanotomy. All presented cases had an electrode insertion through the round window (RW) after intratympanic injection of dexamethasone and hyaluronic acid to the RW. Electrode insertions were carried out with consistent use of the insertion tool of AB after extended RW approach and with an insertion depth of 1 1/4 turns. Electrode tip fold over or kinking were ruled out by postoperative Stenvers view radiograph. The implantations have been performed by two operating surgeons (JEM, ON).

### 2.3. Postoperative Care

The first fitting of the cochlear implant was 2–4 weeks after surgery. All CI-recipients of this study went through an in-patient rehabilitation process in a specialized after-care center for cochlea implantees and received regular implant fittings at 3, 6, 9, 12, 18 and 24 months after activation of the CI. Depending on the hearing development of the patients, additional fittings were included, if necessary. After this period, yearly controls were carried out. Additionally, patients were motivated to train independently using CDs and Apps developed for auditory training.

*2.4. Assessment of Audiological Performance*

The audiometric protocol involved the following test battery: the Freiburger speech recognition test (monosyllables, numbers) was carried out routinely at each hearing measurement, preoperatively using headphones, with hearing aid and with CI postoperatively in free-field condition (signal on the implanted side, 45° azimuth, $S_{45}$).

The HSM (Hochmair–Schulz–Moser) sentence-test with and without noise consists of three training lists and 30 test lists with each 20 daily life sentences in German. The measurements in noise were performed $S_0N_0$ at two levels (65 dB/65 dB or 65 dB/55 dB). The HSM sentence-test was introduced during the study and is not available for each participant of the study. The HSM sentence-test was utilized preoperatively, at 3 and 6 months postoperatively.

The OLSA ("Oldenburger Satztest") or Oldenburger sentence-test with and without noise contains 40 test lists with 30 sentences (alternatively 25 test lists with each 20 sentences) uses an inventory of 50 words which can be randomly selected in a fixed order of noun/verb/number/adjective/grammatical object. The sentences are this way just partially meaningful; thus, not easy to retain and the test can be repeated. The OLSA measures the threshold at which test persons understand the 50% of the sentences in noise ($S_0N_{-90}$). However, if test persons do not achieve at least 80% speech understanding without noise, the measurements in noise are not rational. Additionally, patients having another native language as German have difficulty to understand the test sentences. Consequently, not all participants of the study could be tested preoperatively and at 12 months postoperatively.

The data of HSM und OLSA were not included in the analysis due to the incomplete dataset.

If masking of the better or normal hearing ear of the contralateral side was necessary, it was performed with a headphone and noise covering the speech frequencies.

Preoperative unaided speech reception thresholds ($SRT_{50}$) and speech understanding for monosyllables (SIM) at 70 dB SPL using the Freiburger speech recognition test were compared with the postoperative aided thresholds at 1, 3, 6 and 12 months after cochlear implantation.

*2.5. Measurements of the Quality of Life (QoL)*

The Nijmegen Cochlear Implant Questionnaire (NCIQ) was used to assess the development of patients' basic and advanced sound perception, speech production (so-called physical domains), self-esteem (psychological domain), activity limitations and social interactions (social domains) [2]. Each of the six subdomains of NCIQ contains ten items covering a total of 60 questions, prepared in a 5-point Liker scale. The first 55 questions can be answered with "never" (1), "sometimes" (2), regularly (3), "usually" (4) and "always" (5), and the last five items with "no" (1), "poor" (2), "moderate" (3), "good" (4) and "fairly good" (5). Participants can choose a sixth answer category "not applicable" in the case the item is not suitable. The total score for each subdomain is calculated as 1 = 0, 2 = 25, 3 = 50, 4 = 75 and 5 = 100, then the scores of each subdomain are summed and divided by the number of answers. The global score is the mean of the scores of the six subdomains. A higher score means a better QoL.

*2.6. Statistical Analysis*

Quantitative variables were expressed as means (±standard deviations). Data were summarized by descriptive statistics and normality was confirmed by the D'Agostino-Pearson test. Multiple comparisons were performed by one-way ANOVA (repeated measures, Tukey's post-hoc test). Relationships between variables (QoL/SIM and deafness duration/SIM) were analyzed by correlation analysis (Pearson). Results were considered significant for $p < 0.05$. All calculations were performed using Microsoft Excel (version 15.29, Microsoft Corporation, Redmond, WA, USA) and GraphPad Prism8 (GraphPad Software, San Diego, CA, USA).

## 3. Results

Individual epidemiological data, hearing results and quality of life scores are presented in Table 2.

### 3.1. Audiological Outcome

The functional results are presented in Table 2. The wearing time of the cochlear implant was less than 1 year in $n = 2$ (6.3%) ears, between 1 and 2 years in $n = 22$ (68.8%) ears and more than 2 years in $n = 8$ (25%) ears.

### 3.2. Freiburger Speech Recognition Test for Monosyllables (SIM) at 70 dB SPL

The SIM values were as follows: preoperative (pre) $3.1 \pm 7.0\%$ ($n = 32$), at 1 month (1M) postoperatively $8.3 \pm 15.43\%$ ($n = 32$), at 3 months (3M) $29.7 \pm 25.0\%$, at 6 months (6M) $48.5 \pm 27.9\%$ ($n = 30$) and at 12 months (12M) $54.8 \pm 29.1\%$ ($n = 29$). There was a significant and continuous improvement of SIM in Tukey's multiple comparisons test, from 3 to 12 months with the use of the cochlear implant (pre vs. 3M: $p < 0.0001$, 95% CI $-38.16$ to 13.72; pre vs. 6M: $p < 0.0001$, 95% CI $-58.71$ to $-31.10$; pre vs. 12M: $p < 0.0001$, 95% CI $-66.16$ to $-37.90$; 1M vs. 3M: $p < 0.0001$, 95% CI $-30.87$ to $-10.06$; 1M vs. 6M: $p < 0.0001$, 95% CI $-52.94$ to $-25.93$; 1M vs. 12M: $p < 0.0001$, 95% CI $-60.37$ to $-32.75$; 3M vs. 6M: $p = 0.0006$, 95% CI $-30.91$ to $-7.026$; 3M vs. 12M: $p < 0.0001$, 95% CI $-39.39$ to $-12.79$; 6M vs. 12M: $p = 0.0319$, 95% CI $-13.80$ to $-0.4468$) (Figure 1). Only the preoperative SIM and the values at one month postoperatively did not significantly differ (pre vs. 1M: $p = 0.1825$, 95% CI $-12.45$ to 1.512).

For the group of patients with long-term (>10 years) deafness ($n = 12$, 42.9%) and for the cohort with short-term (<10 years) deafness ($n = 16.57.1\%$) the following SIM values were measured: pre-OP $1 \pm 3.2\%$ and $4.4 \pm 8.38\%$ ($p = 0.99$), 1M $6.7 \pm 15.4\%$ and $8.9 \pm 16.1\%$ ($p = 0.99$), 3M $27.1 \pm 30.7\%$ and $30 \pm 21.3\%$ ($p = 0.99$), 6M $40.8 \pm 32.1\%$ and $51.8 \pm 24.4\%$ ($p = 0.68$), 12M $47.9 \pm 33.6\%$ and $57.1 \pm 25.3\%$ ($p = 0.82$), respectively. No significant differences were found between the groups.

For the group of patients having single-sided deafness (SSD $n = 5$, 17.9%) with normal hearing on the contralateral side and for the rest of the patients were the following SIM values measured: pre-OP $7.5 \pm 15\%$ and $2.5 \pm 5.11\%$ ($p = 0.99$), 1M $2 \pm 4.5\%$ and $9.2 \pm 16.8\%$ ($p = 0.97$), 3M $23 \pm 19.2\%$ and $30 \pm 26.2\%$ ($p = 0.97$), 6M $40 \pm 22.9\%$ and $48.8 \pm 28.8\%$ ($p = 0.94$), 12M $51 \pm 27.9\%$ and $54 \pm 29.3\%$ ($p = 0.99$), respectively. No significant differences were found between the groups.

### 3.3. Speech Reception Thresholds ($SRT_{50}$)

If the $SRT_{50}$ was not measurable due to patient' deafness, the value was calculated with 120 dB. The following speech reception thresholds were measured: preoperative $113.6 \pm 12.8$ dB SPL ($n = 32$, measurable: $n = 9$, 28.1%), at 1 month postoperatively $82.4 \pm 26.8$ dB ($n = 32$, measurable: $n = 22$, 68.7%), at 3 months $63.5 \pm 21.1$ dB ($n = 32$, measurable: $n = 30$, 93.8%), at 6 months $55.1 \pm 16.4$ dB ($n = 30$), at 12 months $47.5 \pm 7.8$ dB ($n = 29$). (Figure 2). The $SRT_{50}$ decreased significantly after 1 month postoperatively (pre vs. 1M: $p < 0.0001$, 95% CI 16.93 to 45.47), after 3 months (1M vs. 3M: $p < 0.0001$, 95% CI 6.212 to 31.60; pre vs. 3M: $p < 0.0001$, 95% CI 38.33 to 61.88) and up to 12 months (pre vs. 6M: $p < 0.0001$, 95% CI 47.89 to 69.17; pre vs. 12M: $p < 0.0001$, 95% CI 55.84 to 72.63; 3M vs. 6M: $p = 0.1844$, 95% CI $-2.354$ to 19.20; 3M vs. 12M: $p = 0.0007$, 95% CI 5.172 to 23.08; 6M to 12M: $p = 0.1135$, 95% CI $-0.8647$ to 12.27).

Table 2. Epidemiological data, hearing results and quality of life scores of all patients in the study.

| Patient | Epidemiological Data | | | | Hearing Performance Post-Op 12 Months (n = 32 Ears) | | | Quality of Life Pre-Op/Post-Op 12 Months (n = 20 Ears) | | | | | |
|---|---|---|---|---|---|---|---|---|---|---|---|---|---|
| | Age | Contralateral Ear | Cause of Deafness | Duration of Deafness (Years) | SRT$_{50}$ (dB) | SIM at 70 dB (%) | Sound Perception Basic | Sound Perception Advanced | Speech Production | Self-Esteem | Activity | Social Interactions | Global Score |
| 1 | 34 | normal hearing | SHL, SSD | 1 | 50 | 30 | | | | | | | |
| 2 | 81 | moderate hearing loss | PSHL | 1 | 47 | 80 | 25/58.3 | 50/50 | 45.8/62.5 | 55/43.8 | 25/30 | 25/50 | 37.6/49.1 |
| 3 | 59 | profound hearing loss | congenital, Gusher | >10 | 57 | 45 | 22.5/77.5 | 47.5/75 | 20/62.5 | 37.5/70 | 57.5/85 | 55/72.5 | 40/73.8 |
| 4 | 50 | profound hearing loss | congenital | >10 | 58 | 60 | | | | | | | |
| 5 | 64 (65) | first implanted ear, contralateral profound hearing loss / second implanted ear (bilateral cochlear implantation) | PSHL | 1 | 43 / 40 | 75 / 70 | 17.5/63.9 / 37.5/90 | 30.6/36.1 / 37.5/75 | 20/50 / 40/70 | 30/37.5 / 47.5/60 | 8.3/50 / 44.4/65.6 | 22.2/41.7 / 50/63.9 | 21.4/46.5 / 42.8/70.8 |
| 6 | 38 | profound hearing loss | congenital | >10 | 63 | 0 | | | | | | | |
| 7 | 52 | deafness | congenital | >10 | 67 | 0 | 15/32.5 | 30/32.5 | 2.5/15 | 27.5/45 | 41.7/22.5 | 35/21.4 | 25.3/28.2 |
| 8 | 59 | normal hearing | PSHL, SSD | 2 | 50 | 70 | 80.6/77.5 | 82.5/82.5 | 80/75 | 45/63.9 | 69.4/75 | 50/69.4 | 67.9/73.9 |
| 9 | 47 | deafness | congenital | >10 | 43 | 65 | | | | | | | |
| 10 | 43 | profound hearing loss | Genetic | 4 | 42 | 85 | 47.5/72.5 | 95/100 | 50/72.5 | 44.4/66.7 | 37.5/50 | 41.7/66.7 | 52.7/71.4 |
| 11 | 63 | moderate hearing loss | SHL | >10 | 47 | 75 | 58.3/70 | 97.5/100 | 72.5/90 | 40/75 | 38.9/61.1 | 40.6/57.5 | 58/75.6 |
| 12 | 79 | profound hearing loss | PSHL | 2 | 43 | 65 | 41.7/78.1 | 62.5/80 | 16.7/62.5 | 42.5/52.5 | 32.1/63.9 | 27.8/45 | 37.2/63.7 |
| 13 | 44 | normal hearing | SHL, SSD | 7 | 50 | 40 | 32.5/52.5 | 47.2/63.9 | 38.9/67.5 | 33.3/57.5 | 25/52.5 | 27.8/45 | 34.1/56.5 |
| 14 | 47 | severe hearing loss | PSHL | 1 | 55 | 45 | | | | | | | |
| 15 | 41 (42) | first implanted ear severe hearing loss / second implanted ear (bilateral cochlear implantation) | congenital / SHL | >10 / 1 | 72 / 39 | 0 / 95 | 52.5/75 / 58.3/72.5 | 52.5/75 / 80/80 | 62.5/82.5 / 57.5/87.5 | 72.5/90 / 80/92.5 | 75/88.9 / 67.5/87.5 | 62.5/75 / 72.5/87.5 | 62.9/81.1 / 69.3/84.6 |
| 16 | 28 | simultaneous bilateral cochlear implantation, profound hearing loss on both sides | Accident | 4 | 58 / 62 | 45 / 35 | | | | | | | |
| 17 | 76 | profound hearing loss | PSHL | 1 | 32 | 95 | | | | | | | |
| 18 | 62 | moderate hearing loss | SHL | 1 | 47 | 55 | | | | | | | |
| 19 | 46 | bilaterally implanted within 1 week profound hearing loss on both sides | PSHL | >10 / 1 | 40 / 32 | 95 / 95 | 7.5/97.5 | 63.9/81.3 | 17.5/90 | 22.5/75 | 30.6/86.1 | 19.4/67.5 | 26.9/82.9 |
| 20 | 53 | normal hearing | meningitis, SSD | 1 | 42 | 90 | 80/85 | 92.5/91.7 | 80/87.5 | 62.5/80 | 55.6/90 | 55.6/97.2 | 71/88.6 |
| 21 | 23 | moderate hearing loss | surgical removal of vestibular schwannoma | 1 | 50 | 25 | | | | | | | |

Table 2. Cont.

| Patient | Age | Epidemiological Data | | | | Hearing Performance Post-Op 12 Months (n = 32 Ears) | | | | | Quality of Life Pre-Op/Post-Op 12 Months (n = 20 Ears) | | | | |
|---|---|---|---|---|---|---|---|---|---|---|---|---|---|---|---|
| | | Contralateral Ear | Cause of Deafness | Duration of Deafness (Years) | $SRT_{50}$ (dB) | SIM at 70 dB (%) | Sound Perception Basic | Sound Perception Advanced | Speech Production | Self-Esteem | Activity | Social Interactions | Global Score | | |
| 22 | 49 | profound hearing loss | PSHL | >10 | 55 | 25 | 60/72.5 | 63.9/75 | 60/66.7 | 27.5/35 | 57.5/44.4 | 46.8/44.4 | 52.6/56.3 | | |
| 23 | 65 | profound hearing loss | PSHL | >10 | 40 | 75 | 15.6/82.5 | 33.3/82.5 | 18.8/77.8 | 8.3/45 | 0/56.3 | 21.9/61.1 | 16.3/67.5 | | |
| 24 | 68 | normal hearing | SIHL, SSD | 6 | 55 | 25 | 55/75 | 94.4/97.5 | 35.7/62.5 | 20/27.5 | 30/44.4 | 25/30.6 | 43.4/56.3 | | |
| 25 | 60 | severe hearing loss | PSHL | >10 | 46 | 60 | 77.8/67.5 | 91.7/100 | 88.9/75 | 72.5/65 | 70/65 | 62.5/72.5 | 77.2/74.2 | | |
| 26 | 82 | moderate hearing loss | Surgery | >10 | 43 | 75 | 57.5/92.5 | 82.1/90.6 | 70/87.5 | 55/87.5 | 58.3/91.7 | 27.8/65.6 | 58.5/85.9 | | |
| 27 | 78 | severe hearing loss | PSHL | 1 | 58 | 20 | 71.4/96.4 | 91.7/89.3 | 78.1/87.5 | 66.7/71.9 | 43.8/82.1 | 37.5/83.3 | 64.9/85.1 | | |
| 28 | 61 | profound hearing loss | PSHL | 1 | 53 | 40 | | | | | | 39.7/60.89 | 45.6/68.58 | | |
| For the whole patient cohort: | | | | | 47.5 ± 7.84 | 54.8 ± 29.09 | 42.1/74.46 | 61.4/77.89 | 46.2/71.60 | 41.5/62.06 | 42.4/64.60 | | | | |

Table 2. Patient-level data with epidemiologic characteristics, functional results and quality of life scores of Nijmegen Cochlear Implant Questionnaire. SIHL: sudden idiopathic hearing loss, SSD: single-sided deafness, PSHL: progressive sensorineural hearing loss.

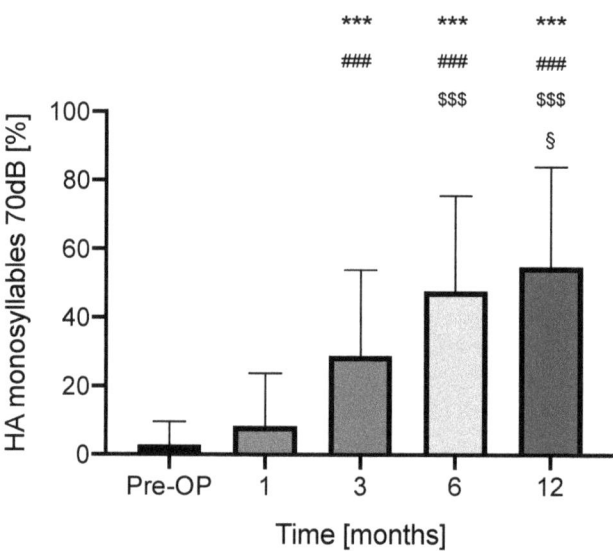

**Figure 1.** Aided (HA) speech understanding at 70 dB (Freiburger monosyllable test) preoperatively (with hearing aid), at 1, 3, 6 and 12 months postoperatively (with CI) in the whole patient cohort. Significant differences ($p < 0.05$) are indicated in comparison with * vs. Pre-OP, # vs. 1 month, $ vs. 3 months, § vs. 6 months. Significance levels are indicated as **/##/$$/§§ if $p < 0.005$ and as ***/###/$$$/§§§ if $p < 0.0001$.

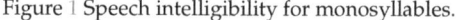

Figure 1 Speech intelligibility for monosyllables.

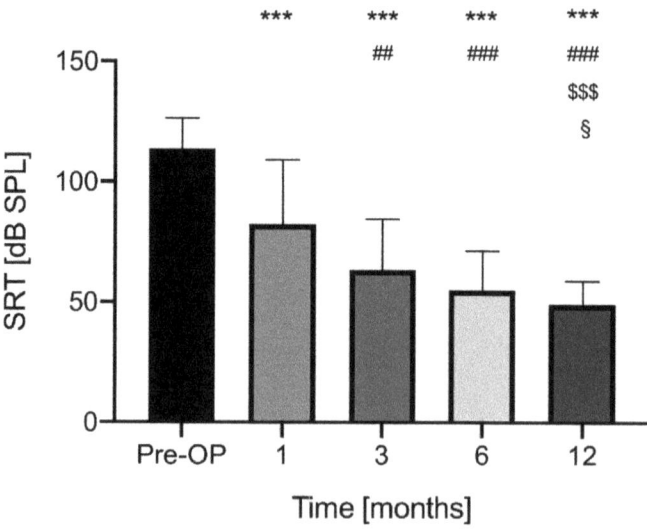

**Figure 2.** Speech reception thresholds (Freiburger speech test) preoperatively, at 1, 3, 6 and 12 months postoperatively in the whole patient cohort. Significant differences ($p < 0.05$) are indicated in comparison with * vs. Pre-OP, # vs. 1 month, $ vs. 3 months, § vs. 6 months. Significance levels are indicated as **/##/$$/§§ if $p < 0.005$ and as ***/###/$$$/§§§ if $p < 0.0005$.

For the group of patients with long-term (>10 years) deafness and for the cohort with short-term (<10 years) deafness the following $SRT_{50}$ values were measured: pre-OP not measurable and $94.3 \pm 12.6$ dB, 1M $64.2 \pm 12.8$ dB and $66.3 \pm 7.4$ dB ($p = 0.97$), 3M $60.7 \pm 14.7$ dB and $56.5 \pm 7.6$ dB ($p = 0.75$), 6M $57.0 \pm 13.9$ dB and $51.1 \pm 8.8$ dB ($p = 0.46$), 12M $52.6 \pm 11$ dB and $48.2 \pm 7.7$ dB ($p = 0.72$), respectively. No significant differences were found between the groups.

For the group of patients having single-sided deafness (SSD, $n = 5$, 17.9%) with normal hearing on the contralateral side and for the rest of the patients were the following $SRT_{50}$ values were measured: pre-OP $102.5 \pm 10.6$ dB and $91.6 \pm 12.8$ dB ($p = 0.18$), 1M $68.5 \pm 6.6$ dB and $65.1 \pm 9.1$ dB ($p = 0.97$), 3M $58.4 \pm 7.5$ dB and $57.9 \pm 11.3$ dB ($p = 0.99$), 6M $53 \pm 9.1$ dB and $53.5 \pm 11.9$ dB ($p = 0.99$), 12M $49.4 \pm 4.7$ dB and $50 \pm 9.9$ dB ($p = 0.99$), respectively. No significant differences were found between the groups.

Figure 2 Speech reception thresholds.

There were $n = 3$ (10.1%) patients with a long history (>20 years) of deafness who had no speech intelligibility 12 months postoperatively. However, all three patients had SIM at the last control (patient 6: 45% SIM after 5 years, patient 7: 10% SIM after 4 years, and first implanted ear of patient 15: 40% SIM after 3 years of CI use, respectively). If these patients with long-time deafness excluded, SIM and $SRT_{50}$ reached 12 months postoperatively $60.5 \pm 24.1$% and $47.5 \pm 7.8$ dB, respectively. No correlation between deafness time and SIM was found. Looking at the distribution of the whole cohort, $n = 13$ (40.6%) ears achieved a SIM of at least 70% after 12 months of CI wearing time. Five ears (15.6%) developed a SIM of 55–65%, another $n = 5$ (15.6%) ears 40–45%, respectively. Nine ears (28.1%) had a SIM of less than 40% (Table 2).

### 3.4. Measurements of Quality of Life

The hearing-related quality of life was registered with the Nijmegen Cochlear Implant Questionnaire (NCIQ). Preoperatively, $n = 24$ (85.7%) patients ($n = 28$, 87.5% of implanted ears) filled out the NCIQ. Nineteen patients (67.9%; $n = 20$ ears, 62.5%) and eighteen patients (64.3%; $n = 20$ ears, 71.4%) were eligible at the control at 6 and 12 months, respectively.

### 3.5. NCIQ Subdomain Scores

In general, QoL subdomain scores significantly improved between the preoperative and postoperative period (Figure 3). We observe a progressive and significant improvement of QoL up to 12 months in the basic sound perception subdomain (pre vs. 6M: $p = 0.0082$, 95% CI $-31.91$ to $-4.261$; pre vs. 12M: $p < 0.0001$, 95% CI $-45.40$ to $-19.27$; 6M vs. 12M: $p = 0.0011$, 95% CI $-22.08$ to $-6.057$), in speech production (pre vs. 6M: $p = 0.0307$, 95% CI $-26.02$ to $-1.176$; pre vs. 12M: $p < 0.0001$, 95% CI $-36.35$ to $-14.51$; 6M vs. 12M: $p < 0.0001$, 95% CI $-16.76$ to $-6.905$) and in social interactions (pre vs. 6M: $p = 0.0057$, 95% CI $-21.78$ to $-3.667$; pre vs. 12M: $p < 0.0001$, 95% CI $-29.62$ to $-12.72$; 6M vs. 12M: $p = 0.0410$, 95% CI $-16.55$ to $-0.3299$).in The advanced sound perception reached its plateau at 6 months postoperatively (pre vs. 6M: $p = 0.0094$, 95% CI $-18.00$ to $-2.444$, pre vs. 12M: $p = 0.0455$, 95% CI $-25.81$ to $-0.2333$6M vs. 12M: $p = 0.7822$, 95% CI $-13.66$ to $8.067$), similar to the self-esteem (pre vs. 6M: $p = 0.0055$, 95% CI $-20.91$ to $-3.557$, pre vs. 12M: $p < 0.0001$, 95% CI $-28.89$ to $-12.24$, 6M vs. 12M: $p = 0.0693$, 95% CI $-17.27$ to $0.6097$). The activity score showed a slow but significant increase up to 12 months postoperatively (pre vs. 6M: $p = 0.0944$, 95% CI $-20.70$ to $1.431$, pre vs. 12M: $p < 0.0001$, 95% CI $-33.06$ to $-11.37$, 6M vs. 12M: $p = 0.0097$, 95% CI $-22.06$ to $-3.107$).

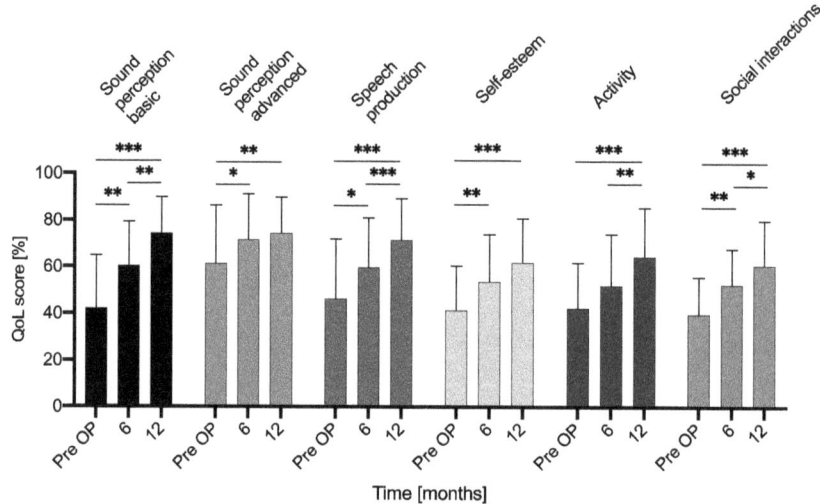

**Figure 3.** Results of Nijmegen Cochlear Implant Questionnaire before and 6 or 12 months after cochlear implantation in the whole patient cohort. Asterisks indicate a significant difference: * $p < 0.05$, ** $p < 0.005$, *** $p < 0.0005$.

Figure 3 NCIQ QoL subdomain scores.

### 3.6. NCIQ Global Score

The preoperative global QoL score (45.6 ± 17.2) increased progressively at both 6 months (58.6 ± 16.5, pre vs. 6M: $p = 0.0014$, 95% CI −21.32 to −5.241) and 12 months (68.6 ± 15.8, pre vs. 12M: $p < 0.0001$, 95% CI −30.73 to −15.33, 6M vs. 12M: $p = 0.001$, 95% CI −15.26 to −4.234) postoperatively in our patient group (Figure 4).

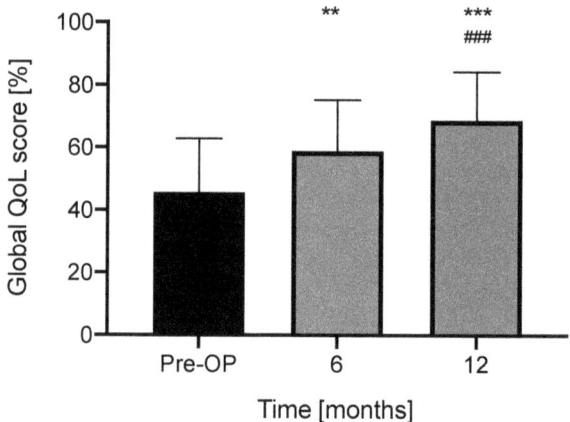

**Figure 4.** NCIQ global QoL scores preoperatively, and at 6 and 12 postoperative months. Asterisks indicate a significant difference in comparison with pre-OP: ** $p < 0.005$, *** $p < 0.0005$. Hashes indicate a significant difference in comparison with 6M: ### $p < 0.0005$ (for exact values see text).

In the patient group with long-term deafness, out of 12 participants $n = 9$ (75%) filled out the NCIQ, in the patient cohort with short-term deafness out of 16 $n = 14$ (87.5%). The following global QoL scores were measured (long vs. short-term deafness): pre-OP 46.4 ± 20.4 and 45.1 ± 15.9 ($p = 0.99$), 6M 62.8 ± 20.6 and 55.1 ± 12.6 ($p = 0.63$), 12M

69.5 ± 17.8 and 67.8 ± 14.7 (*p* = 0.99), respectively. No significant differences were found between the groups.

In the patient group of SSD, out of five *n* = 4 participants (80%) filled out the NCIQ, in the rest of the patient cohort out of 23 participants *n* = 15 (65.2%). In the latter cohort, patients 5 and 15 filled out the NCIQ twice (sequential bilateral implantation). The following global QoL scores were measured (SSD vs. rest of the patient cohort): pre-OP 54.1 ± 18.2 and 44.0 ± 17 (*p* = 0.63), 6M 64.1 ± 14.4 and 56.8 ± 17 (*p* = 0.82), 12M 68.8 ± 15.6 and 68.5 ± 16.3 (*p* = 0.99), respectively. No significant differences were found between the groups.

Figure 4 NCIQ global QoL scores.

The global QoL score correlated with the SIM of the whole patient cohort (Pearson correlation analysis, $r = 0.3821$, $p = 0.0482$) (Figure 5).

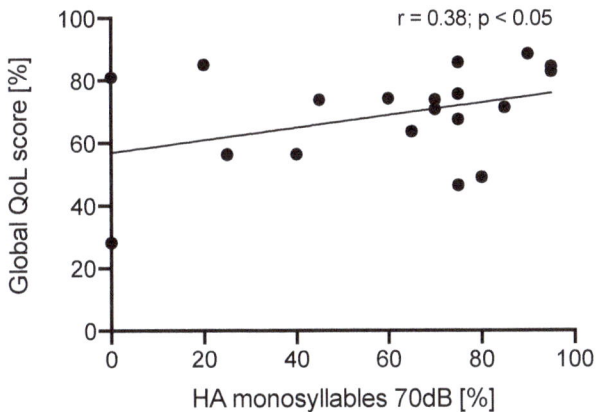

**Figure 5.** Correlation of global Quality of Life (QoL) scores of the Nijmegen Cochlear Implant Questionnaire with the CI-aided (HA) speech understanding at 70 dB SPL (Freiburger monosyllable test) postoperatively at 12 months.

Figure 5 Correlation of SIM and NCIQ global QoL scores.

All data of this study are available as Supplementary Material (File S1, Excel-table).

## 4. Discussion

### 4.1. Summary of the Goals and Main Results of the Study

In this study, the development of speech recognition and QoL scores should be analyzed over time and the relation of these two measures should be examined. We found that in this patient cohort speech understanding for monosyllables (SIM) developed progressively up to one year after cochlear implantation. Some patients with a long history of deafness and with no speech recognition after one year follow-up developed a usable SIM after several years. All subdomain scores of the NCIQ increased significantly up to the end of the follow-up period of 12 months and the NCIQ global score increased significantly at both 6 and 12 postoperative months, either. We demonstrated a low correlation of SIM and global QoL score after 12 months CI wearing time in the whole patient cohort. Hearing-related QoL after cochlear implantation was in some cases high despite poor results of standard speech understanding tests.

### 4.2. Audiological Outcomes and Quality of Life after Cochlear Implantation

Eighteen (56.3%) ears in our study achieved a SIM of at least 50% after 12 months of CI wearing time. Nevertheless, nine ears (28.1%) underperformed having less than 40% SIM after 1 year of CI use. Looking closer at the cause of deafness and at the hearing of the contralateral side in this patient group, we can observe that three patients had a congenital or early-onset deafness and one patient had a removal of a vestibular schwannoma on the implanted side. These conditions are usually associated with a slower post-implantation hearing development and often result in a poor hearing performance after one year of CI use [17]. Interestingly, two patients of the congenital deafness group developed a usable speech understanding with the CI only after several years. High motivation and consequent CI use may have contributed to this hearing performance. Contrary to these cases, two patients in the underperforming group had single side deafness (patients 1 and 24, SIM at 12 months postoperatively 30 and 25%, respectively; Table 2). The latter patients may more rely on the contralateral side with a good hearing and therefore are less motivated to train with the CI, a possible reason for their poor speech understanding scores on the implanted ear. According to Muigg et. al, patients with SSD and long-term deafness are at higher risk to abandon the CI but if they do not discontinue CI use, they can have equal QoL benefit measured with NCIQ as implanted SSD patients with short-term (<10 years) deafness [44]. However, there is a bias in analyzing QoL results of patients with single-sided deafness as NCIQ measures QoL of both ears at the same time. Accordingly, patients with SSD having poor performance on the implanted ear and with normal contralateral hearing could have a good quality of life. In our study, those five patients with SSD (1, 8, 13, 20 and 24) were compared with the rest of the cohort and they had actually no difference regarding SIM at 12 months postoperatively ($51 \pm 27.9\%$ vs. $54 \pm 29.2\%$ in the other 23 patients, $p = 0.99$) or global QoL score at 12 months ($68.8 \pm 15.6$ vs. $68.5 \pm 16.3$, $p = 0.99$). We hypothesize that the masking of the normal hearing ear may be used during hearing training with the CI to achieve better audiological results on the implanted side, but we are not aware of a study that analyzed this theory.

The subgroup of early-deafened, late implanted patients in our cohort ($n = 6$) shows, in accordance with the literature, very heterogeneous audiological results postoperatively [17,29,31]. Three patients had usable (45 to 65%) SIM, the remaining three patients had no measurable benefit in terms of speech understanding after one year of CI wearing time. Nevertheless, two initial poor performer patients of this group achieved 40% and 45% SIM after 3 and 5 years, respectively.

Comparing the patient groups with long-term (>10 years) and short-term (<10 years) deafness, the latter showed by tendency a better SIM after 12 months CI wearing time ($47.9 \pm 33.6\%$ vs. $57.1 \pm 25.3\%$, $p = 0.82$), but the global QoL scores were after 1 year follow-up very similar ($69.5 \pm 17.8$ vs. $67.9 \pm 14.7$). Accordingly, patients with a long-term deafness in our study had similar subjective benefit of the use of their cochlear implant as patients with short-term deafness.

With the use of CI, QoL scores increased significantly at the last measurement at 12 months in our whole patient group in all six subdomains of the NCIQ. The improvement of the global QoL score was in our study significant at both 6 and 12 months, either. Hirschfelder et al. published significant improvements in the global score and in all subdomain scores using NCIQ in 56 adult CI users [7]. The improvement of QoL concerns not only audiological aspects such as sound perception and speech production, but also psychosocial aspects such as self-esteem, activity level and social interaction. A significant improvement of QoL scores except for "activity" can be seen already after a wearing period of six months (Figures 3 and 4). Furthermore, QoL scores at 12 months improved significantly in comparison with both preoperative and 6 months postoperative values, except for "sound perception advanced" and "self-esteem", which reached their plateau after 6 months. Accordingly, the mean activity level and social interaction rose after implantation, which reinforces the thesis of postoperative re-socialization. In 2015, Mosnier reported in their study using the NCIQ a significant improvement of the QoL scores in all six subdomains after 6 months of CI use in elderly (65–85 years) patients. In contrast to our data, they measured stable results in QoL between 6 to 12 months after cochlear implantation [45]. Mean age at implantation of our cohort was $54.2 \pm 15.9$ years (range: 23–82) but the significant improvement of QoL scores in our study cannot be explained by implantees' age alone. Notably, Plath et al. published recently their results of patients with a very similar age distribution (mean $55.3 \pm 16.9$ years, $n = 100$) at implantation and they reported no significant improvement of both global QoL score and NCIQ subdomain scores between 6 and 12 months postoperatively [15].

It would be interesting to determine the benefits of bilateral cochlear implantation compared to unilateral ones. Rader et al. reported that QoL measured with NCIQ increased by 23.7% after second CI in their patient cohort [46]. Unfortunately, there were only four bilaterally implanted patients in this study and only three of them filled out the NCIQ. Interestingly, the intrapersonal comparison demonstrated that two patients in our cohort who had been implanted sequentially showed gradual improvement of QoL scores after each cochlear implantation (patients 5 and 15, Table 2). This result is in line with the literature data and indicates the higher benefit of bilateral over unilateral cochlear implantation in patients with profound bilateral hearing loss or deafness [11,46].

Our data showed a low correlation of Freiburger SIM and global QoL score after one year CI wearing time ($r = 0.384$). Similarly, Hirschfelder et al. found a correlation of NCIQ total score, advanced sound perception, speech production subscore and speech recognition using the Freiburger SIM and HSM sentence-test [7]. Using the NCIQ and postoperative sentence or word recognition in quiet, Capretta found no broad correlation of hearing outcome and QoL in adult postlingually deafened CI users, significant correlations were only in speech related subscales of QoL measures [8]. A recent meta-analysis of QoL improvement after CI and associations with speech recognition abilities showed a very strong improvement of all hearing-related QoL measures, but the positive correlation was low between hearing-specific QoL and word recognition in quiet ($r = 0.213$), sentence recognition in quiet ($r = 0.241$), or sentence recognition in noise ($r = 0.238$) [47]. Apparently, traditional open-set speech tests may not fully capture the self-perceived benefit of a so-called poor performer CI-recipient. A good example in our cohort for this ambiguity is the patient 15 who had one year postoperatively 0% SIM on the first implanted ear but showed a considerable improvement of QoL scores which were near to (advanced sound perception) or higher than the mean scores of the subdomains in the cohort. In contrast, patient 7 with no measurable SIM 1 year postoperatively showed just minimal improvement of QoL scores. Our data appears to indicate that in early-deafened CI users, the benefit in terms of QoL scores is generally independent of auditory gains. Therefore, the assessment of subjective experiences after CI should be an integral component of the evaluation protocol, given that an individually experienced benefit is not fully captured by the auditory tests.

*4.3. Strengths and Limitations of the Study*

To our knowledge, our study is the first to demonstrate the audiological results together with the benefit on hearing-related QoL of the MSE. Furthermore, it is of advantage that data were collected with a specific CI to reduce the confounding effect of different CI systems using different algorithms, speech processors, or electrode arrays in performance analysis. The drawback of the study is the retrospective design, the incomplete QoL database and the low number of patients included. Further limitation of the study is the assessment of QOL which records the quality of life regarding both ears at the same time.

## 5. Conclusions

In our patient cohort, both hearing performance and hearing-related QoL scores improved progressively up to the last control at 12 months postoperatively. Early-deafened, late implanted patients may need several years for speech understanding development. Further studies with a prospective multi-centric design are needed to identify factors influencing post-implantation functional results and QoL in this special patient group. As self-perceived benefits of patients with CI can be high despite poor results of standard speech understanding tests, hearing-related QoL should also be routinely used as an outcome measure.

**Supplementary Materials:** The following supporting information can be downloaded at: https://www.mdpi.com/article/10.3390/jcm11175156/s1, File S1: Dataset of the study title.

**Author Contributions:** Conceptualization: J.E.M., D.N.-D., O.N. and A.O.; Methodology: D.N.-D., D.F.S. and A.O.; Software: D.N.-D. and D.F.S.; Validation: D.N.-D., J.E.M., O.N., C.K., L.H. and A.O.; Formal analysis: D.N.-D., J.E.M., O.N., C.K., L.H. and A.O.; Investigation: D.N.-D., O.N., L.H. and A.O.; Resources: D.N.-D., D.F.S., O.N., C.K. and J.E.M.; Data Curation: D.N.-D.; Writing—Original Draft Preparation: A.O.; Writing—Review and Editing: L.H., D.N.-D., D.F.S., C.K., O.N. and J.E.M.; Visualization: D.N.-D., D.F.S. and A.O.; Supervision: J.E.M., Project Administration: J.E.M., Funding Acquisition: not applicable. All authors have read and agreed to the published version of the manuscript.

**Funding:** This research has received no external founding.

**Institutional Review Board Statement:** The retrospective chart review was performed in accordance with the ethical standards as laid down in the 1964 Declaration of Helsinki and its later amendments. The Ethic Committee of the Lübeck University, Germany approved the study (registry number: 20-076A). The principal investigator was JEM. All patients signed an informed consent before surgery and a consent for transfer their pseudonymized data for scientific analysis. All data were collected during the regular pre-implantation processes with follow-up care after surgery and were analyzed retrospectively. The final decision about cochlear implantation was met interdisciplinary involving audiologists, a psychologist and the operating surgeon. The patients had co-decision right in the choice of cochlear implant type.

**Informed Consent Statement:** All patients signed an informed consent before surgery and a consent for transfer their pseudonymized data for scientific analysis. Patients´ consent to publish this paper was waived as this retrospective study included only pseudonymized data and the participating patients cannot be identified by other persons or by the patients themselves.

**Data Availability Statement:** Data are contained within the article.

**Conflicts of Interest:** The authors declare no conflict of interest.

## References

1. Schramm, D.; Fitzpatrick, E.; Séguin, C. Cochlear implantation for adolescents and adults with prelinguistic deafness. *Otol. Neurotol.* **2002**, *23*, 698–703. [CrossRef] [PubMed]
2. Klop, W.M.; Boermans, P.P.; Ferrier, M.B.; van den Hout, W.B.; Stiggelbout, A.M.; Frijns, J.H. Clinical relevance of quality of life outcome in cochlear implantation in postlingually deafened adults. *Otol. Neurotol.* **2008**, *29*, 615–621. [CrossRef]
3. Most, T.; Shrem, H.; Duvdevani, I. Cochlear implantation in late-implanted adults with prelingual deafness. *Am. J. Otolaryngol.* **2010**, *31*, 418–423. [CrossRef] [PubMed]
4. Van Dijkhuizen, J.N.; Beers, M.; Boermans, P.B.M.; Briaire, J.J.; Frijns, J.H.M. Speech intelligibility as a predictor of cochlear implant outcome in prelingually deafened adults. *Ear Hear.* **2011**, *32*, 445–458. [CrossRef]
5. Straatman, L.V.; Huinck, W.J.; Langereis, M.C.; Snik, A.F.M.; Mulder, J.J. Cochlear implantation in late-implanted prelingually deafened adults: Changes in quality of life. *Otol. Neurotol.* **2014**, *35*, 253–259. [CrossRef] [PubMed]
6. Hinderink, J.B.; Krabbe, P.F.; Van Den Broek, P. Development and application of a health-related quality-of-life instrument for adults with cochlear implants: The Nijmegen cochlear implant questionnaire. *Otolaryngol.-Head Neck Surg.* **2000**, *123*, 756–765. [CrossRef]
7. Hirschfelder, A.; Gräbel, S.; Olze, H. The impact of cochlear implantation on quality of life: The role audiologic performance and variables. *Otolaryngol. Head Neck Surg.* **2008**, *138*, 357–362. [CrossRef]
8. Capretta, N.R.; Moberly, A.C. Does quality of life depend on speech recognition performance for adult cochlear implant users? *Laryngoscope* **2016**, *126*, 699–706. [CrossRef]
9. Knopke, S.; Gräbel, S.; Förster-Ruhrmann, U.; Mazurek, B.; Szczepek, A.J.; Olze, H. Impact of cochlear implantation on quality of life and mental comorbidity in patients aged 80 years. *Laryngoscope* **2016**, *126*, 2811–2816. [CrossRef]
10. Olze, H.; Knopke, S.; Gräbel, S.; Szczepek, A.J. Rapid positive influence of cochlear implantation on the quality of life in adults 70 years and older. *Audiol. Neurotol.* **2016**, *21* (Suppl. S1), 43–47. [CrossRef]
11. van Zon, A.; Smulders, Y.E.; Stegeman, I.; Ramakers, G.G.; Kraaijenga, V.J.; Koenraads, S.P.; Zanten, G.A.; Rinia, A.B.; Stokroos, R.J.; Free, R.H.; et al. Stable benefits of bilateral over unilateral cochlear implantation after two years: A randomized controlled trial. *Laryngoscope* **2017**, *127*, 1161–1168. [CrossRef] [PubMed]
12. Sladen, D.P.; Peterson, A.; Schmitt, M.; Olund, A.; Teece, K.; Dowling, B.; DeJong, M.; Breneman, A.; Beatty, C.W.; Carlson, M.L.; et al. Hughes-Borst B, Driscoll CL Health-related quality of life outcomes following adult cochlear implantation: A prospective cohort study. *Cochlear Implant. Int.* **2017**, *18*, 130–135. [CrossRef] [PubMed]
13. Ketterer, M.C.; Knopke, S.; Häußler, S.M.; Hildenbrand, T.; Becker, C.; Gräbel, S.; Olze, H. Asymmetric hearing loss and the benefit of cochlear implantation regarding speech perception, tinnitus burden and psychological comorbidities: A prospective follow-up study. *Eur. Arch. Otorhinolaryngol.* **2018**, *275*, 2683–2693. [CrossRef] [PubMed]

14. Häußler, S.M.; Knopke, S.; Wiltner, P.; Ketterer, M.; Gräbel, S.; Olze, H. Long term benefit of unilateral cochlear implantation on quality of life and speech perception in bilaterally deafened patients. *Otol. Neurotol.* **2019**, *40*, e430–e440. [CrossRef]
15. Plath, M.; Marienfeld, T.; Sand, M.; van de Weyer, P.S.; Praetorius, M.; Plinkert, P.K.; Baumann, I.; Zaoui, K. Prospective study on health-related quality of life in patients before and after cochlear implantation. *Eur. Arch. Otorhinolaryngol.* **2022**, *279*, 115–125. [CrossRef]
16. McRackan, T.R.; Hand, B.N.; Velozo, C.A.; Dubno, J.R. Cochlear Implant Quality of Life Consortium. Validity and reliability of the Cochlear Implant Quality of Life (CIQOL)-35 Profile and CIQOL-10 Global instruments in comparison to legacy instruments. *Ear Hear.* **2021**, *42*, 896–908. [CrossRef]
17. Caposecco, A.; Hickson, L.; Pedley, K. Cochlear implant outcomes in adults and adolescents with early-onset hearing loss. *Ear Hear.* **2012**, *33*, 209–220. [CrossRef]
18. Hinderink, J.B.; Mens, L.H.; Brokx, J.P.; van den Broek, P. Performance of prelingually and postlingually deaf patients using single-channel or multichannel cochlear implants. *Laryngoscope* **1995**, *105*, 618–622. [CrossRef]
19. Zwolan, T.A.; Kileny, P.R.; Telian, S.A. Self-report of cochlear implant use and satisfaction by prelingually deafened adults. *Ear Hear.* **1996**, *17*, 198–210. [CrossRef]
20. Peasgood, A.; Brookes, N.; Graham, J. Performance and benefit as outcome measures following cochlear implantation in non-traditional adult candidates: A pilot study. *Cochlear Implant. Int.* **2003**, *4*, 171–190. [CrossRef]
21. Kaplan, D.M.; Shipp, D.B.; Chen, J.M.; Ng, A.H.C.; Nedzelski, J.M. Early-deafened adult cochlear implant users: Assessment of outcomes. *J. Otolaryngol.* **2003**, *32*, 245–249. [CrossRef] [PubMed]
22. Bosco, E.; Nicastri, M.; Ballantyne, D.; Viccaro, M.; Ruoppolo, G.; Ionescu Maddalena, A.; Mancini, P. Long-term results in late implanted adolescent and adult CI recipients. *Eur. Arch. Otorhinolaryngol.* **2013**, *270*, 2611–2620. [CrossRef] [PubMed]
23. van Dijkhuizen, J.N.; Boermans, P.P.; Briaire, J.J.; Frijns, J.H. Intelligibility of the patient´s speech predicts the likelihood of cochlear implant success in prelingually deaf adults. *Ear Hear.* **2016**, *37*, e302–e310. [CrossRef]
24. Yang, W.S.; Moon, I.S.; Kim, H.N.; Lee, W.S.; Lee, S.E.; Choi, J.Y. Delayed cochlear implantation in adults with prelingual severe-to-profound hearing loss. *Otol Neurotol.* **2011**, *32*, 223–228. [CrossRef]
25. Zeitler, D.M.; Anwar, A.; Green, J.E.; Babb, J.S.; Friedmann, D.R.; Roland, J.T., Jr.; Waltzman, S.B. Cochlear implantation in prelingually deafened adolescents. *Arch. Pediatr. Adolesc. Med.* **2012**, *166*, 35–41. [CrossRef] [PubMed]
26. Rousset, A.; Dowell, R.; Leigh, J. Receptive language as a predictor of cochlear implant outcome for prelingually deaf adults. *Int. J. Audiol.* **2016**, *55* (Suppl. S2), S24–S30. [CrossRef] [PubMed]
27. Kraaijenga, V.J.; Smit, A.L.; Stegeman, I.; Smilde, J.J.; van Zanten, G.A.; Grolman, W. Factors that influence outcomes in cochlear implantation in adults, based on patient-related characteristics—A retrospective study. *Clin. Otolaryngol.* **2016**, *41*, 585–592. [CrossRef]
28. Lenarz, M.; Sönmez, H.; Joseph, G.; Büchner, A.; Lenarz, T. Long-term performance of cochlear implants in postlingually deafened adults. *Otolaryngol. Head Neck Surg.* **2012**, *147*, 112–118. [CrossRef]
29. Santarelli, R.; De Filippi, R.; Genovese, E.; Arslan, E. Cochlear implantation outcome in prelingually deafened young adults. A speech perception study. *Audiol. Neuro-Otol.* **2008**, *13*, 257–265. [CrossRef]
30. Craddock, L.; Cooper, H.; Riley, A.; Wright, T. Cochlear implants for pre-lingually profoundly deaf adults. *Cochlear Implant. Int.* **2016**, *17* (Suppl. S1), 26–30. [CrossRef]
31. Debruyne, J.; Janssen, M.; Brokx, J. Late cochlear implantation in early-deafened adults: A detailed analysis of auditory and self-perceived benefits. *Audiol. Neuro-Otol.* **2017**, *22*, 364–376. [CrossRef]
32. Global AB 2020 Reliability Report. AB Technical Reports. Advanced Bionics. Available online: https://www.advancedbionics.com/content/dam/advancedbionics/Documents/Global/en_ce/Professional/Technical-Reports/Reliability/Global-AB-Reliability-Report-Autumn-2021.pdf (accessed on 25 March 2022).
33. Gibson, P.; Boyd, P. Optimal electrode design: Straight versus perimodiolar. *Eur. Ann. Otorhinolaryngol. Head Neck Dis.* **2016**, *166* (Suppl. S1), S63–S65. [CrossRef] [PubMed]
34. Boyle, P.J. The rational for a mid-scala electrode array. *Eur. Ann. Otorhinolaryngol. Head Neck Dis.* **2016**, *133* (Suppl. 1), S61–S62. [CrossRef]
35. Zelener, F.; Majdani, O.; Roemer, A.; Lexow, G.J.; Giesemann, A.; Lenarz, T.; Warnecke, A. Relation between scalar shift and insertion depth in human cochlear implantation. *Otol. Neurotol.* **2020**, *41*, 178–185. [CrossRef]
36. O'Connell, B.P.; Cakir, A.; Hunter, J.B.; Francis, D.O.; Noble, J.H.; Labadie, R.F.; Zuniga, G.; Dawant, B.M.; Rivas, A.; Wanna, G.B. Electrode Location and Angular Insertion Depth Are Predictors of Audiologic Outcomes in Cochlear Implantation. *Otol. Neurotol.* **2016**, *37*, 1016–1023. [CrossRef] [PubMed]
37. Downing, M. Electrode designs for protection of the delicate cochlear structures. *J. Int. Adv. Otol.* **2018**, *14*, 401–403. [CrossRef] [PubMed]
38. Kamali, A.; Gahm, C.; Palmgren, B.; Marklund, L.; Halle, M.; Hammarstedt-Nordenvall, L. Use of a mid-scala and a lateral wall electrode in children: Insertion depth and hearing preservation. *Acta Oto-Laryngol.* **2017**, *137*, 1–7. [CrossRef]
39. Svrakic, M.; Roland, J.T., Jr.; McMenomey, S.O.; Svirsky, M.A. Initial operative experience and short-term hearing preservation results with a mid-scala cochlear implant electrode array. *Otol. Neurotol.* **2016**, *37*, 1549–1554. [CrossRef] [PubMed]

40. Wanna, G.B.; O'Connell, B.P.; Francis, D.O.; Gifford, R.H.; Hunter, J.B.; Holder, J.T.; Bennett, M.L.; Rivas, A.; Labadie, R.F.; Haynes, D.S. Predictive factors for short- and long-term hearing preservation in cochlear implantation with conventional-length electrodes. *Laryngoscope* **2018**, *128*, 482–489. [CrossRef]
41. Van der Jagt, M.A.; Briaire, J.J.; Verbist, B.M.; Frijns, J.H. Comparison of the HiFocus mid-scala and HiFocus 1J electrode array: Angular insertion depths and speech perception outcomes. *Audiol. Neurotol.* **2016**, *21*, 316–325. [CrossRef]
42. Battmer, R.D.; Scholz, S.; Gazibegovic, D.; Ernst, A.; Seidl, R.O. Comparison of a Mid Scala and a Perimodiolar Electrode in Adults: Performance, Impedances, and Psychophysics. *Otol. Neurotol.* **2020**, *41*, 467–475. [CrossRef] [PubMed]
43. Fabie, J.E.; Keller, R.G.; Hatch, J.L.; Holcomb, M.A.; Camposeo, E.L.; Lambert, P.R.; Meyer, T.A.; McRackan, T.R. Evaluation of Outcome Variability Associated with Lateral Wall, Mid-scalar, and Perimodiolar Electrode Arrays When Controlling for Preoperative Patient Characteristics. *Otol. Neurotol.* **2018**, *39*, 1122–1128. [CrossRef]
44. Muigg, F.; Bliem, H.R.; Kühn, H.; Seebacher, J.; Holzner, B.; Weichbold, V.W. Cochlear implantation in adults with single-sided deafness: Generic and disease-specific long-term quality of life. *Eur. Arch. Otorhinolaryngol.* **2020**, *277*, 695–704. [CrossRef] [PubMed]
45. Mosnier, I.; Bebear, J.P.; Marx, M.; Fraysse, B.; Truy, E.; Lina-Granade, G. Improvement of cognitive function after cochlear implantation in elderly patients. *JAMA Otolaryngol. Head Neck Surg.* **2015**, *141*, 442–450. [CrossRef] [PubMed]
46. Rader, T.; Haerterich, M.; Ernst, B.P.; Stöver, T.; Strieth, S. Quality of life and vertigo after bilateral cochlear implantation: Questionnaires as tools for quality assurance. *HNO* **2018**, *66*, 219–228. [CrossRef]
47. McRackan, T.R.; Bauschard, M.; Hatch, J.L.; Franko-Tobin, E.; Droghini, H.R.; Nguyen, S.A.; Dubno, J.R. Meta-analysis of quality-of-life improvement after cochlear implantation and associations with speech recognition abilities. *Laryngoscope* **2018**, *128*, 982–990. [CrossRef]

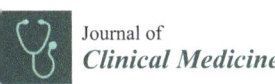

Article

# Prognostic Factors Associated with Recovery from Recurrent Idiopathic Sudden Sensorineural Hearing Loss: Retrospective Analysis and Systematic Review

So Young Jeon, Dae Woong Kang, Sang Hoon Kim, Jae Yong Byun and Seung Geun Yeo *

Department of Otorhinolaryngology-Head & Neck Surgery, School of Medicine, Kyung Hee University, 23 Kyungheedae-ro, Dongdaemun-gu, Seoul 02447, Korea; iamjsy89@gmail.com (S.Y.J.); kkang814@naver.com (D.W.K.); hoon0700@naver.com (S.H.K.); otorhioo512@naver.com (J.Y.B.)
* Correspondence: yeo2park@gmail.com; Tel.: +82-2-958-8980; Fax: +82-2-958-8470

**Citation:** Jeon, S.Y.; Kang, D.W.; Kim, S.H.; Byun, J.Y.; Yeo, S.G. Prognostic Factors Associated with Recovery from Recurrent Idiopathic Sudden Sensorineural Hearing Loss: Retrospective Analysis and Systematic Review. *J. Clin. Med.* **2022**, *11*, 1453. https://doi.org/10.3390/jcm11051453

Academic Editor: George Psillas

Received: 4 February 2022
Accepted: 5 March 2022
Published: 7 March 2022

**Publisher's Note:** MDPI stays neutral with regard to jurisdictional claims in published maps and institutional affiliations.

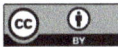

**Copyright:** © 2022 by the authors. Licensee MDPI, Basel, Switzerland. This article is an open access article distributed under the terms and conditions of the Creative Commons Attribution (CC BY) license (https:// creativecommons.org/licenses/by/ 4.0/).

**Abstract:** Although idiopathic sudden sensorineural hearing loss (ISSNHL) is uncommon, recurrent ISSNHL is even rarer. The knowledge about factors associated with patient recovery from recurrent episodes is needed to counsel and treat the patients. Medical records of patients admitted for high dose oral steroid therapy for recurrent ISSNHL between January 2009 and December 2021 were reviewed. Their demographic and clinical characteristics, co-morbid symptoms, and audiologic results were analyzed. The 38 patients admitted for treatment of recurrent ISSNHL included 14 men and 24 women. Recovery rates after the first and recurrent episodes of ISSNHL were 78.9% and 63.2%, respectively. Patients who recovered after recurrent episodes showed significantly higher rates of ear fullness symptoms and early treatment onset than those who did not recover ($p < 0.05$ each). Of the 30 patients who recovered after the first episode, those who had ear fullness symptoms ($p < 0.05$, odds ratio (OR) 0.1, 95% confidence interval (CI) 0.01–0.76) and who showed a lower initial hearing threshold ($p < 0.05$, OR 1.06, 95% CI 1.01–1.12) during the recurrent episode showed significantly better or similar recovery than after the first episode. Ear fullness symptoms and less initial hearing loss were associated with a more favorable prognosis after intial than after recurrent ISSNHL.

**Keywords:** sudden; idiopathic sensorineural hearing loss; recurrent

## 1. Introduction

Idiopathic sudden sensorineural hearing loss (ISSNHL) is typically defined as a sensorineural hearing loss greater than 30 dB over at least three consecutive frequencies within three days [1]. Its incidence is 5 to 20 per 100,000 people per year [2]. Studies analyzing long-term outcomes of ISSNHL have found that recurrence rates vary widely, ranging between 0.8% and 47% [3–8].

There is no known single cause of ISSNHL, but factors may include viral infection, vascular disturbance, cochlear membrane rupture, immune-mediated mechanisms, tumor, autonomic nervous disease, ototoxic drugs, and congenital anomaly, or it may be idiopathic [9]. Although many studies have assessed the causes, pathogenesis, diagnostic criteria, treatment, and prognostic factors of ISSNHL [10–12], few have analyzed the clinical features and prognostic factors associated with recurrent ISSNHL. Furthermore, to our knowledge, no study has compared the clinical features or factors associated with recovery from initial and recurrent episodes of ISSNHL. This study retrospectively analyzed 38 patients with recurrent ISSNHL and compared the clinical features and prognostic factors associated with recovery from initial and recurrent episodes of ISSNHL.

## 2. Subjects and Methods

### 2.1. Study Design

This retrospective study included patients with recurrent ISSNHL who visited the ear, nose, and throat (ENT) clinic at Kyung-Hee Medical Center and Gang-dong Kyung-Hee Medical Center for SSNHL and were admitted for high dose steroid therapy between January 2009 and December 2021. Patients were excluded if they had vertigo, chronic otitis media, a history of middle ear cavity surgery, disorders of the central nervous system, tumors, or progressive sensorineural hearing loss.

The medical records of the patients were reviewed, and their demographic and clinical characteristics were recorded, including age, sex, body mass index, medical history, comorbid symptoms, days from onset to treatment, time to recovery, and duration of recurrence. Only current alcohol use and smoking were considered, respectively. Following admission, all patients underwent daily pure tone audiometry (PTA) tests in a sound-treated audiology booth in the ENT clinic by qualified and experienced audiologists, with hearing thresholds calculated using the six-division method (($500$ Hz + ($1000$ Hz $\times$ 2) + ($2000$ Hz $\times$ 2) + $4000$ Hz)/6).

High dose steroid therapy consisted of 1 mg/kg/day oral methylprednisolone for four days, followed by tapering. Patients were discharged after tapering and followed in the outpatient clinic. Hearing threshold at recovery was defined as the threshold observed when PTA tests showed no improvement for two weeks. Hearing recovery was assessed using Siegel's classification [13], with patients categorized as experiencing complete, partial, slight, and no recovery for both episodes of ISSNHL. Complete, partial, and slight recovery were grouped as the recovery group. Factors were compared in patients who did and did not recover after both episodes (Table 1). To analyze factors associated with poorer outcomes after the recurrent than after the first episode of ISSNHL, patients who recovered after the first episode were divided into those who experienced similar or better recovery and those who experienced poorer recovery after the recurrent than after the first episode. In this analysis, patients who did not recover after the first episode were excluded (Table 2).

Table 1. Characteristics of patients who did and not recover after the first and recurrent episodes of idiopathic sudden sensorineural hearing loss.

| Variables | | First Episode | | | Recurrent Episode | | |
|---|---|---|---|---|---|---|---|
| | | Recovery (n = 30) | No Recovery (n = 8) | p-Value | Recovery (n = 24) | No Recovery (n = 14) | p-Value |
| | | n (%) or Mean ± SD | n (%) or Mean ± SD | | n (%) or Mean ± SD | n (%) or Mean ± SD | |
| Age (year) mean ± SD | | 48.90 ± 16.40 | 48.75 ± 18.11 | 0.7489 | 53.63 ± 14.13 | 51.00 ± 19.52 | 0.9880 |
| Sex | Male | 12 (40.00%) | 2 (25.00%) | 0.6836 | 8 (3.33%) | 6 (42.86%) | 0.7293 |
| | Female | 18 (60.00%) | 6 (75.00%) | | 16 (66.67%) | 8 (57.14%) | |
| BMI (kg/m$^2$), mean ± SD | | 22.89 ± 2.57 | 22.42 ± 2.78 | 0.6605 | 22.78 ± 2.75 | 22.80 ± 2.37 | 0.8373 |
| Alcohol | | 4 (13.33%) | 3 (37.50%) | 0.1461 | 5 (20.83%) | 2 (14.29%) | 1.0000 |
| Smoking | | 8 (26.67%) | 2 (25.00%) | 1.0000 | 5 (20.83%) | 5 (35.71%) | 0.4485 |
| HTN | | 5 (16.67%) | 2 (25.00%) | 0.6236 | 3 (12.50%) | 4 (28.57%) | 0.3870 |
| DM | | 7 (23.33%) | 1 (12.50%) | 0.6600 | 6 (25.00%) | 2 (14.29%) | 0.6836 |
| Tinnitus | | 19 (63.33%) | 6 (75.00%) | 0.6893 | 16 (66.67%) | 12 (85.71%) | 0.2685 |
| Ear fullness | | 20 (66.67%) | 8 (100.00%) | 0.0821 | 22 (91.67%) | 4 (28.57%) | 0.0001 * |
| Treatment onset (days), mean ± SD | | 7.17 ± 16.07 | 5.50 ± 5.01 | 0.5193 | 5.58 ± 11.99 | 16.71 ± 20.73 | 0.0361 * |
| Recovery time (months), mean ± SD | | 0.95 ± 1.04 | 4.57 ± 10.29 | 0.2630 | 1.31 ± 2.04 | 3.01 ± 5.07 | 0.0303 * |
| Hearing level of the affected ear before treatment (dB), mean ± SD | | 48.44 ± 25.45 | 47.60 ± 16.27 | 0.8588 | 44.58 ± 21.94 | 49.17 ± 11.92 | 0.5686 |
| Hearing level of the affected ear after treatment (dB), mean ± SD | | 21.00 ± 14.87 | 41.56 ± 15.88 | 0.0023 * | 23.13 ± 13.60 | 53.39 ± 15.35 | <0.0001 * |
| Time to recurrence (days), mean ± SD | | - | - | - | 43.22 ± 54.31 | 44.86 ± 37.84 | 0.3697 |

Abbreviation SD, standard deviation; BMI, body mass index; HTN, hypertension; DM, Diabetes mellitus. * $p < 0.05$.

**Table 2.** Distribution of patients according to types of recovery after the first and recurrent episodes of idiopathic sudden sensorineural hearing loss. Complete, partial, slight and no recovery were determined according to the Siegel's criteria [13].

|  | Recovery Type | Recurrent Episode | | | | |
|---|---|---|---|---|---|---|
|  |  | Complete | Partial | Slight | No | Total |
| First episode | Complete | 15 | 0 | 1 | 5 | 21 |
|  | Partial | 1 | 2 | 2 | 3 | 8 |
|  | Slight | 0 | 0 | 0 | 1 | 1 |
|  | No | 2 | 1 | 0 | 5 | 8 |
|  | Total | 18 | 3 | 3 | 14 | 38 |

*2.2. Statistical Analysis*

Categorical variables were compared using Fisher's exact tests and continuous variables were compared using Wilcoxon rank sum tests. Factors associated with recovery were assessed by multiple ordinal logistic regression analysis, adjusted by age and sex. All statistical analyses were performed using the SAS9.4 (Statistical Analysis System version, SAS Institute, Cary, NC, USA) software, with a $p$-value < 0.05 defined as statistically significant.

*2.3. Research on Recurrent ISSNHL*

This systematic review was performed in accordance with the Primary Reporting Items for Systematic Review and Meta-analyses (PRISMA) statement [14]. Studies were included if (a) they were retrospective or prospective investigative studies; (b) all patients had been diagnosed with recurrent idiopathic sudden sensorineural hearing loss, with those having other causes of hearing loss excluded; and (c) the studies were published in English. Studies were excluded if they were (a) unpublished data; (b) review articles; (c) grey literature; (d) case reports; or (e) duplicates of published research. Studies published before 1 September 2021 were retrieved by one of the investigators (S.Y.J.) from three electronic databases: SCOPUS, PubMed and the Cochrane Library. Search terms included "recurrent sudden hearing loss".

## 3. Results

During the study period, 38 patients with recurrent ISSNHL were treated for recurrent ISSNHL; their demographic, audiometric, and other clinical characteristics are summarized in Table 1. The 38 patients consisted of 14 (36.8%) men and 24 (63.2%) women. Their mean age at the first episode was 48.9 years (range 7–69 years), and their mean age at the recurrent episode was 52.7 years (range 12–76 years). Recurrences were ipsilateral in thirty-five (92.1%) patients and contralateral in three (7.9%). Thirty (78.9%) patients recovered after the first episode, whereas eight (21.1%) did not. In comparison, 24 (63.2%) patients recovered after the recurrent episode, whereas 14 (36.8%) did not.

A comparison of demographic and clinical characteristics of the patients who did and did not recover after the first episode showed no significant differences. In contrast, a comparison of patients who did and did not recover after the recurrent episode showed that the symptom of ear fullness (91.7% vs. 28.6%; $p < 0.05$) was significantly more frequent, time to treatment onset significantly shorter (5.6 days vs. 16.7 days, $p < 0.05$) and recovery time significantly shorter (1.3 months vs. 3.1 months, $p < 0.05$) in patients who did rather than did not recover after the recurrent episode (Table 1).

Of the 30 patients who recovered after the first episode, 18 (60.0%) showed better or similar recovery after the recurrent episode, whereas 12 (40.0%) showed poorer recovery after the recurrent rather than after the first episode (Table 3). Ear fullness symptoms were significantly less frequent (50% vs. 88.9%, $p < 0.05$) and mean initial hearing threshold significantly higher (57.2 dB vs. 40.1 dB, $p < 0.05$) in patients who did rather than did not experience poorer recovery after the recurrent rather than after the first episode of ISSNHL (Table 3).

**Table 3.** Characteristics of patients who did and did not experience a poorer recovery after a recurrent episode than after the first episode of idiopathic sudden sensorineural hearing loss.

| Variables | | No Worse than after the First Episode (n = 18) | Worse than after the First Episode (n = 12) | p-Value |
|---|---|---|---|---|
| | | n (%) or Mean ± SD | n (%) or Mean ± SD | |
| Age (year), mean ± SD | | 52.33 ± 13.81 | 53.00 ± 20.78 | 0.5855 |
| Sex | Male | 7 (38.89%) | 5 (41.67%) | 1.0000 |
| | Female | 11 (61.11%) | 7 (58.33%) | |
| BMI (kg/m$^2$), mean ± SD | | 22.70 ± 2.71 | 23.18 ± 2.42 | 0.3645 |
| Alcohol | | 3 (16.67%) | 1 (8.33%) | 0.6315 |
| Smoking | | 5 (27.78%) | 3 (25.00%) | 1.0000 |
| HTN | | 1 (5.65%) | 4 (33.33%) | 0.1282 |
| DM | | 4 (22.22%) | 3 (25.00%) | 1.0000 |
| Tinnitus | | 12 (66.67%) | 10 (83.33%) | 0.4192 |
| Ear fullness | | 16 (88.89%) | 6 (50.00%) | 0.0342 * |
| Treatment onset (days), mean ± SD | | 5.67 ± 13.69 | 8.33 ± 10.74 | 0.1721 |
| Recovery time (months), mean ± SD | | 1.26 ± 2.25 | 1.47 ± 1.29 | 0.0992 |
| Hearing level of the affected ear before treatment (dB), mean ± SD | | 40.05 ± 20.17 | 57.22 ± 12.92 | 0.0357 * |
| Hearing level of the affected ear after treatment (dB), mean ± SD | | 18.29 ± 8.47 | 52.36 ± 12.08 | <0.0001 * |
| Time to recurrence (days), mean ± SD | | 34.65 ± 37.54 | 53.35 ± 37.46 | 0.1139 |

Abbreviation SD; standard deviation, BMI; body mass index, HTN; hypertension, DM; diabetes mellitus. * $p < 0.05$.

Based on the results of preliminary simple linear regression analysis to determine the factors associated with poorer recovery after the recurrent rather than after the first episode of ISSNHL, multiple regression analysis was performed with adjustment for age and sex (Table 4). Ear fullness symptoms at the time of ISSNHL recurrence were associated with a lower risk of poorer recovery after the recurrent episode ($p < 0.05$, odds ratio (OR) 0.1, 95% confidence interval (CI)] 0.01–0.76). Higher hearing loss at the time of ISSNHL recurrence was associated with a higher risk of poorer recovery after the recurrent episode ($p < 0.05$, OR 1.06, 95% CI 1.01–1.12).

Following ISSNHL recurrence, 23 patients underwent temporal bone MRI scans to rule out brain tumors or other ear abnormalities. None of these patients showed evidence of cerebellopontine angle tumors.

Using the search term "recurrent sudden hearing loss", 35 papers were identified from the three databases. Only nine (25.7%) of these studies fulfilled the inclusion criteria and were reviewed and these are shown in Figure 1. The characteristics of the included studies are shown in Table 5. This review especially focused on recovery rate from recurrent ISSNHL, although two of these studies [7,8] only provided data on the recurrence rate. The nine previous studies reported that the rate of recovery in patients with recurrent ISSNHL ranged from 43.4% to 78.6%. Only one study reported the second recurrence rate, which was 21.4%. In most studies, the proportion of females and males was almost the same. These studies utilized different tests, including electrocochleography (ECohG) and vestibular-evoked myogenic potential (VEMP), and analyzed different parameters, including neutrophil to lymphocyte ratio (NLR) and platelet to lymphocyte ratio (PLR), to identify prognostic factors associated with recurrent ISSNHL.

**Table 4.** Adjusted risk factors for poorer recovery after a recurrent rather than after the first episode of ISSNHL.

| Variables | Simple Logistic Model | | | Multiple Logistic Model * | | |
| --- | --- | --- | --- | --- | --- | --- |
| | OR | 95% CI | *p*-Value | OR | 95% CI | *p*-Value |
| Age (year) | 1.00 | 0.96–1.05 | 0.9128 | adj. | | |
| Female (ref. Male) | 0.89 | 0.20–3.95 | 0.8791 | adj. | | |
| BMI | 1.08 | 0.80–1.45 | 0.6213 | 1.01 | 0.69–1.47 | 0.9703 |
| Alcohol | 0.46 | 0.04–4.98 | 0.5185 | 0.44 | 0.04–4.89 | 0.4997 |
| Smoking | 0.87 | 0.16–4.58 | 0.8662 | 0.69 | 0.09–5.67 | 0.7323 |
| HTN [†] | 6.18 | 0.69–55.18 | 0.1032 | 10.03 | 0.82–123.31 | 0.0717 |
| DM | 1.17 | 0.21–6.48 | 0.8602 | 1.17 | 0.17–8.2 | 0.8761 |
| Tinnitus | 2.50 | 0.41–15.23 | 0.3203 | 2.58 | 0.42–16.04 | 0.3092 |
| Ear fullness | 0.13 | 0.02–0.80 | 0.0280 | 0.10 | 0.01–0.76 | 0.0262 ** |
| Treatment onset (days) | 1.02 | 0.96–1.09 | 0.5032 | 1.03 | 0.96–1.11 | 0.4077 |
| Recovery time (months) | 1.06 | 0.72–1.56 | 0.7698 | 1.06 | 0.72–1.57 | 0.7546 |
| Hearing level of the affected ear before treatment (dB) | 1.06 | 1.01–1.11 | 0.0263 | 1.06 | 1.01–1.12 | 0.0210 ** |
| Time to recurrence (days) | 1.02 | 1.00–1.03 | 0.0442 | 1.02 | 0.99–1.04 | 0.1569 |

Abbreviation OR; odds ratio; BMI; body mass index; HTN; hypertension; DM; diabetes mellitus. [†] Logistic regression with Firth's method (reference: patients not experiencing poorer outcomes after recurrence). * Logistic regression of patients with poorer outcomes after the recurrent than after the first episode (reference: patients not experiencing poorer outcomes after recurrence). * Adjusted by age, gender. ** $p < 0.05$.

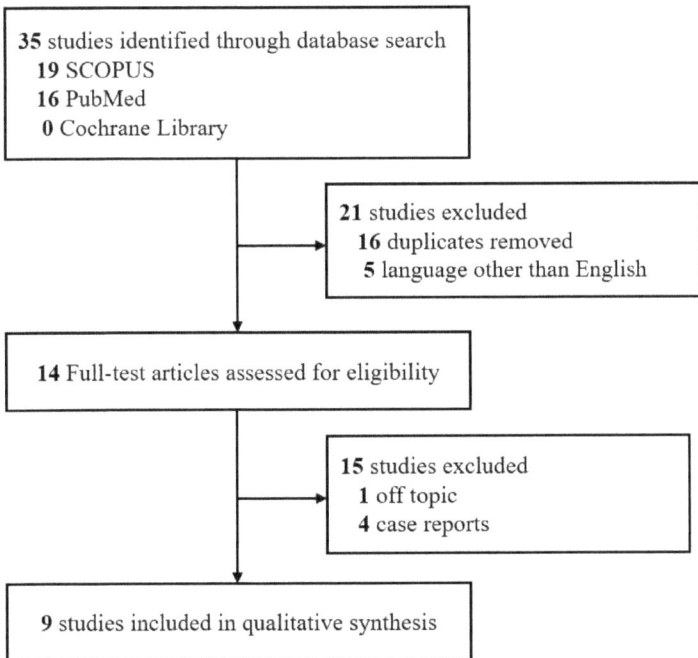

**Figure 1.** PRISMA flow diagram. Abbreviation: PRISMA: Primary Reporting Items for Systematic Review and Meta-analyses.

Table 5. Studies assessing recurrent ISSNHL.

| Reference | Country | Study Design | Number of Patients with Recurrence | Recovery Rate from Recurrence | M:F | Conclusions |
|---|---|---|---|---|---|---|
| Seo et al. [9] | South Korea | Retrospective | First recurrence: 16<br>Second recurrence: 16 | First recurrence: 78.6%<br>Second recurrence: 21.4% | 8:8<br>8:8 | NLR and PLR higher in patients with both recurrent and non-recurrent ISSNHL. |
| Park et al. [5] | South Korea | Retrospective | 11 | 72.7% | 6:5 | Hearing outcomes were poorer after a recurrent than after the first episode, with SSNHL almost always recurring in the same ear. |
| Ohashi et al. [6] | Japan | Retrospective | 23 | 69.5% | NA | Favorable prognostic factors in patients with recurrent ISSNHL included an enhanced SP/AP ratio of ECohG, a low initial AP threshold, a low initial hearing level, and an up-sloping type of audiogram.<br>Initial vertigo was associated with unfavorable outcomes in patients with recurrent ISSNHL. |
| Kuo et al. [15] | Taiwan | Retrospective | Ipsilateral: 7<br>Contralateral: 9 | 50%<br>(Ipsilateral type: 71.4%<br>Contralateral type: 33.3%) | 3:4<br>5:4 | Normal VEMPs in the affected ear of patients with recurrent sudden deafness may indicate a good hearing outcome. |
| † Fushiki et al. [7] | Japan | Retrospective | 33 | * Recurrence rate<br>1 year: 29%<br>5 years: 47%<br>(45% of recurrences occurred within 6 months of the first episode) | - | Recurrence rate higher in patients with elevated SP/AP and spontaneous nystagmus (78.6%) than in patients with normal SP/AP and absence of spontaneous nystagmus (31.8%) |
| Furuhashi et al. [3] | Japan | Retrospective | 14 | 78.5% | 9:5 | Recurrence of sudden deafness rare during long-term follow-up<br>The degree of hearing deterioration on the first affected side was not significantly different from that on the non-affected side |
| † Wu et al. [8] | Taiwan | Retrospective | 2281<br>(Data from the Taiwan NHI) | * Recurrence rate<br>5 years: 4.99% | 1252:1029 | Factors associated with relapse included age 35–64 years, diabetes mellitus, and hypercholesterolemia |
| Pecorari et al. [16] | Italy | Retrospective | 73 | 63%<br>* Recurrence rate<br>2 years: 5.6%<br>5 years: 10.34% | 30:43 | Recurrence correlated only with the presence of tinnitus during follow-up |
| Wu et al. [17] | Taiwan | Retrospective | 30 | 43.44%<br>(First episode: 53.55%) | 16:14 | Hearing recovery after a recurrent episode correlated significantly with hearing outcome after the initial episode. |

Abbreviation: NLR, neutrophil to lymphocyte ratio; PLR, platelet to lymphocyte ratio; ISSNH, idiopathic sudden sensorineural hearing loss; SP, summating potential; AP, action potential; ECohG, electrocochleography; VEMP, vestibular-evoked myogenic potential; NHI, National Health Insurance program * Recurrence rate: cumulative recurrence rate. † These studies only reported about relapse rate.

## 4. Discussion

Many patients who experience recurrent ISSNHL report significant stress relative to the recurrence and are more concerned about recovery than during the first episode of ISSNHL. Clinicians also express concern about the likelihood of recovery relative to the first episode and about the possibility that recurrent ISSNHL is caused by a tumor.

Most cases of SSNHL are idiopathic; other causes, however, can include vestibular schwannoma, acoustic neuroma, stroke, malignancy, Meniere's disease, trauma, autoimmune disease, syphilis, Lyme disease, and peri-lymphatic fistula [1,18]. The prevalence of vestibular schwannomas in patients with SSNHL has been reported to be 3.0% [19].

This study assessed 38 patients with recurrent ISSNHL, focusing on the factors associated with recovery. The control group of the present study consisted of patients who did not recover from recurrent ISSNHL. If the process of relapse consists of a series of clinical steps, then the factors among patients who recovered after the first episode may differ between those who did and did not experience poorer recovery after the recurrent episode. ISSNHL is an uncommon disease, and recurrent ISSNHL is very rare; hence, knowledge about the factors associated with patient recovery from recurrent episodes may help in counseling and treating patients.

In general, patients with ISSNHL are advised to start treatment with oral steroids within two weeks [1], and starting treatment after 10 days is a negative prognostic factor [20]. Among patients who experienced recurrent episodes in the present study, those who recovered started their treatment at a mean 5.6 days, whereas those who did not recover started their treatment at a mean 16.7 days, further indicating that delayed treatment was associated with a decreased recovery rate ($p < 0.05$). During the first episode, however, the mean time to treatment onset was similar in patients who did and did not recover (7.2 days vs. 5.5 days). Patients with previous experience of ISSNHL may delay visits to the hospital because they become empirically accustomed to symptoms such as sudden ear fullness, tinnitus, and hearing loss. This may delay the diagnosis and treatment of recurrent ISSNHL. The present findings indicate that patients who experience symptoms of recurrent ISSNHL should seek treatment as soon as possible.

The present study also showed that the ear fullness symptoms and the initial hearing level of the affected ear differed significantly between patients with and without poorer recovery after the recurrent episode than after the first episode of ISSNHL. Recovery of hearing after the first episode was shown to be prognostic for the subsequent hearing outcomes after the recurrent episode [17]. The present study found that the initial hearing loss of the affected ear at the time of recurrence was significantly higher in poorer recovery after the initial episode, as well as being a risk factor for poorer recovery after the recurrent than after the first episode (OR 1.06, 95% CI 1.01–1.12, $p < 0.05$) after adjustment for age and sex. Initial profound hearing loss was previously shown to be negatively prognostic for recovery from non-recurrent ISSNHL [20]. Similarly, the present study found that higher initial hearing loss at the time of the recurrent episode was prognostic for poorer recovery after the recurrent than after the first episode.

Ear fullness was experienced by six (50.0%) of the twelve patients who experienced poorer recovery after recurrence than after initial ISSNHL and 16 (88.9%) of the 18 patients who did not. Ear fullness is a subjective symptom, expressed as feelings of blockage, plugging, or pressure, that occurs frequently in patients with acute sensorineural hearing loss. For example, the incidence of ear fullness has been reported to be 63.5% in patients with acute low tone sensorineural hearing loss [18], 40.2% in patients with ISSNHL [1], and 61.0% in patients with Meniere's disease [21]. Ear fullness in acute sensorineural hearing loss was not associated with auditory function on audiograms but was associated with the low-frequency region [21]. This association disappeared after the hearing threshold stabilized, and the disappearance of ear fullness has been associated with hearing prognosis. Ear fullness observed in patients with endolymphatic hydrops or Meniere's disease has been associated with a pressure imbalance between the round and oval windows [17,22,23]. Although the mechanisms underlying these associations have not yet been determined, these findings suggest that ear fullness may be due to a functional factor rather than to an anatomical impairment of the cochlea. The mechanism responsible for ear fullness in patients with sensorineural hearing loss needs to be clarified [21,24].

In this study, patients who showed better or similar recovery from the recurrent rather than from the first episode of ISSNHL had more frequent symptoms of ear fullness than those who showed poorer recovery from recurrent ISSNHL. Although the ear fullness symptom was associated with the low-frequency region, however, none of the six patients with poorer recovery after the recurrent episode and only four of the sixteen patients without poorer recovery after the recurrent episode who presented with ear fullness showed a low tone loss pattern, indicating that ear fullness symptom is not present only in patients with low tone sudden sensorineural hearing loss. In some respects, patients with poorer recovery after the recurrent episode showed a higher initial hearing loss and more frequent ear fullness symptom at the same time than did patients without poorer recovery after the recurrent episode, suggesting that ear fullness affected the remaining or early stages of loss of hearing function. Taken together, these findings suggest that ear fullness may be prognostic of recovery from recurrent ISSNHL.

ISSNHL has been reported to be associated with a history of hypertension (HTN), chronic kidney disease, diabetes mellitus (DM), hypercholesterolemia, and stroke [25–29]. Analysis of data from the US National Nutrition Survey showed a link between hearing loss and high blood pressure [30]. HTN can cause hemorrhage in the inner ear, reducing capillary blood flow and oxygen supply, and resulting in progressive or sudden sensorineural hearing loss [31]. Moreover, older age and HTN are significant negative prognostic factors for recovery from ISSNHL [20,32]. In the present study, however, HTN was not a statistically significant risk factor for poorer recovery after a recurrent rather than after the first episode of ISSNHL. However, our finding, that HTN was more frequent in patients with poorer recovery after a recurrent than after a first episode, suggests that HTN may be a risk factor for poorer recovery from recurrent ISSNHL. Moreover, acquired and inherited cardiovascular risk factors were found to be associated with an increased risk of developing ISSNHL [33]. The management of cardiovascular diseases, including HTN, is therefore important in preventing the recurrence of ISSNHL.

The rates of DM in patients showing better or similar recovery compared to poorer recovery after a recurrent episode rather than after a first episode were 22.22% and 25.00%, respectively. Several studies have reported an association between ISSNHL and DM [25–29], although one previous study [34] found no difference in the outer hair cell (OHC) damage, represented by evoked otoacoustic emissions (e-OAEs), between DM patients and healthy subjects in an acute hyperglycemic clamp study which is assumed as a sudden hazardous condition. Sensorineural hearing loss in DM patients has been shown to be associated with longer duration and poor control of DM; however, a higher compromise is observed in DM patients in an acute hyperglycemia condition [34], so it is hard to find the correlation between the acute hyperglycemia condition and ISSNHL. However, it is clear that DM has an effect on hearing loss in the long term, and must be managed appropriately.

The recovery rate of recurrent ISSNHL of our study was 63.2% and it ranged in between the previous studies in the systematic review (43.4~78.6%). Similar to our study, hearing outcomes were found to be poorer after the recurrent rather than after the initial episode [5,17]. A previous study reported that 45% of recurrences occurred within 6 months from the first episode [7]. In comparison, the present study found that the mean times to recurrence were 43.2 days in patients who recovered from the recurrent episode and 44.9 days in those who did not recover. The cumulative relapse rates in studies included in the systematic review ranged from 4.9% to 47% [7,8,16].

Those studies found that statistically significant factors associated with recurrence included diabetes mellitus, hypercholesterolemia, and tinnitus. ISSNHL has also been associated with a history of HTN, chronic kidney disease, and stroke. Although the present study found that HTN was not a statistically significant risk factor for recurrent ISSNHL, its prevalence was higher in patients with than without poorer recovery after the recurrent rather than after the first episode of ISSNHL. Both the neutrophil to lymphocyte ratio (NLR) and platelet to lymphocyte ratio (PLR) were found to be higher in patients experiencing both the first and recurrent episodes of ISSNHL than in a normal control group [9]. Similar to our findings, electrocochleography (ECohG) showed that low initial hearing level is prognostic for recovery from ISSNHL [6]. Moreover, a more normal vestibular-evoked myogenic potential (VEMP) [15] and better hearing outcome after the initial episode [17] were found to be associated with better hearing outcomes in patients with recurrent ISSNHL.

Although few studies to date have assessed prognosis in patients with recurrent ISSNHL, various clinical, serologic, and audiologic factors have been analyzed. Large population studies have failed to identify factors that are prognostic or predictive of the degree of recovery from recurrent ISSNHL, but in general the factors associated with recurrent ISSNHL have been found not to differ significantly from the factors associated with primary ISNSHL. The present study found that the degree of recovery was associated with treatment onset. A lower initial hearing level and presence of ear fullness symptom were associated with better recovery from the recurrent than from the first episode of ISSNHL. Although further research is needed on the mechanisms responsible for ear fullness, ear fullness can likely be recognized during early stages of functional loss, allowing earlier treatment and improved prognosis.

This study had several limitations. First, this study only analyzed patients who experienced recurrent ISSNHL. To more comprehensively analyze factors prognostic of recurrent ISSNHL, the characteristics of patients who experienced ISSNHL once and those who experienced recurrent ISSNHL should be compared. Second, this study was retrospective in design, which may have introduced a potential selection bias. Third, longer-term serial follow up of patients after recovery from recurrent ISSNHL is needed to specifically classify the patients who might experience additional recurrence. Fourth, a small number of subjects were studied and there was a higher proportion of females compared to males.

## 5. Conclusions

Earlier treatment in patients with recurrent ISSNHL is associated with better hearing outcomes. In addition, ear fullness was associated with a more favorable prognosis, whereas higher initial hearing loss was predictive of a poorer recovery after recurrent than after initial ISSNHL.

**Author Contributions:** Data curation, S.Y.J.; Formal analysis, S.Y.J.; Writing—original draft, S.Y.J.; Writing—review & editing, D.W.K., S.H.K., J.Y.B. and S.G.Y. All authors have read and agreed to the published version of the manuscript.

**Funding:** This research did not receive any specific grant from funding agencies in the public, commercial, or not-for-profit sectors.

**Institutional Review Board Statement:** This research protocol was approved by the Institutional Review Board of Kyung Hee Medical Center (2019-07-065).

**Informed Consent Statement:** Not applicable.

**Data Availability Statement:** The data are available from authors by a reasonable request.

**Acknowledgments:** This work was supported by the National Research Foundation of Korea (NRF) grant funded by the Korean (NRF 2018R1A6A1A03025124) (NRF 2019R1F1A1049878).

**Conflicts of Interest:** The authors declare no conflict of interest.

## References

1. Stachler, R.J.; Chandrasekhar, S.S.; Archer, S.M.; Rosenfeld, R.M.; Schwartz, S.R.; Barrs, D.M.; Robertson, P.J. Clinical practice guideline: Sudden hearing loss. *Otolaryngol. Head Neck Surg.* **2012**, *146*, S1–S35. [CrossRef]
2. Byl, F.M., Jr. Sudden hearing loss: Eight years' experience and suggested prognostic table. *Laryngoscope* **1984**, *94*, 647–661. [CrossRef] [PubMed]
3. Furuhashi, A.; Matsuda, K.; Asahi, K.; Nakashima, T. Sudden deafness: Long-term follow-up and recurrence. *Clin. Otolaryngol.* **2002**, *27*, 458–463. [CrossRef] [PubMed]
4. Psifidis, A.D.; Psillas, G.K.; Daniilidis, J.C. Sudden sensorineural hearing loss: Long-term follow-up results. *Otolaryngol. Head Neck Surg.* **2006**, *134*, 809–815. [CrossRef] [PubMed]
5. Park, I.S.; Kim, Y.B.; Choi, S.H.; Hon, S.M. Clinical analysis of recurrent sudden sensorineural hearing loss. *ORL* **2013**, *75*, 245–249. [CrossRef]

6. Ohashi, T.; Nishino, H.; Arai, Y.; Nishimoto, Y.; Kakutani, T.; Koizuka, I. Electrocochleographic findings in recurrent idiopathic sudden sensorineural hearing loss. *Acta Otolaryngol.* **2012**, *132*, 1022–1027. [CrossRef]
7. Fushiki, H.; Junicho, M.; Aso, S.; Watanabe, Y. Recurrence rate of idiopathic sudden low-tone sensorineural hearing loss without vertigo: A long-term follow-up study. *Otol. Neurotol.* **2009**, *30*, 295–298. [CrossRef]
8. Wu, C.M.; Lee, K.J.; Chang, S.L.; Weng, S.F.; Lin, Y.S. Recurrence of idiopathic sudden sensorineural hearing loss: A retrospective cohort study. *Otol. Neurotol.* **2014**, *35*, 1736–1741. [CrossRef]
9. Seo, Y.J.; Park, Y.A.; Bong, J.P.; Park, D.J.; Park, S.Y. Predictive value of neutrophil to lymphocyte ratio in first-time and recurrent idiopathic sudden sensorineural hearing loss. *Auris Nasus Larynx.* **2015**, *42*, 438–442. [CrossRef]
10. Hughes, F.B.; Freedman, M.A.; Haberkamp, T.J.; Guay, M.E. Sudden sensorineural hearing loss. *Otolryngol. Clin. N. Am.* **1996**, *29*, 393–405. [CrossRef]
11. Cvorovic, L.; Deric, D.; Probst, R.; Hegemann, S. Prognostic model for predicting hearing recovery in idiopathic sudden sensorineural hearing loss. *Otol. Neurotol.* **2008**, *29*, 464–469. [CrossRef] [PubMed]
12. Mattox, D.E.; Lyles, C.A. Idiopathic sudden sensorineural hearing loss. *Am. J. Otol.* **1989**, *10*, 242–247. [PubMed]
13. Siegel, L.G. The treatment of idiopathic sudden sensorineural hearing loss. *Otolaryngol. Clin. N. Am.* **1975**, *8*, 467–473. [CrossRef]
14. Liberati, A.; Altman, D.G.; Tetzlaff, J.; Mulrow, C.; Gøtzsche, P.C.; Ioannidis, J.P.; Moher, D. The PRISMA statement for reporting systematic reviews and meta-analyses of studies that evaluate health care interventions: Explanation and elaboration. *J. Clin. Epidemiol.* **2009**, *62*, e1–e34. [CrossRef]
15. Kuo, Y.L.; Young, Y.H. Hearing outcome of recurrent sudden deafness: Ipsilateral versus contralateral types. *Acta Otolaryngol.* **2012**, *132*, 247–254. [CrossRef]
16. Pecorari, G.; Riva, G.; Bruno, G.; Naqe, N.; Nardo, M.; Albera, A.; Albera, R. Recurrences in Sudden Sensorineural Hearing Loss: A Long-Term Observational Study. *Am. J. Audiol.* **2020**, *29*, 18–22. [CrossRef]
17. Wu, P.H.; Lee, C.Y.; Chen, H.C.; Lee, J.C.; Chu, Y.H.; Cheng, L.H.; Shih, C.P. Clinical characteristics and correlation between hearing outcomes after different episodes of recurrent idiopathic sudden sensorineural hearing loss. *Auris Nasus Larynx.* **2021**, *48*, 870–877. [CrossRef]
18. Rauch, S.D. Clinical practice. Idiopathic sudden sensorineural hearing loss. *N. Engl. J. Med.* **2008**, *359*, 833–840. [CrossRef]
19. Fujita, T.; Saito, K.; Kashiwagi, N.; Sato, M.; Seo, T.; Doi, K. The prevalence of vestibular schwannoma among patients treated as sudden sensorineural hearing loss. *Auris Nasus Larynx.* **2019**, *26*, 78–82. [CrossRef]
20. Edizer, D.T.; Çelebi, Ö.; Hamit, B.; Baki, A.; Yiğit, Ö. Recovery of idiopathic sudden sensorineural hearing loss. *J. Int. Adv. Otol.* **2015**, *11*, 122–126. [CrossRef]
21. Sakata, T.; Esaki, Y.; Yamano, T.; Sueta, N.; Nakagawa, T. A comparison between the feeling of ear fullness and tinnitus in acute sensorineural hearing loss. *Int. J. Audiol.* **2008**, *47*, 134–140. [CrossRef] [PubMed]
22. Gorga, M.P.; Kaminski, J.R.; Beauchaine, K.L. Effects of stimulus phase on the latency of the auditory brainstem response. *J. Am. Acad. Audiol.* **1991**, *2*, 1–6. [PubMed]
23. Tonndorf, J.; Tabor, J.R. Closure of th cochlear windows: Its effect upon air- and bone-conduction. *Ann. Otol. Rhinol. Laryngol.* **1962**, *71*, 5–29. [CrossRef] [PubMed]
24. Sakata, T.; Kato, T. Feeling of ear fullness in acute sensorineural hearing loss. *Acta Oto-Laryngol.* **2006**, *126*, 828–833. [CrossRef] [PubMed]
25. Chang, S.L.; Hsieh, C.C.; Tseng, K.S.; Weng, S.F.; Lin, Y.S. Hypercholesterolemia is correlated with an increased risk of idiopathic sudden sensorineural hearing loss: A historical prospective cohort study. *Ear Hear.* **2014**, *35*, 256–261. [CrossRef] [PubMed]
26. Lin, C.; Lin, S.W.; Lin, Y.S.; Weng, S.F.; Lee, T.M. Sudden sensorineural hearing loss is correlated with an increased risk of acute myocardial infarction: A population-based cohort study. *Laryngoscope* **2013**, *123*, 2254–2258. [CrossRef] [PubMed]
27. Lin, S.W.; Lin, Y.S.; Weng, S.F.; Chou, C.W. Risk of developing sudden sensorineural hearing loss in diabetic patients: A population-based cohort study. *Otol. Neurotol.* **2012**, *33*, 1482–1488. [CrossRef]
28. Lin, C.; Hsu, H.T.; Lin, Y.S.; Weng, S.F. Increased risk of getting sudden sensorineural hearing loss in patients with chronic kidney disease: A population-based cohort study. *Laryngoscope* **2013**, *123*, 767–773. [CrossRef]
29. Lin, H.C.; Chao, P.Z.; Lee, H.C. Sudden sensorineural hearing loss increases the risk of stroke: A 5-year follow-up study. *Stroke* **2008**, *39*, 2744–2748. [CrossRef]
30. Agrawal, Y.; Platz, E.A.; Niparko, J.K. Prevalence of hearing loss and differences by demographic characteristics among US adults: Data from the National Health and Nutrition Examination Survey, 1999–2004. *Arch Intern. Med.* **2008**, *168*, 1522–1530. [CrossRef]
31. Siegelaub, A.B.; Friedman, G.D.; Adour, K.; Seltzer, C.C. Hearing loss in adults: Relation to age, sex, exposure to loud noise, and cigarette smoking. *Arch Environ. Occup. Health* **1974**, *29*, 107–109. [CrossRef] [PubMed]
32. Lionello, M.; Staffieri, C.; Breda, S.; Turato, C.; Giacomelli, L.; Magnavita, P.; Marioni, G. Uni-and multivariate models for investigating potential prognostic factors in idiopathic sudden sensorineural hearing loss. *Eur. Arch. Otorhinol.* **2015**, *272*, 1899–1906. [CrossRef] [PubMed]
33. Lin, R.J.; Krall, R.; Westerberg, B.D.; Chadha, N.K.; Chau, J.K. Systematic review and meta-analysis of the risk factors for sudden sensorineural hearing loss in adults. *Laryngoscope* **2012**, *122*, 624–635. [CrossRef] [PubMed]
34. Sasso, F.C.; Salvatore, T.; Tranchino, G.; Cozzolino, D.; Caruso, A.A.; Persico, M.; Torella, R. Cochlear Dysfunction in Type 2 Diabetes: A complication Independent of Neuropathy and Acute Hyperglycemia. *Metabolism* **1999**, *48*, 1346–1350. [CrossRef]

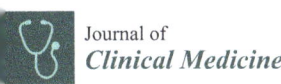

Article

# Correlation of Neutrophil-to-Lymphocyte Ratio and the Dilation of the Basilar Artery with the Potential Role of Vascular Compromise in the Pathophysiology of Idiopathic Sudden Sensorineural Hearing Loss

Dae-Woong Kang [1], Seul Kim [2] and Woongsang Sunwoo [2],*

[1] Department of Otorhinolaryngology, Seoul National University Hospital, Seoul National University College of Medicine, Seoul 03080, Korea
[2] Department of Otorhinolaryngology, Gil Medical Center, Gachon University College of Medicine, Incheon 21565, Korea
* Correspondence: sunwoowoongsang@gmail.com or sunwoow@gachon.ac.kr

**Abstract:** Idiopathic sudden sensorineural hearing loss (SSNHL) currently lacks a clear etiology, as well as an effective treatment. One of the most probable explanations for SSNHL is impairment of the cochlear blood flow. However, dissimilar to a fundoscopic examination, direct observation of cochlear blood vessels is not possible. To indirectly support an ischemic etiology of SSNHL, we investigated whether the degree of initial hearing loss is associated with two atherosclerotic risk factors: dilatation of the basilar artery (BA) and a chronic subclinical inflammatory status measured by the neutrophil-to-lymphocyte ratio (NLR). This retrospective study collected data from 105 consecutive patients diagnosed with idiopathic SSNHL. Then, the patients were divided into two groups according to their NLR as "abnormally high NLR (>3.53, $n = 22$)" and "NLR within the normal range (0.78–3.53, $n = 83$)". The BA diameter and severity of initial hearing loss were significantly correlated with each other in the abnormally high NLR group ($p < 0.001$). However, there was no significant correlation between initial hearing loss and the BA diameter in the normal NLR group ($p = 0.299$). Therefore, the NLR may serve as a marker for SSNHL of vascular etiology and a rationale for magnetic resonance imaging examinations based on the pathophysiology.

**Keywords:** sudden sensorineural hearing loss; neutrophil-to-lymphocyte ratio; etiology; basilar artery

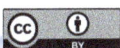

## 1. Introduction

Sudden sensorineural hearing loss (SSNHL) is defined as sensorineural hearing loss of 30 dB or more at three consecutive frequencies within 3 days and is often accompanied by tinnitus, dizziness, ear fullness, nausea, and vomiting [1]. Although the annual prevalence of sudden hearing loss has been reported to be 5–20 per 100,000, the actual prevalence is expected to be higher, considering that the spontaneous recovery rate is approximately 32–65% [2,3]. Viral or bacterial infection, vascular disturbance, microcirculatory failure, trauma, autoimmune disease, and neoplasm are possible etiologies of SSNHL [4,5]. However, most cases of SSNHL have no identified etiology and are commonly termed idiopathic.

Circulatory disturbance has been speculated to be a possible cause of SSNHL, because the cochlea receives a limited blood supply without collateral circulation. The inner ear is an end organ supplied only by the cochlear artery, which branches out from the internal auditory artery (IAA). As expected from this vulnerable anatomical condition, the occurrence of unilateral SSNHL has been reported as an early presentation of ischemic stroke of the anterior inferior cerebellar artery (AICA), where the IAA is branched [6,7]. Consistent with these case reports, animal studies have shown that disruption of the cochlear blood flow can immediately lead to cochlear dysfunction [8,9]. In addition, several studies have suggested that defibrinogenation therapy or adjuvant heparin therapy could be more beneficial than steroid monotherapy in some patients with profound hearing loss [10–12]. Accordingly, these previous findings indicate the importance of considering the vascular etiology when evaluating SSNHL of an unknown cause.

Recently, the neutrophil-to-lymphocyte ratio (NLR) has been widely used not only as an inflammatory marker but also as a predictive marker in various diseases, including diabetes mellitus, chronic pulmonary disease, autoimmune disease, and cardiovascular disease [13–16]. Several studies have also investigated the association between NLR and SSNHL. These studies revealed that a high NLR is associated with the development and poor prognosis of SSNHL [17–20]. However, the reason a high NLR is correlated with a higher risk in patients with SSNHL remains unknown. To the best of our knowledge, the detailed role of the NLR in the pathogenesis of SSNHL has not yet been studied. Therefore, there is a need for evidence to elucidate the role of an elevated NLR in the high incidence and poor outcome of SSNHL. Based on the relationship between an elevated NLR and atherosclerotic events in cardiovascular disease, it has been postulated that endothelial dysfunction caused by chronic subclinical inflammatory conditions may play a role in the initiation and progression of atherosclerosis [13,21]. Thus, we hypothesized that an elevated NLR may be related to a diminished cochlear blood flow or cochlear ischemia caused by endothelial dysfunction or microvascular inflammation in the blood vessels supplying the cochlea.

To investigate the etiological role of an elevated NLR in SSNHL, we focused on the vascular etiology and evaluated the radiological findings of the basilar artery (BA) as the origin of the AICA using magnetic resonance imaging (MRI). It has been suggested that morphological deformation of the BA, including angulation and dilatation, may be associated with atherogenesis in the vertebrobasilar system and contribute to the development of SSNHL by decreasing blood flow to the cochlea and generating microemboli or microthrombi [22–25]. Therefore, we aimed to investigate whether a high NLR in SSNHL is associated with BA dilatation. Specifically, we hypothesized that if the etiology of SSNHL is vascular, the degree of reduction in the cochlear blood flow may be associated with the degree of initial hearing loss.

## 2. Materials and Methods

The Institutional Review Board of Gachon University Gil Medical Center approved this study (IRB No. GFIRB2021-243) and waived the need for informed consent owing to the retrospective nature of the study and the use of anonymous clinical data for analysis. This study complied with the Declaration of Helsinki and was performed according to ethics committee approval.

This retrospective single-center study included patients diagnosed with idiopathic SSNHL at the Gachon University Gil Medical Center between January 2014 and December 2018. Patients were included if they had undergone (1) pure-tone audiometry, (2) laboratory tests including a complete blood count (CBC) with differential, and (3) an MRI of the temporal bone within 2 weeks of hearing loss onset. Patients meeting any of the following criteria were excluded: age $\leq 18$ years, white blood cell (WBC) count >10,000 cells/mm$^3$, and lesions on the MRI causally or potentially related to hearing loss. After exclusion, 105 patients (54 men and 51 women aged 27–81 years) were included in the final analysis.

The initial hearing levels were measured using pure-tone audiometry at the time of diagnosis. Using the average hearing threshold level at speech frequencies (500, 1000, 2000, and 4000 Hz) in the affected ear, we computed the pure-tone average (PTA) to estimate the hearing loss. The pure-tone audiogram shapes were classified as follows: "up-sloping" or "down-sloping" (minimum difference of 20 dB between the 500-Hz and 4000-Hz thresholds), "flat" (difference between the 500-Hz and 4000-Hz thresholds <20 dB), and "profound" (PTA >90 dB) [26,27].

The CBC with differential reported counts for five main types of WBCs, either as percentages or as the absolute number of cells (cells/mm$^3$). The NLR was calculated by dividing the absolute neutrophil count by the absolute lymphocyte count. Based on the normal NLR values for healthy adults reported by Forget et al., an NLR > 3.53 was considered abnormal [28]. Patients were classified into two groups: those with normal NLR ($\leq$3.5) and those with abnormally high NLR (>3.5).

All MRI data were acquired using a 3-Tesla MRI scanner (Skyra; Siemens Medical System, Erlangen, Germany). The diameter of the BA was measured at the mid-pons level on the axial view of a 3-dimensional (3D) T2-weighted image. The parameters of the T2-weighted sampling perfection with application-optimized contrasts using different flip angle evolutions sequence were as follows: repetition time, 1000 ms; echo time, 140 ms; flip angle, 120°; field of view, 208 × 230; matrix size, 384 × 345; and slice thickness, 0.8 mm. When the BA displays angulation in its course, its longitudinal axis can be tilted to the measured plane. Thus, the short axis of the elliptical BA at the level of entry of the trigeminal nerve into the anterolateral aspect of the pons was considered the diameter of the BA (Figure 1). The MRI scans were analyzed while blinded to all clinical information.

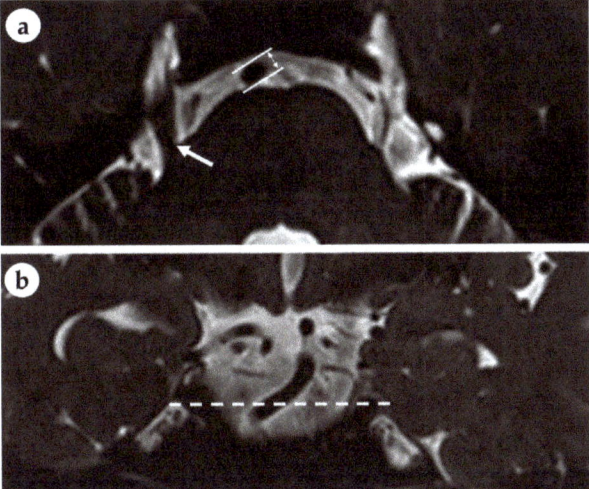

**Figure 1.** Measurement of the short axis of the basilar artery (BA) diameter (double arrow) on the axial T2-weighted magnetic resonance image at the mid-pons level; the level of the trigeminal nerve (arrow) emerging from the anterolateral aspect of the pons (**a**). Coronal T2-weighted image shows the tortuous BA that courses transversely at the mid-pons level (dotted line) (**b**).

Descriptive data were reported as the median (range) or count (percentage). The chi-square test or Fisher's exact test were used to compare categorical variables. Continuous variables were compared using the Student's *t*-test, and groups for skewed variables were compared using the Mann–Whitney *U* test. A one-way analysis of variance (ANOVA) was performed to compare the effect of four different audiometric curves on the NLR values. Audiometric types were compared between the normal NLR and abnormally high NLR groups using a linear-by-linear association test. The Spearman rank correlation coefficient was used to evaluate the correlation between the BA diameter, NLR, and initial PTA. To test whether the effect of the initial PTA on the NLR is dependent on the value of the BA diameter, a multiple linear regression was calculated, including the interaction terms of the initial PTA and BA diameter. Statistical significance was set at $p < 0.05$. All statistical analyses were performed using IBM SPSS software (IBM Corp., Armonk, NY, USA).

## 3. Results

The demographic and general characteristics of the study population are summarized in Table 1. The mean age of the 105 patients (54 men and 51 women) in the study population was $52.1 \pm 11.6$ years. The mean WBC count was $6.73 \pm 1.36 \times 10^3$ cells/mm$^3$, and the NLR value ranged from 0.8 to 11.75 (median, 2.05). The median PTA at diagnosis was 68.8 dB (range: 20–120 dB). The flat type ($n$ = 38, 36.2%) was the most common configuration of the audiogram, followed by the up-sloping ($n$ = 23, 21.9%) and down-sloping ($n$ = 18, 17.2%) types. Twenty-six patients with PTA > 90 dB (24.8%) were classified as the profound type. There were no statistically significant differences in the NLR values between groups, as determined by one-way ANOVA ($F(3, 101)$ = 0.508, $p$ = 0.678). The median BA diameter was 3.44 mm (range, 2.29–5.16 mm). There were only five cases (4.8%) of BA dolichoectasia in which the diameter of the BA was >4.5 mm.

Table 1. General characteristics of the study groups.

| | Total (N = 105) | NLR ≤ 3.53 (n = 83) | NLR > 3.53 (n = 22) | p |
|---|---|---|---|---|
| Age (years) | 52 (27–81) | 52 (27–79) | 51.5 (34–81) | 0.816 [1] |
| Sex (male/female) | 54/51 | 45/38 | 9/13 | 0.267 [2] |
| Body mass index (kg/m$^2$) | 24.8 (17.4–51.0) | 24.8 (17.4–51.0) | 24.2 (19.1–35.2) | 0.634 [3] |
| Hypertension | 27 (25.7%) | 62 (74.7%) | 6 (27.3%) | 0.851 [2] |
| Diabetes mellitus | 17 (16.2%) | 15 (18.1%) | 2 (9.1%) | 0.515 [4] |
| Cardiovascular disease | 6 (5.7%) | 5 (6.0%) | 1 (4.5%) | 1.000 [4] |
| Affected side (right/left) | 56/49 | 48/35 | 8/14 | 0.073 [2] |
| Initial PTA (dB) | 68.8 (20.0–120.0) | 70.0 (20.0–118.8) | 67.5 (37.5–120.0) | 0.595 [3] |
| Vertigo | 21 (20%) | 13 (15.7%) | 8 (36.4%) | 0.040 [4] |
| Audiometric curves<br>Up-sloping type<br>Down-sloping type<br>Flat type<br>Profound | <br>23 (21.9%)<br>18 (17.1%)<br>38 (36.2%)<br>26 (24.8%) | <br>17 (20.5%)<br>16 (19.3%)<br>30 (36.1%)<br>20 (24.1%) | <br>6 (27.3%)<br>2 (9.1%)<br>8 (36.4%)<br>6 (27.3%) | 1.000 [5] |
| BA diameter (mm) | 3.44 (2.29–5.16) | 3.44 (2.29–4.83) | 3.50 (2.58–5.16) | 0.850 [3] |
| BA dolichoectasia | 5 (4.8%) | 4 (4.8%) | 1 (4.5%) | 1.000 [4] |
| WBC ($\times 10^3$ cells/mm$^3$) | 6.73 (3.57–9.72) | 6.57 (3.57–9.40) | 7.35 (4.64–9.72) | 0.015 [1] |
| Neutrophil ($\times 10^3$ cells/mm$^3$) | 4.21 (1.46–8.02) | 3.78 (1.46–6.44) | 5.83 (3.37–8.02) | <0.001 [3] |
| Lymphocyte ($\times 10^3$ cells/mm$^3$) | 1.96 (0.50–4.00) | 2.17 (1.26–4.00) | 1.15 (0.50–1.88) | <0.001 [3] |
| Platelet ($\times 10^3$ cells/mm$^3$) | 250.5 (130–522) | 250.3 (130–522) | 251.4 (148–329) | 0.471 [3] |
| MPV (fL) | 10.1 (6.6–12.6) | 10.2 (7.5–12.6) | 9.8 (6.6–12.0) | 0.125 [1] |

Values are presented as the median (range) or count (%). PTA, pure-tone average of the thresholds at 500, 1000, 2000, and 4000 Hz; BA, the basilar artery; NLR, neutrophil-to-lymphocyte ratio; WBC, white blood cell; and MPV, mean platelet volume. The $p$-values are computed from the [1] Student's $t$-test, [2] chi-square test, [3] Mann–Whitney $U$ test, [4] Fisher's exact test, and [5] linear-by-linear association.

There was no correlation between the NLR and initial PTA and BA diameter (Figure 2). Specifically, the Spearman correlation coefficient of the NLR with the initial PTA and BA diameter was $r_S = -0.003$ ($p$ = 0.976) and $r_S = -0.027$ ($p$ = 0.781), respectively.

Patients were divided into two groups according to their NLR. Twenty-two patients had an abnormally high NLR value (NLR > 3.53), and eighty-three had an NLR value within the normal range (NLR between 0.78 and 3.53) [28]. A comparison of the general data between the two groups is shown in Table 1. In the univariate analysis, patients with vertigo showed a higher probability of having an abnormally high NLR ($p$ = 0.040).

None of the other clinical characteristics, including the initial PTA and BA diameter, were statistically associated with the NLR.

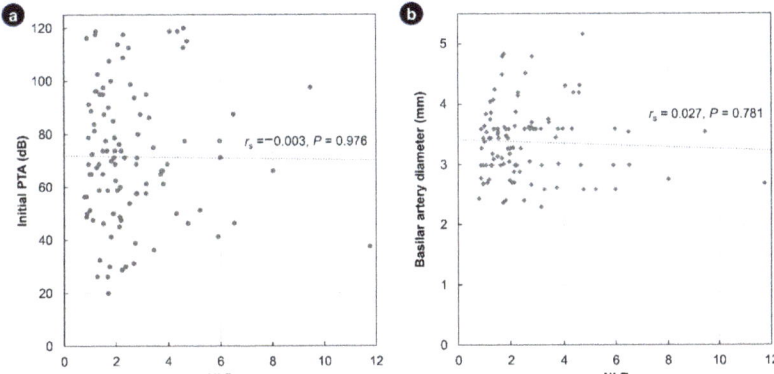

**Figure 2.** Scatter plots showing the correlation between the neutrophil-to-lymphocyte ratio (NLR) and the initial pure-tone average of the thresholds (PTA) (**a**) and the basilar artery diameter (**b**). Spearman's correlation coefficient ($r_s$) and corresponding *p*-value are reported alongside the regression lines.

A multiple linear regression was run to predict the NLR from age, sex, initial PTA, BA diameter, and the two-way interaction term of the initial PTA and BA diameter. These variables statistically significantly predicted the NLR, $F(5, 99) = 1.44$, $p = 0.216$, $R^2 = 0.068$. Age and sex did not significantly predict the NLR ($p = 0.9$ and $0.2$, respectively). The initial PTA and BA diameter were significant predictors of the NLR ($p = 0.044$ and $0.049$, respectively). It was found that the interaction between the initial PTA and BA diameter was significant ($p = 0.042$). This means that the effect of the initial PTA on NLR depends on the BA diameter and vice versa.

Assuming that the increased risk of atherosclerotic events and cochlear ischemia would be better described by the combination of the NLR and BA diameter, we analyzed the etiological value of the NLR/BA diameter combination in idiopathic SSNHL. First, we assessed the relationship between the BA diameter and the initial PTA level for each group separately. As shown in Figure 3, a significant positive correlation was observed between the initial PTA and BA diameter in the high NLR group ($r_s = 0.702$, $p < 0.001$), suggesting that, for idiopathic SSNHL of vascular etiology, a dilated BA would increase susceptibility to an insufficient cochlear blood supply and increase the initial level of hearing loss. However, there was no significant link between the initial PTA and BA diameter in the normal NLR group ($r_s = 0.115$, $p = 0.299$).

Spearman's correlation coefficient was used to examine the cutoff of NLR in predicted cases of vascular etiology based on our hypothesis. Figure 4 illustrates Spearman's rho values between the BA diameter and the initial PTA level in the high NLR group as the NLR cutoff value varies from 1.0 to 6.0. The Spearman's correlation coefficients were between 0.70 and 0.82, which indicate a high degree of correlation, when the NTR cutoff values of 3.44–4.60 were applied. Since there were only twelve patients with values of the NLR higher than 4.61 in this study, the higher the NLR cutoff value at 4.60 or more, the lower the degree of correlation. In addition, 3.69 was the lowest NLR value among patients with NLRs higher than 3.44, so applying 3.53 as the NLR cutoff value was considered to be appropriate.

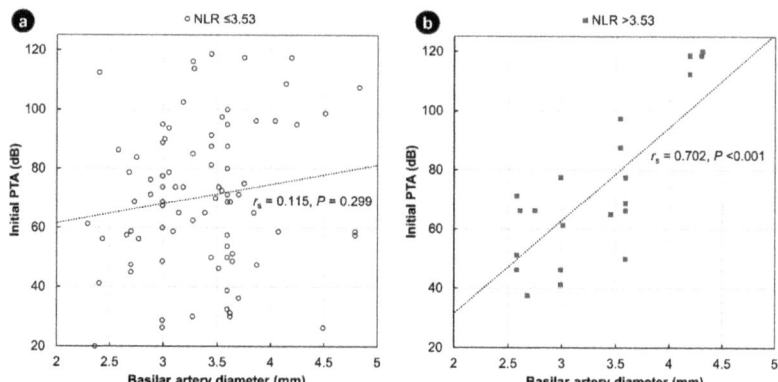

**Figure 3.** Scatter plots showing the relationship between the basilar artery diameter and the initial pure-tone average of the thresholds (PTA) in the normal neutrophil-to-lymphocyte ratio (NLR) group (**a**) and the high NLR group (**b**). Spearman's correlation coefficient ($r_s$) and the corresponding $p$-value are shown alongside the regression lines.

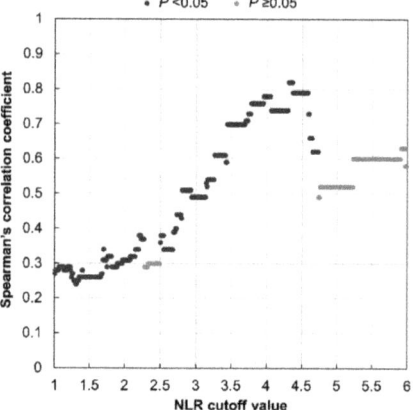

**Figure 4.** Scatter plots showing the Spearman's correlation coefficient between the basilar artery diameter and the initial pure-tone average of the thresholds in the high neutrophil-to-lymphocyte ratio group according to the NLR cutoff value. Dark gray marks represent statistical significance ($p < 0.05$).

## 4. Discussion

Various potential etiological factors and a lack of helpful etiological markers in idiopathic SSNHL make a pathophysiology-based approach to the treatment of SSNHL difficult. Recently, the NLR has been proposed as an easily accessible and reliable biomarker of vascular etiology in a variety of diseases. In this study, we investigated the association between the severity of the initial hearing loss and BA diameter using temporal bone MRI and investigated the etiological value of the NLR by classifying patients with SSNHL into two groups based on normal NLR reference values. The main findings of the present study were as follows: (1) neither the degree of BA dilatation or the severity of the initial hearing loss showed a quantitative relationship with the NLR itself, and (2) in SSNHL patients with abnormally high NLR values, the initial hearing loss was more severe as the BA diameter increased, a significant correlation that was not observed in SSNHL patients with normal NLR values.

Table 1 shows the demographic and clinical characteristics of the patients with SSNHL included in this study. We obtained not only sociodemographic factors such as age and sex but also conventional risk factors associated with vascular occlusion and circulatory disturbances, including hypertension and diabetes mellitus. These factors can contribute to the vascular etiology of SSNHL, regardless of the NLR, by accelerating the prothrombotic events in the BA [22]. As presented in Table 1, because there were no significant differences in the risk factors between the high NLR group and the normal NLR group, they were not adjusted for in further analyses. In this study, the proportion of patients with vertigo was higher in the high NLR group. Since the inner ear has a blood supply from the labyrinthine artery, which branches into the anterior vestibular artery and the common cochlear artery, vestibular symptoms can occur frequently in AICA infarctions [29]. In addition, previous studies have interpreted vertigo symptoms in SSNHL to result from an ischemic etiology [30,31]. Therefore, considering that both SSNHL with vertigo and SSNHL with high NLR are related to a poor prognosis, we believe that a higher proportion of vertigo symptoms in the high NLR group arises from dysfunction of the audio–vestibular system due to vascular causes [17,32].

The severity of the initial hearing loss, measured by the initial PTA as an indicator of vascular dysfunction, was used to evaluate the vascular etiological value of the NLR in this study. Electrophysiological studies have revealed that the extent of cochlear blood flow reduction during circulatory blockage in the BA system correlates with cochlear dysfunction [9]. Based on these experiments, we assumed that the more severe the reduction in cochlear blood flow, the greater the initial PTA. Consistent with this assumption, clinical studies have reported that patients with a higher initial PTA, which means more severe hearing impairment at the time of diagnosis, had a poor response to conventional steroid therapy, resulting in poorer hearing outcomes [27,33]. Considering the possible action of steroids to reduce inflammation and edema in the hearing organs, the administration of steroids to treat patients with SSNHL caused mainly by vascular pathology may not be effective. In addition, other treatment modalities proposed to improve cochlear microcirculation based on vascular pathogenesis, including defibrinogenation, adjuvant heparin, and hyperbaric oxygen therapy, have shown potential benefits in patients with severe or profound initial hearing loss [10–12,34]. We believe that revascularization of the ischemic cochlea could help improve hearing in patients whose steroid treatment alone was ineffective.

The BA that supplies blood to the inner ear arises from the intersection of the two vertebral arteries (VAs). Since only 6–26% of people have both VAs with the same diameter, the BA receives an unbalanced mechanical force from the VAs on both sides [35]. This unstable and unbalanced mechanical force causes angulation and dilatation of the BA through shear stress on the vessel wall. This dilatation of the BA can cause an ischemic effect by reducing blood flow to the AICA. In addition, increased prothrombotic states in the vessel wall of the dilated BA can cause microemboli and lead to ischemia of the AICA territory [36]. Furthermore, an increased BA diameter is associated with cerebral small-vessel diseases, as well as large-vessel atherosclerosis, such as intracranial arterial stenosis [24]. Therefore, it can be expected that the BA diameter may be associated with the blood supply to the cochlea. Based on the above findings, we hypothesized that the BA diameter would be correlated with the severity of the initial hearing loss in cases of SSNHL of vascular etiology.

In the group of all subjects, significant correlations between either the BA diameter or initial PTA and the NLR were not observed. The pathophysiological heterogeneity of SSNHL may have contributed to these negative results. The inclusion of patients with SSNHL not caused by a vascular etiology may potentially render this biomarker analysis invalid. Another possible reason is the high proportion of subjects within the normal range of the NLR (83/105, 79%). In general, the prognostic and diagnostic efficacy of a marker depends on the established cutoff, which determines its effectiveness, specificity, and sensitivity. However, the optimal NLR cutoff value has not been clarified in patients with SSNHL. In previous studies, the suggested cutoff values of the NLR for predicting prognoses varied between 3.42 and 6.66 [37,38]. Accordingly, we classified all SSNHL patients into a high NLR group and a normal NLR group based on the commonly used normal reference NLR values for further analysis. However, similar to the results in the overall study population, neither the BA diameter or the initial PTA individually correlated significantly with the NLR values in either subgroup.

To improve the diagnostic efficacy of the NLR as an etiological marker in SSNHL, we used a combination of a dilated BA diameter with a high NLR value, which individually had no significant correlations with the initial hearing loss level. Interestingly, the severity of the initial hearing loss showed a significant positive correlation with the BA diameter only in the group of patients with abnormally high NLR values (Figure 3). These findings support our hypothesis that the combination of BA dilatation and an elevated NLR could indicate vascular pathogenesis in idiopathic SSNHL, such as atherosclerotic events and cochlear ischemia. As mentioned above, dilatation of the BA can reduce the blood flow through the AICA and cause ischemic damage to the cochlea. Similarly, hearing loss has been reported as one of the main symptoms in patients with BA dolichoectasia, whose BA diameter is excessively dilated by vascular remodeling [39,40]. Wang et al. suggested that mural thrombi and atherosclerotic plaques generated by slowed blood flow and turbulence in dilated and tortuous vessels could cause changes in the hemodynamics of the posterior circulation [41]. By indirectly proving the etiological value of the NLR in this study, we believe that it could be helpful to interpret the results of previous and future studies of NLR values in idiopathic SSNHL in terms of the vascular etiology.

This study had several limitations. First, our study suggests only presumptive evidence that indirectly supports the etiological value of NLR as a vascular origin in idiopathic SSNHL. To measure changes in the hemodynamics or demonstrate ischemic effects, the blood flow must be directly measured and analyzed. However, as there is still no imaging modality that can directly measure cochlear blood flow, we used an indirect method that can reflect the blood flow. Recently, several studies have reported that the use of 3D fluid-attenuated inversion-recovery MRI can provide information on pathologic conditions in the cochlea, especially intracochlear hemorrhage, a common pathological finding observed after vascular occlusion in SSNHL [8,42,43]. Therefore, further analysis of 3D fluid-attenuated inversion-recovery MRI findings combined with NLR in future studies may contribute to the elucidation of the etiological value of the NLR. Second, because the aim of this study was to evaluate the etiological value of the NLR related to vascular causes, the treatment outcomes were not analyzed. The vascular pattern in the BA system has been reported to have various anastomoses between the AICA and collateral blood vessels [44,45]. In addition, the severity of degenerative changes in the cochlea caused by vascular occlusion is affected by the presence of collateral blood vessels or anatomical variations of the IAA [8]. Therefore, this anatomical variation and the presence of collateral circulation can affect the prognosis of SSNHL of vascular etiology. Since it may not be possible to distinguish whether the outcome of hearing recovery is a response to steroid treatment or due to collateral circulation in the case of partial occlusion, analyses of the prognostic efficacy of the NLR were not conducted in the current study.

## 5. Conclusions

Idiopathic SSNHL currently lacks a clear etiology, as well as an effective treatment. One of the most probable explanations for SSNHL is impairment of the cochlear blood flow. However, dissimilar to a fundoscopic examination, direct observation of the cochlear blood vessels is not possible in patients with SSNHL. Our results indirectly support an ischemic etiology of SSNHL originating in branches of the BA and is associated with two atherosclerotic risk factors: dilatation of the BA and a chronic subclinical inflammatory status measured by the NLR. In this study, the BA diameter and severity of the initial hearing loss, which reflects the degree of reduced cochlear blood flow, were significantly correlated with each other only in patients with abnormally high NLR values. Therefore, the NLR may serve as a marker for SSNHL of vascular etiology and a rationale for an MRI examination based on the pathophysiology.

**Author Contributions:** Conceptualization, W.S. and S.K.; methodology, W.S.; formal analysis, D.-W.K.; investigation, S.K.; data curation, D.-W.K.; writing—original draft preparation, D.-W.K. and S.K.; writing—review and editing, W.S.; visualization, D.-W.K.; supervision, W.S.; and funding acquisition, W.S. All authors have read and agreed to the published version of the manuscript.

**Funding:** This research was supported by the National Research Foundation of Korea (NRF) grant funded by the Korea government (MSIT) (No. 2020R1C1C1005488); by the Gachon University Gil Medical Center (No. FRD2022-04); and the Korea Medical Device Development Fund grant funded by the Korea government (MSIT, MOTIE, and MFDS) (KMDF-PR-20200901-0147). The APC was funded by the Korea government (MSIT, MOTIE, and MFDS).

**Institutional Review Board Statement:** This study was conducted in accordance with the Declaration of Helsinki and approved by the Institutional Review Board of Gachon University Gil Medical Center (protocol code GFIRB2021-243, approved 6 July 2021).

**Informed Consent Statement:** Patient consent was waived due to the retrospective nature of the study and the use of anonymous clinical data for analysis.

**Data Availability Statement:** The data that support the findings of this study are available from the corresponding author upon reasonable request.

**Acknowledgments:** We would like to thank Zarathu (www.zarathu.com, accessed on 30 September 2022) for the statistical consulting.

**Conflicts of Interest:** The authors declare no conflict of interest.

# References

1. Hughes, G.B.; Freedman, M.A.; Haberkamp, T.J.; Guay, M.E. Sudden sensorineural hearing loss. *Otolaryngol. Clin. N. Am.* **1996**, *29*, 393–405.
2. Stachler, R.J.; Chandrasekhar, S.S.; Archer, S.M.; Rosenfeld, R.M.; Schwartz, S.R.; Barrs, D.M.; Brown, S.R.; Fife, T.D.; Ford, P.; Ganiats, T.G.; et al. Clinical practice guideline: Sudden hearing loss. *Otolaryngol. Head Neck Surg.* **2012**, *146*, S1–S35. [CrossRef]
3. Schreiber, B.E.; Agrup, C.; Haskard, D.O.; Luxon, L.M. Sudden sensorineural hearing loss. *Lancet* **2010**, *375*, 1203–1211. [CrossRef]
4. Masuda, M.; Kanzaki, S.; Minami, S.; Kikuchi, J.; Kanzaki, J.; Sato, H.; Ogawa, K. Correlations of inflammatory biomarkers with the onset and prognosis of idiopathic sudden sensorineural hearing loss. *Otol. Neurotol.* **2012**, *33*, 1142–1150. [CrossRef]
5. Merchant, S.N.; Durand, M.L.; Adams, J.C. Sudden deafness: Is it viral? *ORL J. Otorhinolaryngol. Relat. Spec.* **2008**, *70*, 52–60. [CrossRef]
6. Ito, H.; Hibino, M.; Iino, M.; Matsuura, K.; Kamei, T. Unilateral hearing disturbance could be an isolated manifestation prior to ipsilateral anterior inferior cerebellar artery infarction. *Intern. Med.* **2008**, *47*, 795–796. [CrossRef]
7. Amarenco, P.; Rosengart, A.; DeWitt, L.D.; Pessin, M.S.; Caplan, L.R. Anterior inferior cerebellar artery territory infarcts. Mechanisms and clinical features. *Arch. Neurol.* **1993**, *50*, 154–161. [CrossRef]
8. Belal, A., Jr. Pathology of vascular sensorineural hearing impairment. *Laryngoscope* **1980**, *90*, 1831–1839. [CrossRef]
9. Ito, H. Effects of circulatory disturbance on the cochlea. *ORL J. Otorhinolaryngol. Relat. Spec.* **1991**, *53*, 265–269. [CrossRef]
10. Suzuki, H.; Furukawa, M.; Kumagai, M.; Takahashi, E.; Matsuura, K.; Katori, Y.; Shimomura, A.; Kobayashi, T. Defibrinogenation therapy for idiopathic sudden sensorineural hearing loss in comparison with high-dose steroid therapy. *Acta Oto-Laryngol.* **2003**, *123*, 46–50. [CrossRef]
11. Kim, J.; Jeong, J.; Ha, R.; Sunwoo, W. Heparin therapy as adjuvant treatment for profound idiopathic sudden sensorineural hearing loss. *Laryngoscope* **2020**, *130*, 1310–1315. [CrossRef]
12. Shiraishi, T.; Kubo, T.; Okumura, S.; Naramura, H.; Nishimura, M.; Okusa, M.; Matsunaga, T. Hearing recovery in sudden deafness patients using a modified defibrinogenation therapy. *Acta Otolaryngol. Suppl.* **1993**, *501*, 46–50. [CrossRef]
13. Balta, S.; Celik, T.; Mikhailidis, D.P.; Ozturk, C.; Demirkol, S.; Aparci, M.; Iyisoy, A. The Relation Between Atherosclerosis and the Neutrophil-Lymphocyte Ratio. *Clin. Appl. Thromb./Hemost. Off. J. Int. Acad. Clin. Appl. Thromb./Hemost.* **2016**, *22*, 405–411. [CrossRef]
14. Chollangi, S.; Rout, N.K.; Patro, S. A Study on Correlation of Neutrophil to Lymphocyte Ratio and Red Cell Distribution Width with Microalbuminuria in Type 2 Diabetes Mellitus. *J. Assoc. Physicians India* **2022**, *70*, 11–12.
15. Zinellu, A.; Zinellu, E.; Pau, M.C.; Carru, C.; Pirina, P.; Fois, A.G.; Mangoni, A.A. A Comprehensive Systematic Review and Meta-Analysis of the Association between the Neutrophil-to-Lymphocyte Ratio and Adverse Outcomes in Patients with Acute Exacerbation of Chronic Obstructive Pulmonary Disease. *J. Clin. Med.* **2022**, *11*, 3365. [CrossRef]

16. Buonacera, A.; Stancanelli, B.; Colaci, M.; Malatino, L. Neutrophil to Lymphocyte Ratio: An Emerging Marker of the Relationships between the Immune System and Diseases. *Int. J. Mol. Sci.* **2022**, *23*, 3636. [CrossRef]
17. Ni, W.; Song, S.P.; Jiang, Y.D. Association between routine hematological parameters and sudden sensorineural hearing loss: A meta-analysis. *J. Otol.* **2021**, *16*, 47–54. [CrossRef]
18. Chen, L.; Zhang, G.; Zhang, Z.; Wang, Y.; Hu, L.; Wu, J. Neutrophil-to-lymphocyte ratio predicts diagnosis and prognosis of idiopathic sudden sensorineural hearing loss: A systematic review and meta-analysis. *Medicine* **2018**, *97*, e12492. [CrossRef]
19. Guo, Y.; Liu, J. The Roles Played by Blood Inflammatory Parameters in Sudden Sensorineural Hearing Loss. *Ear. Nose Throat J.* **2021**. ahead of print. [CrossRef]
20. Lee, J.S.; Hong, S.K.; Kim, D.H.; Lee, J.H.; Lee, H.J.; Park, B.; Choi, H.G.; Kong, I.G.; Song, H.J.; Kim, H.J. The neutrophil-to-lymphocyte ratio in children with sudden sensorineural hearing loss: A retrospective study. *Acta Oto-Laryngol.* **2017**, *137*, 35–38. [CrossRef]
21. Bhat, T.; Teli, S.; Rijal, J.; Bhat, H.; Raza, M.; Khoueiry, G.; Meghani, M.; Akhtar, M.; Costantino, T. Neutrophil to lymphocyte ratio and cardiovascular diseases: A review. *Expert Rev. Cardiovasc. Ther.* **2013**, *11*, 55–59. [CrossRef]
22. Kim, C.; Sohn, J.H.; Choi, H.C. Vertebrobasilar angulation and its association with sudden sensorineural hearing loss. *Med. Hypotheses* **2012**, *79*, 202–203. [CrossRef]
23. Hong, J.M.; Chung, C.-S.; Bang, O.Y.; Yong, S.W.; Joo, I.S.; Huh, K. Vertebral artery dominance contributes to basilar artery curvature and peri-vertebrobasilar junctional infarcts. *J. Neurol. Neurosurg. Psychiatry* **2009**, *80*, 1087–1092. [CrossRef]
24. Tanaka, M.; Sakaguchi, M.; Miwa, K.; Okazaki, S.; Furukado, S.; Yagita, Y.; Mochizuki, H.; Kitagawa, K. Basilar artery diameter is an independent predictor of incident cardiovascular events. *Arterioscler. Thromb. Vasc. Biol.* **2013**, *33*, 2240–2244. [CrossRef]
25. Kim, C.; Sohn, J.-H.; Jang, M.U.; Hong, S.-K.; Lee, J.-S.; Kim, H.-J.; Choi, H.-C.; Lee, J.H. Ischemia as a potential etiologic factor in idiopathic unilateral sudden sensorineural hearing loss: Analysis of posterior circulation arteries. *Hear. Res.* **2016**, *331*, 144–151. [CrossRef]
26. Huy, P.T.; Sauvaget, E. Idiopathic sudden sensorineural hearing loss is not an otologic emergency. *Otol. Neurotol.* **2005**, *26*, 896–902. [CrossRef]
27. Kuhn, M.; Heman-Ackah, S.E.; Shaikh, J.A.; Roehm, P.C. Sudden sensorineural hearing loss: A review of diagnosis, treatment, and prognosis. *Trends Amplif.* **2011**, *15*, 91–105. [CrossRef]
28. Forget, P.; Khalifa, C.; Defour, J.P.; Latinne, D.; Van Pel, M.C.; De Kock, M. What is the normal value of the neutrophil-to-lymphocyte ratio? *BMC Res. Notes* **2017**, *10*, 12. [CrossRef]
29. Lee, H.; Sohn, S.I.; Jung, D.K.; Cho, Y.W.; Lim, J.G.; Yi, S.D.; Lee, S.R.; Sohn, C.H.; Baloh, R.W. Sudden deafness and anterior inferior cerebellar artery infarction. *Stroke* **2002**, *33*, 2807–2812. [CrossRef]
30. Pogson, J.M.; Taylor, R.L.; Young, A.S.; McGarvie, L.A.; Flanagan, S.; Halmagyi, G.M.; Welgampola, M.S. Vertigo with sudden hearing loss: Audio-vestibular characteristics. *J. Neurol.* **2016**, *263*, 2086–2096. [CrossRef]
31. Murofushi, T.; Tsubota, M.; Suzuki, D. Idiopathic acute high-tone sensorineural hearing loss accompanied by vertigo: Vestibulo-cochlear artery syndrome? Consideration based on VEMP and vHIT. *J. Neurol.* **2019**, *266*, 2066–2067. [CrossRef]
32. Vofo, G.; de Jong, M.A.; Kaufman, M.; Meyler, J.; Eliashar, R.; Gross, M. The impact of vestibular symptoms and electronystagmography results on recovery from sudden sensorineural hearing loss. *J. Basic Clin. Physiol. Pharmacol.* **2021**, ahead of print. [CrossRef]
33. Sajid, T.; Ali, S.M.; Shah, M.I.; Hussain, A.; Zaman, A.; Qamar Naqvi, S.R.; Sajid, Z. Oral Corticosteroid Therapy for Sudden Sensorineural Hearing Loss and Factors Affecting Prognosis. *J. Ayub Med. Coll. Abbottabad JAMC* **2021**, *33*, 279–282.
34. Eryigit, B.; Ziylan, F.; Yaz, F.; Thomeer, H. The effectiveness of hyperbaric oxygen in patients with idiopathic sudden sensorineural hearing loss: A systematic review. *Eur. Arch. Otorhinolaryngol.* **2018**, *275*, 2893–2904. [CrossRef]
35. Jeng, J.S.; Yip, P.K. Evaluation of vertebral artery hypoplasia and asymmetry by color-coded duplex ultrasonography. *Ultrasound Med. Biol.* **2004**, *30*, 605–609. [CrossRef]
36. Cunningham, K.S.; Gotlieb, A.I. The role of shear stress in the pathogenesis of atherosclerosis. *Lab. Investig. A J. Tech. Methods Pathol.* **2005**, *85*, 9–23. [CrossRef]
37. Wu, S.; Cao, Z.; Shi, F.; Chen, B. Investigation of the prognostic role of neutrophil-to-lymphocyte ratio in Idiopathic Sudden Sensorineural Hearing Loss based on propensity score matching: A retrospective observational study. *Eur. Arch. Oto-Rhino-Laryngol.* **2020**, *277*, 2107–2113. [CrossRef]
38. Kang, J.W.; Kim, M.G.; Kim, S.S.; Im, H.I.; Dong, S.H.; Kim, S.H.; Yeo, S.G. Neutrophil-lymphocyte ratio as a valuable prognostic marker in idiopathic sudden sensorineural hearing loss. *Acta Oto-Laryngol.* **2020**, *140*, 307–313. [CrossRef]
39. Huh, G.; Bae, Y.J.; Woo, H.J.; Park, J.H.; Koo, J.W.; Song, J.J. Vestibulocochlear Symptoms Caused by Vertebrobasilar Dolichoectasia. *Clin. Exp. Otorhinolaryngol.* **2020**, *13*, 123–132. [CrossRef]
40. Gilbow, R.C.; Ruhl, D.S.; Hashisaki, G.T. Unilateral Sensorineural Hearing Loss Associated with Vertebrobasilar Dolichoectasia. *Otol. Neurotol.* **2018**, *39*, e56–e57. [CrossRef]
41. Wang, Y.; Huang, J.; Qian, G.; Jiang, S.; Miao, C. Study on the Correlation between different Levels of Patients with Vertebrobasilar Dolichoectasia and Posterior Circulation Blood Perfusion. *J. Stroke Cerebrovasc. Dis.* **2022**, *31*, 106378. [CrossRef]
42. Berrettini, S.; Seccia, V.; Fortunato, S.; Forli, F.; Bruschini, L.; Piaggi, P.; Canapicchi, R. Analysis of the 3-dimensional fluid-attenuated inversion-recovery (3D-FLAIR) sequence in idiopathic sudden sensorineural hearing loss. *JAMA Otolaryngol. Head Neck Surg.* **2013**, *139*, 456–464. [CrossRef]

43. Gao, Z.; Chi, F.L. The clinical value of three-dimensional fluid-attenuated inversion recovery magnetic resonance imaging in patients with idiopathic sudden sensorineural hearing loss: A meta-analysis. *Otol. Neurotol.* **2014**, *35*, 1730–1735. [CrossRef]
44. Hassler, O. Arterial pattern of human brainstem. Normal appearance and deformation in expanding supratentorial conditions. *Neurology* **1967**, *17*, 368–375. [CrossRef]
45. Nishijima, Y. Anatomical analysis of the basilar artery and its branches with special reference to the arterial anastomosis, and its course and distribution on the pontine ventral surface. *Nihon Ika Daigaku Zasshi* **1994**, *61*, 529–547. [CrossRef]

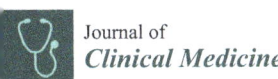 

Article

# Clinical and Cytokine Profile in Patients with Early and Late Onset Meniere Disease

Maria-Del-Carmen Moleon [1,2,3,†], Estrella Martinez-Gomez [1,3,†], Marisa Flook [1,3], Andreina Peralta-Leal [1], Juan Antonio Gallego [4], Hortensia Sanchez-Gomez [5], Maria Alharilla Montilla-Ibañez [6], Emilio Dominguez-Durán [7], Andres Soto-Varela [8], Ismael Aran [9], Lidia Frejo [1,3,‡] and Jose A. Lopez-Escamez [1,2,3,10,*,‡]

1. Otology and Neurotology Group CTS495, Department of Genomic Medicine, GENYO—Centre for Genomics and Oncological Research—Pfizer/University of Granada/Junta de Andalucía, PTS, 18016 Granada, Spain; mcarmenmoleon@gmail.com (M.-D.-C.M.); estrella.martinez@genyo.es (E.M.-G.); marisa.flook@genyo.es (M.F.); andreina.peralta@genyo.es (A.P.-L.); lidia.frejo@genyo.es (L.F.)
2. Department of Otolaryngology, Instituto de Investigación Biosanitaria ibs.Granada, Hospital Universitario Virgen de las Nieves, Universidad de Granada, 18014 Granada, Spain
3. Sensorineural Pathology Programme, Centro de Investigación Biomédica en Red en Enfermedades Raras, CIBERER, 28029 Madrid, Spain
4. Department of Neurology, Hospital Universitario Virgen de las Nieves, Universidad de Granada, 18014 Granada, Spain; jagaza16@correo.ugr.es
5. Otoneurology Unit, Department of Otorhinolaryngology, University Hospital of Salamanca, IBSAL, 37007 Salamanca, Spain; hortensiasanchez1@hotmail.com
6. Department of Otorhinolaryngology, Complejo Hospitalario de Jaén, 23007 Jaen, Spain; alharillamontilla@gmail.com
7. Department of Otolaryngology, Hospital Virgen Macarena, 41009 Sevilla, Spain; emiliodominguezorl@gmail.com
8. Division of Neurotology, Department of Otorhinolaryngology, Complexo Hospitalario Universitario, 15706 Santiago de Compostela, Spain; andres.soto@usc.es
9. Department of Otolaryngology, Complexo Hospitalario de Pontevedra, 36071 Pontevedra, Spain; ismaelaran2000@yahoo.com
10. Department of Surgery, Division of Otolaryngology, Facultad de Medicina, Universidad de Granada, 18006 Granada, Spain
* Correspondence: jalopezescamez@ugr.es; Tel.: +34-958-715-500-160
† M.-D.-C.M. and E.M.-G. shared co-first authorship.
‡ L.F. and J.A.L.-E. should be considered joint senior authors.

**Abstract:** Background: Meniere disease (MD) is an inner ear disorder associated with comorbidities such as autoimmune diseases or migraine. This study describes clinical and cytokine profiles in MD according to the age of onset of the condition. Methods: A cross-sectional study including 83 MD patients: 44 with early-onset MD (EOMD, <35 years old), and 39 with late-onset MD (LOMD, >50 years old), 64 patients with migraine and 55 controls was carried out. Clinical variables and cytokines levels of CCL3, CCL4, CCL18, CCL22, CXCL,1 and IL-1β were compared among the different groups. Results: CCL18 levels were higher in patients with migraine or MD than in controls. Elevated levels of IL-1β were observed in 11.4% EOMD and in 10.3% LOMD patients and these levels were not dependent on the age of individuals. EOMD had a longer duration of the disease ($p = 0.004$) and a higher prevalence of migraine than LOMD ($p = 0.045$). Conclusions: Patients with EOMD have a higher prevalence of migraine than LOMD, but migraine is not associated with any cytokine profile in patients with MD. The levels of CCL18, CCL3, and CXCL4 were different between patients with MD or migraine and controls.

**Keywords:** hearing loss; vertigo; migraine; cytokines; inflammation; vestibular disorders

## 1. Introduction

Patients with acute vertigo and a history of episodic vestibular symptoms represent a diagnostic challenge for clinicians [1,2]. Particularly, Meniere disease (MD), an inner ear

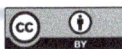

disorder characterized by sensorineural hearing loss (SNHL), attacks of episodic vertigo, is usually associated with tinnitus [3]. Some patients with MD also have migraine headaches and they usually show an early onset of auditory and vestibular symptoms [4,5].

Although the majority of MD patients are considered sporadic [3], familial clustering has been reported in 8% and 6% of cases in the Spanish [6] and South Korean populations [7]. Several genes have been identified in familial MD by exome sequencing, the most common being *OTOG*, found in 30% of familial cases [8]. Familial cases usually show early age of onset, but some non-familial cases (sporadic) may also develop the disease in the third decade of life. The mechanisms leading to this early onset of symptoms are not well understood and they may involve genetic, epigenetic, and environmental factors.

The epidemiological association of MD with migraine and some autoimmune diseases, supports the hypothesis of a wide clinical spectrum with a cochleo-vestibular phenotype. However, the effect of autoimmunity or migraine on the onset of the condition has not been investigated. Previous studies have shown that MD can be classified according to few clinical predictors, and it is possible to define subsets within unilateral MD (UMD) and bilateral MD (BMD) patients (Table 1) [4,5].

**Table 1.** Clinical subgroups of patients with unilateral and bilateral Meniere disease. Modified from Frejo et al. [4,5].

| **Unilateral Ménière's Disease (UMD)** |
| --- |
| Type 1: Sporadic and classical MD. |
| Type 2: Delayed MD |
| (hearing loss precedes vertigo attacks in months or years). |
| Type 3: Familial MD |
| (at least two individuals with MD related in the first or second degree). |
| Type 4: Sporadic MD with migraine |
| (temporal relationship not required). |
| Type 5: Sporadic MD plus an autoimmune disease. |
| **Bilateral Ménière's Disease (BMD)** |
| Type 1: Unilateral hearing loss becomes bilateral. |
| Type 2: Sporadic, simultaneous hearing loss (usually symmetric). |
| Type 3: Familial MD |
| (most families have bilateral hearing loss, but unilateral and bilateral cases may coexist in the same family). |
| Type 4: Sporadic MD with migraine. |
| Type 5: Sporadic MD with an autoimmune disease. |

The age of onset in patients with MD may differ according to the clinical subgroup. Interestingly, patients with MD and migraine (type 4) and individuals with MD with a co-morbid autoimmune condition (type 5) have an earlier age of onset than MD type 1 or 2 [5]. Moreover, it was also observed that MD types 4 and 5 have more vertigo attacks than the other groups [5]. Thereby, individuals with BMD showed an earlier age of onset, associated with a worse score in the AAO-HNS functional scale than patients with UMD among familial cases [6].

Previous studies have reported that basal levels of proinflammatory cytokines may be increased in some patients with MD [9], but the relationship between cytokine levels with the age of onset, migraine, or autoimmunity has not been investigated. The cytokine profile may represent two subgroups of MD patients with intrinsic differences in the immune response or two functional states of the immune system in patients with MD [9,10]. The studies mentioned before had defined different clinical subgroups in patients with UMD or BMD, but patients with MD and increased basal levels of cytokines and negative autoantibodies may be considered as an autoinflammatory condition of the inner ear [11].

The aim of the study is to characterize the clinical and cytokine profile, according to the age of onset in MD.

## 2. Experimental Section

### 2.1. Patient Assessment and Selection

A cross-sectional study was designed to recruit a total of 83 patients with MD. Eighteen of them were also included in a previous study [10]. Forty-four patients were considered as early-onset MD (EOMD, age of onset < 35 years old), 39 patients were classified as late-onset MD (LOMD, age of onset > 50 years old). We also recruited 64 migraine patients and 55 healthy controls that were selected from the MeDiC database to compare clinical and cytokine profiles among the different groups. All patients with MD were diagnosed according to the diagnostic criteria for MD described by the International Committee for the Classification Vestibular Disorders of the Barany Society [3], and a clinical evaluation was performed after obtaining informed consent. Patients with migraine were diagnosed according to the diagnostic criteria for migraine of the International Headache Society [12]. Patients with diagnostic criteria for vestibular migraine [13] were excluded from this study.

The experimental protocol of this study was approved by the Institutional Review Board in all participating hospitals, and each participant signed a written informed consent before donating blood samples (PE-0356-2018). The study was carried out according to the principles of the Declaration of Helsinki revised in 2013 for investigation with humans.

A complete audiological and vestibular assessment was carried out in all MD cases, including the following variables, sex, age, age of onset, duration of the disease, type of MD (uni/bilateral), main associated comorbidities (migraine, autoimmune disorders), and cytokine levels in peripheral venous blood. Serial pure-tone audiograms were retrieved from clinical records to assess hearing loss since the initial diagnosis. Clinical features of migraine patients recruited in the study are included in Table S1.

### 2.2. Peripheral Blood Mononuclear Cell (PBMC) Isolation and Incubation

Peripheral blood was diluted 1:1 with 1× PBS and disposed carefully into the corresponding 20:12 volume of Lymphosep, lymphocyte separation media (Biowest, Nuaillé, France). Samples were centrifuged for 20 min at 2000 rpm to separate blood content. PBMCs were collected and washed with 1× PBS twice and cultured in RPMI 1640 supplemented with 10% (v/v) fetal bovine serum (Biowest, Nuaillé, France) and plated at a concentration of $1 \times 10^6$ cells/mL in 6-well plates. PBMCs were incubated overnight at 37 °C in 7% $CO_2$. After the incubation, PBMCs were centrifuged, and supernatants were collected and stored at −80 °C until enough samples were acquired.

### 2.3. Cytokine Measurement

Frozen samples were thawed immediately prior to analysis and none of the samples underwent more than two freeze–thaw cycles prior to analysis. One cytokine (IL-1β) and five chemokines (CCL3, CCL4, CXCL1, CCL22, and CCL18) were measured using the commercially available Multiplex Bead-Based Kits (EMD Millipore, Billerica, MA, USA). The measurements were performed in accordance with the kit-specific protocols provided by Millipore, using a Luminex 200 platform (Luminex Corp., Austin, TX, USA) and read with Luminex x PONENT 3.1 software (Luminex Corp.). Two quality controls for each cytokine were run in duplicate.

### 2.4. Statistic and Data Analysis

A descriptive analysis was conducted using GraphPad Prism v8.0 (GraphPad Software, San Diego, CA, USA) for the clinical and cytokine data. Quantitative variables were displayed as the mean and standard deviation (SD). Qualitative variables were compared using Chi-square and Fisher exact test. Quantitative variables were compared using U Mann–Whitney test and the Pearson correlation coefficient. Analysis of variance (ANOVA) was used to compare the three groups of the study (MD, migraine patients, and healthy controls). The level of significance considered was $p < 0.05$. To find and remove the cytokines outlier values, we considered outlier values that were:

$$1.5 \times IQR > Q3$$

$$1.5 \times IQR < Q1,$$

where Q1 is the median of the lower half of the data set, Q3 is the median of the upper half of the data set, and IQR is the interquartile range, the difference from Q3 to Q1, [14]. Thus, from the total cytokines' measures of 61 MD patients, 64 migraine patients, and 55 control, we used 56, 59, and 42 measures respectively.

## 3. Results

### 3.1. Clinical Profile in Early and Late Onset MD

Table 2 includes all patients with EOMD. Twenty-three patients had been diagnosed as unilateral MD (54.5%) and 21 were considered bilateral MD (45.5%). Twenty-six (59%) were women and 18 (41%) were men.

**Table 2.** Clinical features and basal levels of IL-1β cytokine in patients with EOMD ($n$ = 44). Elevated levels of IL-1β are highlighted in bold type.

| Patient | Gender | Ear | Age of Onset | Duration of Disease (y) | FMD | Migraine | MD Subgroup | IL-1β Level |
|---|---|---|---|---|---|---|---|---|
| 1 | Woman | Bilateral | 34 | 8 | Yes | Yes | 3 | 3.68 |
| 2 | Woman | Bilateral | 33 | 8 | Yes | Yes | 3 | 1.24 |
| 3 | Woman | Unilateral | 28 | 12 | No | Yes | 4 | 0.82 |
| 4 | Man | Unilateral | 29 | 9 | No | No | 1 | 1.57 |
| 5 | Woman | Bilateral | 33 | 24 | No | Yes | 4 | 3.20 |
| 6 | Woman | Bilateral | 18 | 34 | Yes | No | 3 | 4.74 |
| 7 | Woman | Unilateral | 28 | 27 | No | X | 4 | 1.41 |
| 8 | Woman | Unilateral | 20 | 1 | Yes | Yes | 3 | **18.64** |
| 9 | Woman | Unilateral | 28 | 8 | No | No | 2 | 3.69 |
| 10 | Woman | Unilateral | 29 | 20 | Yes | Yes | 3 | 2.79 |
| 11 | Man | Bilateral | 27 | 16 | No | No | 2 | 2.64 |
| 12 | Woman | Bilateral | 33 | 8 | No | Yes | 4 | 2.10 |
| 13 | Woman | Bilateral | 24 | 15 | No | Yes | 4 | **28.45** |
| 14 | Woman | Bilateral | 33 | 17 | No | No | 5 | 1.66 |
| 15 | Woman | Bilateral | 23 | 18 | No | Yes | 4 | 1.59 |
| 16 | Man | Bilateral | 31 | 15 | No | Yes | 1 | 1.25 |
| 17 | Man | Unilateral | 34 | 8 | No | No | 1 | 0.49 |
| 18 | Woman | Unilateral | 27 | 17 | No | No | 1 | 2.11 |
| 19 | Man | Bilateral | 35 | 16 | No | No | 1 | 0.92 |
| 20 | Woman | Bilateral | 34 | 20 | No | No | 1 | 3.68 |
| 21 | Woman | Unilateral | 35 | 20 | Yes | No | 3 | 0.01 |
| 22 | Man | Bilateral | 29 | 15 | No | No | 2 | 0.18 |
| 23 | Man | Unilateral | 29 | 11 | No | No | 1 | 0 |
| 24 | Man | Unilateral | 24 | 1 | No | No | 1 | 1.84 |
| 25 | Man | Unilateral | 30 | 27 | No | Yes | 1 | **46.41** |
| 26 | Man | Bilateral | 27 | 22 | No | No | 1 | 0 |
| 27 | Man | Unilateral | 32 | 3 | No | No | 1 | 2.77 |
| 28 | Man | Bilateral | 22 | 23 | Yes | Yes | 1 | 0.44 |
| 29 | Woman | Bilateral | 31 | 5 | No | Yes | 1 | 1.14 |
| 30 | Man | Bilateral | 22 | 22 | No | No | 1 | 1.57 |
| 31 | Man | Bilateral | 25 | 25 | No | No | 1 | 0.31 |
| 32 | Man | Bilateral | 34 | 34 | No | No | 1 | 1.14 |
| 33 | Man | Bilateral | 28 | 18 | No | No | 1 | **18.18** |
| 34 | Woman | Unilateral | 28 | 25 | No | No | 5 | 2.19 |
| 35 | Woman | Unilateral | 23 | 50 | No | No | 1 | 3.14 |
| 36 | Woman | Unilateral | 29 | 30 | No | No | 5 | **6.66** |
| 37 | Woman | Unilateral | 23 | 50 | No | No | 1 | 3.07 |
| 38 | Man | Unilateral | 27 | 5 | No | No | 1 | 1.79 |
| 39 | Woman | Unilateral | 18 | 18 | Yes | Yes | 3 | 4.68 |
| 40 | Woman | Unilateral | 35 | 20 | No | No | 1 | 0 |

Table 2. Cont.

| Patient | Gender | Ear | Age of Onset | Duration of Disease (y) | FMD | Migraine | MD Subgroup | IL-1β Level |
|---|---|---|---|---|---|---|---|---|
| 41 | Woman | Unilateral | 21 | 2 | Yes | No | 3 | 0 |
| 42 | Man | Unilateral | 24 | 28 | Yes | No | 3 | 0.80 |
| 43 | Woman | Unilateral | 18 | 9 | Yes | Yes | 2 | 0.69 |
| 44 | Woman | Unilateral | 24 | 28 | No | Yes | 4 | 1.37 |

Table 3 shows all individuals with LOMD. Twenty-six (67%) had been diagnosed as unilateral MD and 13 had bilateral MD (33.3%). Twenty-one (54%) were women and 18 (46%) men.

**Table 3.** Clinical features and basal levels of IL-1β cytokine in patients with LOMD (*n* = 39). Elevated levels of IL-1β are highlighted in bold type.

| Patient | Gender | Ear | Age of Onset | Duration of Disease (y) | FMD | Migraine | MD Subgroup | IL-1β Level |
|---|---|---|---|---|---|---|---|---|
| 1 | Man | Bilateral | 55 | 20 | No | No | 2 | 0.83 |
| 2 | Woman | Unilateral | 65 | 8 | Yes | No | 3 | 1.23 |
| 3 | Man | Unilateral | 50 | 13 | No | No | 1 | 1.56 |
| 4 | Man | Bilateral | 55 | 30 | No | No | 2 | 2.24 |
| 5 | Man | Unilateral | 61 | 16 | No | No | 1 | 2.64 |
| 6 | Woman | Unilateral | 50 | 23 | Yes | No | 3 | 2.10 |
| 7 | Man | Bilateral | 53 | 16 | No | No | 2 | 3.14 |
| 8 | Woman | Unilateral | 50 | 8 | No | No | 1 | 2.67 |
| 9 | Man | Bilateral | 53 | 30 | No | No | 2 | 4.34 |
| 10 | Man | Unilateral | 50 | 14 | Yes | No | 3 | **6.93** |
| 11 | Man | Unilateral | 62 | 1 | No | Yes | 4 | 0.01 |
| 12 | Woman | Unilateral | 52 | 17 | No | Yes | 4 | 0.57 |
| 13 | Woman | Bilateral | 56 | 24 | No | No | 2 | 2.27 |
| 14 | Woman | Unilateral | 55 | 10 | No | No | 1 | 2.06 |
| 15 | Woman | Unilateral | 63 | 13 | Yes | Yes | 3 | 1.07 |
| 16 | Man | Bilateral | 56 | 5 | No | No | 2 | 0.58 |
| 17 | Man | Unilateral | 53 | 2 | Yes | Yes | 3 | 0.01 |
| 18 | Man | Bilateral | 54 | 3 | No | No | 2 | 1.03 |
| 19 | Woman | Bilateral | 53 | 4 | No | Yes | 4 | 2.67 |
| 20 | Man | Bilateral | 55 | 17 | Yes | No | 3 | 1.27 |
| 21 | Woman | Unilateral | 50 | 20 | Yes | No | 3 | 1.73 |
| 22 | Woman | Bilateral | 55 | 9 | Yes | Yes | 3 | **5.95** |
| 23 | Woman | Unilateral | 50 | 8 | No | No | 1 | 3.07 |
| 24 | Woman | Bilateral | 52 | 6 | No | No | 2 | 1.03 |
| 25 | Man | Bilateral | 53 | 2 | Yes | Yes | 3 | 3.68 |
| 26 | Woman | Unilateral | 56 | 2 | No | No | 1 | 0.83 |
| 27 | Man | Unilateral | 57 | 2 | No | No | 1 | 1.66 |
| 28 | Man | Bilateral | 53 | 7 | No | No | 2 | 0.39 |
| 29 | Woman | Unilateral | 65 | 1 | No | Yes | 4 | **4.96** |
| 30 | Man | Unilateral | 69 | 2 | No | No | 1 | 0.76 |
| 31 | Man | Unilateral | 66 | 5 | No | No | 1 | 2.33 |
| 32 | Woman | Unilateral | 51 | 5 | No | No | 1 | 4.67 |
| 33 | Woman | Unilateral | 63 | 6 | No | No | 1 | 3.94 |
| 34 | Woman | Unilateral | 61 | 6 | No | No | 1 | 1.25 |
| 35 | Man | Unilateral | 51 | 7 | No | No | 1 | 1.52 |
| 36 | Woman | Unilateral | 50 | 8 | No | No | 1 | **5.79** |
| 37 | Woman | Unilateral | 54 | 1 | Yes | No | 3 | 1.32 |
| 38 | Woman | Unilateral | 57 | 6 | Yes | No | 3 | 1.47 |
| 39 | Woman | Unilateral | 54 | 7 | No | Yes | 1 | 3.47 |

There was no difference in the frequency of FMD between patients with EOMD (11 patients, 25%) and LOMD (11 patients, 28%). Eighteen years was the mean duration of the disease in EOMD patients, whereas in LOMD patients the mean was 9.8 years old. In our series, elevated levels of IL-1β (>4.78 pg/mL) were observed in 5 of 44 (11.3%) patients with EOMD and in 4 of 39 (10.3%) patients with LOMD.

### 3.2. EOMD Has a Higher Prevalence of Migraine Than LOMD Patients

Table 4 compares the clinical features of patients with EOMD and LOMD. Patients with EOMD had a longer duration of the disease, defined as the time since the onset of the symptoms than patients with LOMD ($p = 0.004$). As expected, both groups of MD patients had similar hearing loss thresholds, familial history of hearing loss, and prevalence of vascular risk factors. However, EOMD patients presented a higher frequency of migraine than LOMD patients ($p = 0.045$), but no differences were found for any type of headache between both groups.

**Table 4.** Clinical features of patients with EOMD and LOMD included in the study. Migraine was more frequently observed in patients with EOMD.

| Variable | EOMD ($n = 44$) | LOMD ($n = 39$) | $p$-Value |
|---|---|---|---|
| Duration of the disease (mean ± SD) | 18.0 ± 11.4 | 9.8 ± 7.9 | **0.0004** |
| Age of onset (mean ± SD) | 27.7 ± 4.9 | 55.6 ± 5.2 | **<0.0001** |
| Sex (% female) | 59.0 | 53.8 | 0.195 |
| Bilateral hearing loss (%) | 45.5 | 33.3 | 0.545 |
| Hearing loss (% synchronic) | 29.5 | 12.8 | 0.338 |
| MD type | | | 0.589 |
| 1 | 21 | 15 | |
| 2 | 4 | 9 | |
| 3 | 9 | 4 | |
| 4 | 7 | 3 | |
| 5 | 3 | 0 | |
| Hearing loss (%) | | | 0.357 |
| High frequency | 61.4 | 69.2 | |
| Low frequency | 38.6 | 30.8 | |
| Family History of hearing loss (%) | 25.0 | 28.2 | 0.999 |
| Any Headache (%) | 59.0 | 56.4 | 0.440 |
| Migraine (%) | **38.6** | **23.0** | **0.045** |
| Arterial Hypertension (%) | 22.7 | 25.6 | 0.948 |
| Smoking (%) | 13.6 | 10.3 | 0.532 |
| Dyslipidemia (%) | 18.2 | 28.2 | 0.400 |
| Diabetes Mellitus (%) | 25.0 | 25.6 | 0.854 |

Significant differences ($p < 0.05$) are highlighted in bold.

### 3.3. Cytokine Levels Do Not Allow to Distinguish between EOMD and LOMD Patients

Cytokines were measured in 56 MD patients (40 EOMD and 16 LOMD). We did not observe any differences between the levels of IL-1β or any of the chemokines CCL3, CCL4, CXCL1, CCL22, CCL8 (all $p$-values > 0.1, (Figure S1). However, when we performed a sex-specific analysis, there were significant differences in EOMD for IL-1β, with higher values in men ($p = 0.039$), and for CXCL1 with higher values in women ($p = 0.007$, Figure 1). Moreover, CCL3 levels were significantly higher in LOMD women than men ($p = 0.04$).

### 3.4. Cytokines Levels Do Not Differ between Patients with and without Migraine in MD

Since patients with EOMD presented a higher prevalence of migraine than LOMD ($p = 0.045$), we compared cytokines levels considering migraine as a clinical covariable. However, none of the cytokines or chemokines measured showed significant differences between patients with and without migraine in MD (Figure 2). Interestingly, the prevalence of a comorbid autoimmune disease was significantly higher in patients with MD and migraine compared to patients without migraine ($p < 0.001$).

We also separated MD patients according to IL-1β levels into two groups: MD with high levels of IL-1β (MDH) and low levels of IL-1β (MDL) (Figure 3). However, we found no difference in the relative frequency of patients according to the clinical subgroups and IL-1β levels (Table 5).

**Table 5.** Frequency distribution of patients with MD according to the clinical subgroup and IL-1β levels.

| Variable | MDH (n = 9) | MDL (n = 74) | p-Value |
|---|---|---|---|
| MD type (%) | | | 0.9924 |
| 1 | 3 (33.3) | 33 (44) | |
| 2 | 0 (0) | 13 (14.6) | |
| 3 | 3 (33.3) | 17 (22.9) | |
| 4 | 2 (22.2) | 9 (12.1) | |
| 5 | 1 (11.1) | 2 (2.7) | |

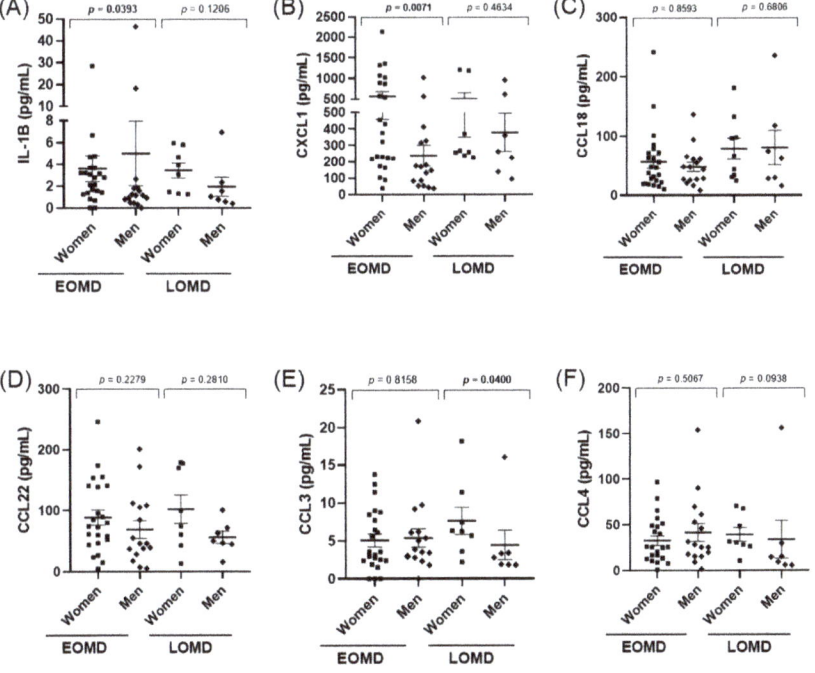

**Figure 1.** Scatter plots showing medians and IQRs for IL-1β (**A**), CXCL1(**B**), CCL18 (**C**), CCL22 (**D**), CCL3 (**E**), CCL4 (**F**), levels measured in PBMC's supernatant in patients with EOMD and LOMD. Cytokine and chemokine levels were compared between men and women by the Mann–Whitney test and p-values are shown for each comparison. Significant differences ($p < 0.05$) are highlighted in bold.

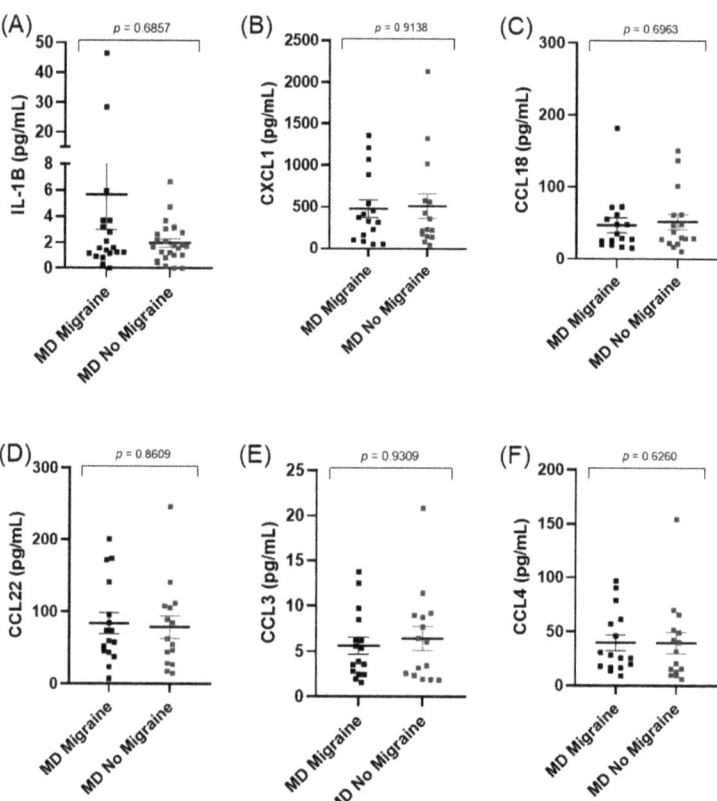

**Figure 2.** Scatter plots showing cytokine and chemokines levels in patients with MD (**A–F**), stratified according to the presence of migraine.

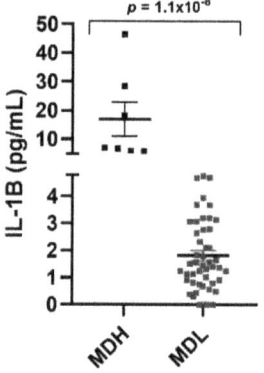

**Figure 3.** MD patients separated according to their IL-1β levels (MDH (>4.78 pg/mL) and MDL (<4.78 pg/mL)).

*3.5. Cytokines Levels Do Not Differ between Familial (FMD) and Sporadic (SMD) MD Patients*

We observed that the IL-1β levels were not different between familial and sporadic MD, however, significant differences were found in CXCL1 ($p = 0.024$) and CCL22 ($p = 0.012$), (Figure 4). Moreover, CXCL1 and CCL22 levels showed a higher correlation in FMD ($r = 0.62$) than in sporadic cases ($r = 0.37$).

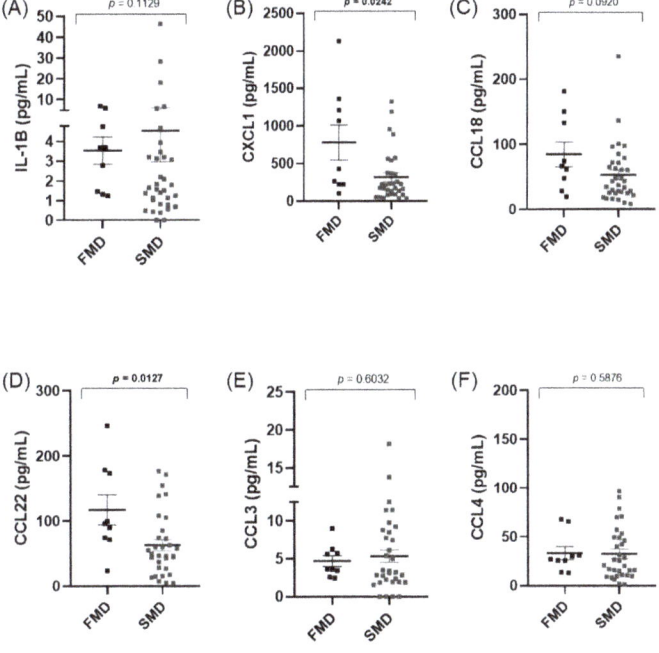

**Figure 4.** Cytokines and chemokine levels in patients with familial or sporadic MD (**A–F**). FMD: Familial Meniere disease Significant differences; SMD: Sporadic Meniere disease; ($p < 0.05$) are highlighted in bold.

*3.6. CCL18, CCL22, and CCL4 Levels Are Different between Patients with MD, Migraine, and Controls*

Levels of IL-1β, CCL3, CCL4, CXCL1, CCL22, and CCL8 were also measured in 55 healthy controls and 64 migraine patients. Significant differences were found in the levels of CCL18 ($p = 0.001$), CCL22 ($p = 0.03$), and CCL4 ($p = 0.02$) when we compared MD, migraine, and controls; however, no differences were found in IL-1β or CCL18 levels of MD vs. migraine patients (Figure 5).

We could observe that the levels of CCL18 were higher in patients with MD or migraine when they were compared to controls. However, CCL18 levels did not allow to distinguish between MD and migraine ($p = 0.74$). Moreover, no correlation was found in CCL18 levels and the age of the patients, either in controls ($p = 0.59$), patients with MD ($p = 0.43$), or migraine ($p = 0.23$) (Figure S2).

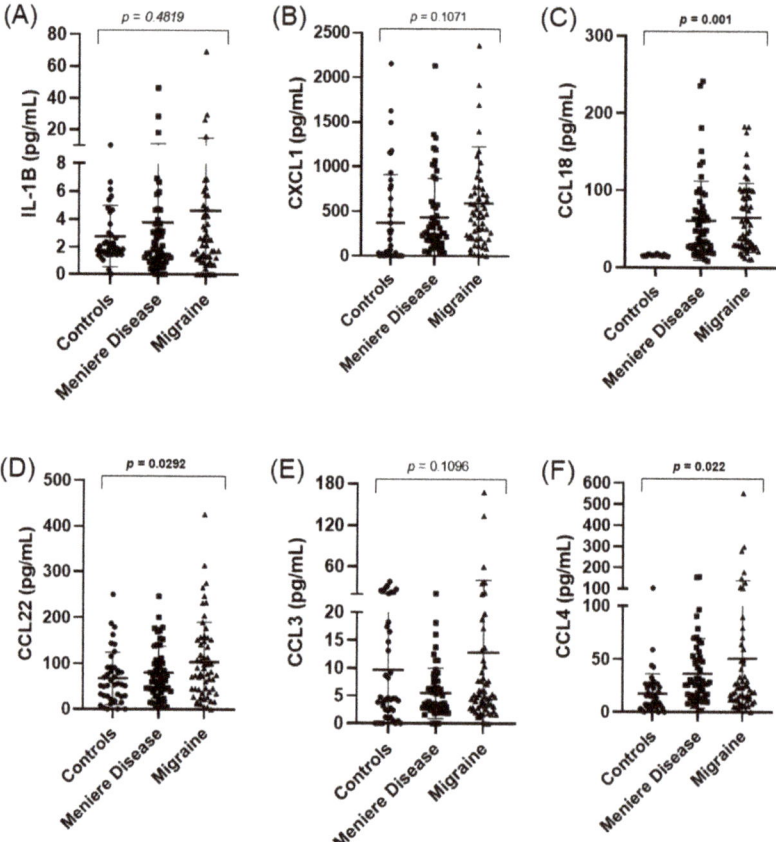

**Figure 5.** Scatter plots showing cytokines with the concentrations of IL-1β (**A**), CXCL1 (**B**), CCL18 (**C**), CCL22 (**D**), CCL3 (**E**), and CCL4 (**F**) in healthy controls, patients with MD, and migraine. Significant differences ($p < 0.05$) are highlighted in bold.

## 4. Discussion

This study analyzes the clinical profile and the levels of several cytokines and chemokines (IL-1β, CCL3, CCL4, CCL22, CCL18, and CXCL1) in patients with MD, according to the age of onset of the disease. The age of onset in MD follows a normal distribution [4,5] with a mean of ~43 years old. We selected Spanish MD patients < 35 and >50 years from the Meniere Disease Consortium to investigate clinical features in patients with early- and late-onset, respectively. The time of onset was confirmed from the medical records

The main finding is that migraine is more frequently observed in patients with EOMD than in LOMD, but the levels of cytokines are not related to the age of onset in MD.

Previous studies have reported that ~20% of patients with MD show high levels of pro-inflammatory cytokines, including IL-1β, TNF-α, and IL-6 [9]. Moreover, Flook et al. (2019) revealed significant differences in several cytokines and chemokines between patients with MD and vestibular migraine, suggesting that this set of protein biomarkers could distinguish MD and vestibular migraine [10].

The findings in this study do not support the hypothesis that the peripheral profile of immune molecules is related to the age of onset in MD or the presence of migraine. Therefore, we measured the levels of IL-1β, CCL3, CCL4, CXCL1, CCL22, and CCL18 in a cohort of 83 patients with MD, which included 44 EOMD and 39 LOMD, and 64 patients with migraine without vestibular symptoms to control the effect of migraine itself on cytokine levels.

We tested the hypothesis that activation of IL-1β signaling contributes to maintaining an autoinflammatory response in MD, however, this response is not age-dependent. Considering that we observed a cytokine increase in PBMCs extracted from peripheral blood, this could indicate that a subgroup of patients with MD has a systemic pro-inflammatory response, which could explain some patient's responses to anti-inflammatory drugs [15,16]. Our study shows that IL-1β concentrations are not age-dependent, neither in MD patients nor healthy controls. Of note, we also found that IL-1β levels are higher in a subgroup of patients with migraine, suggesting a pro-inflammatory state in these patients.

We observed that EOMD patients have a higher prevalence of migraine as a comorbid condition compared to LOMD. This finding confirms the observation reported by Frejo et al. that patients with MD and migraine (type 4) presented an earlier onset than the rest of patients with MD [4,5].

In addition, the clinical association between autoimmunity and MD suggests the possibility of an autoimmune endophenotype according to the immune role of the endolymphatic sac or the synthesis of cytokines [17]. There are two different endotypes of MD patients, according to the pathology of the endolymphatic sac: one endotype characterized by the epithelial degeneration of the endolymphatic sac and a second endotype showing hypoplasia of the endolymphatic sac [18]; however, the cytokine profile or the association with migraine with the hypoplastic or degenerative endolymphatic sac has not been investigated.

To our knowledge, this is the first study in which inflammatory biomarkers and clinical phenotypes were simultaneously assessed both in adult men and women with early-onset as well as late-onset MD. We found an overall reduction in the systemic levels of inflammatory markers in men with EOMD or LOMD, where significant differences were observed for IL-1β, CXCL1, and CCL3. Moreover, we observed no significant differences in other inflammatory biomarkers between groups.

Familial MD has an earlier onset than sporadic cases, suggesting that early-onset patients might have a higher genetic burden, including patients with a potential recessive inheritance. Previous studies have shown that there is an enrichment of rare missense variants in some genes related to hearing loss, such as: *GJB2*, *USH1G*, *SLC26A*, *USH1G*, *ESRRB*, and *CLDN14*, as well as in some genes implicated in the "axonal guidance signaling" signaling pathway such as *NTN4* and *NOX3*, in patients with sporadic MD [19]. This excess of missense variants in some genes may increase the risk of developing hearing loss in MD [20]. We have found higher levels of CXCL1 and CCL22 in familial MD, but the relevance of this finding is unclear. The chemokine CXCL1 recruits and activates neutrophils to the site of infection [21], and it is essential for the expression of pro-inflammatory mediators, activation of NF-kB, and MAPKs [22]. CCL22 is a macrophage-derived chemokine and a potent chemoattractant for chronically activated T-lymphocytes [23,24]. CCL22 is thought to be involved in several conditions, including allergy, autoimmunity, and tumor growth [24], and increased CCL22 expression has been reported in autoinflammatory skin diseases [25].

There are several mechanisms that may drive the onset of MD. A persistent inflammatory response may affect one or both ears and local factors could be involved. The accumulation of endolymph is the result of inner ear damage usually associated with sensorineural hearing loss [26].

The autoinflammatory disease of the inner ear might include an innate immune response mediated by monocytes, IL-1β, and non-specific autoantibodies [27]. In healthy individuals, IL-1 RA is detectable in plasma and IL-1β levels are usually not detectable. IL-1 RA levels were more elevated in most patients with MD regardless of the levels of IL-1β [9]. It was also observed that only 58 genes were differentially expressed in MD patients with high basal levels of IL-1β, supporting the hypothesis that this abnormal response may facilitate the identification of a subgroup of MD patients with a specific gene expression profile [9].

Cytokines are considered as pain mediators in neurovascular inflammation, and therefore, they may cause the generation of migraine pain [28]. Changes in inflammatory activity in migraine patients may be one of the main causes of endothelial dysfunction. The increase in endothelial cell permeability leads to an increase in the paracellular leakage of plasma fluid and proteins [29].

Different findings have been reported in the clinical studies measuring cytokine levels in migraine patients [30–33]. These studies have indicated that immunological changes could play a role in the pathophysiology of migraine. We can speculate that increased release of CCL18 observed in patients with migraine in combination with other pro-inflammatory mediators is likely to contribute to a persistent inflammatory state that may trigger the onset of MD in susceptible individuals. This subgroup of patients with MD and migraine may have an earlier onset and higher risk of autoinflammation.

In addition, the lack of correlation between age and IL-1β plasma levels, regardless of the important role of aging in the immune response, suggests that genetic or epigenetic factors are needed to develop MD in patients with migraine [34].

Our study shows that a better understanding of how the immune mediators could influence the age of onset in MD disease is of great relevance to provide clues on potential strategies to delay the onset of MD in susceptible individuals in an increasingly aged population.

## 5. Limitations of the Study

The main limitation of our study is that the number of investigated patients was low ($n = 83$), and further patients will be needed to validate our findings. Our study is limited by the cross-sectional design and the small number of cytokines and clinical data collected, so it may be not enough to classify patients with MD according to the age of onset. Moreover, the lack of correlation between the age of individuals and IL-1β or CCL18 levels suggest inter-individual differences associated with multiple factors, including migraine.

## 6. Conclusions

1. Patients with EOMD have a higher prevalence of migraine than patients with LOMD.
2. The levels of IL-1β or chemokines were not dependent on the age of the individuals or the presence of migraine in patients with MD.
3. The levels of CCL18, CCL22, and CCL4 were different between patients with MD or migraine and controls.

**Supplementary Materials:** The following are available online at https://www.mdpi.com/article/10.3390/jcm10184052/s1. Table S1. Clinical features and basal levels of IL-1β cytokine in migraine patients ($n = 64$); Figure S1. Distribution of cytokines levels in patients with EOMD and LOMD; Figure S2. Scattered plot showing CCL18 levels as a function of age of patients and years of disease evolution in healthy controls. patients with MD and migraine.

**Author Contributions:** J.A.L.-E. designed the study; M.-D.-C.M., E.M.-G., L.F. and J.A.L.-E. drafted the manuscript; M.-D.-C.M., M.A.M.-I., J.A.G., H.S.-G., E.D.-D., A.S.-V. and I.A. retrieved all clinical data; E.M.-G., M.F. and A.P.-L. carried out experimental work and cytokine measurements; M.-D.-C.M. and E.M.-G. contributed equally and have the right to list their names first in their CV; L.F. and J.A.L.-E. have revised all statistical analyses and approved the final version of the manuscript, and they are prepared to take total responsibility for the integrity of the content. All authors have read and agreed to the published version of the manuscript.

**Funding:** J.A.L.-E. has received funds from ISCIII and European Regional Funds (Grants PI17/01644 and PI20/01126) and Andalusian Health Government (Grant PE-0356-2018). J.A.L.-E. and E.M.-G. have also received funds from the Andalusian Health Government (Grant PI-0027-2020).

**Institutional Review Board Statement:** The experimental protocol of this study was approved by the Institutional Review Board in all participating hospitals (PE-0356-2018).

**Informed Consent Statement:** Informed consent was obtained from all subjects involved in the study.

**Data Availability Statement:** All data generated or analysed during this study are included in this article and its Supplementary Information files.

**Acknowledgments:** Maria-Del-Carmen Moleon is a student in the Biomedicine Program at the Doctorate School at the University of Granada and this work is part of her Doctoral Thesis. We would like to thank all patients for their participation in this study.

**Conflicts of Interest:** The authors declare no conflict of interest.

## References

1. Teggi, R.; Colombo, B.; Albera, R.; Libonati, G.A.; Balzanelli, C.; Caletrio, A.B.; Casani, A.; Espinoza-Sanchez, J.M.; Gamba, P.; Lopez-Escamez, J.A.; et al. Clinical Features, Familial History, and Migraine Precursors in Patients with Definite Vestibular Migraine: The VM-Phenotypes Projects. *Headache J. Head Face Pain* **2018**, *58*, 534–544. [CrossRef]
2. Seemungal, B.; Kaski, D.; Lopez-Escamez, J.A. Early Diagnosis and Management of Acute Vertigo from Vestibular Migraine and Ménière's Disease. *Neurol. Clin.* **2015**, *33*, 619–628. [CrossRef]
3. Lopez-Escamez, J.A.; Carey, J.; Chung, W.H.; Goebel, J.A.; Magnusson, M.; Mandala, M.; Newman-Toker, D.E.; Strupp, M.; Suzuki, M.; Trabalzini, F.; et al. Diagnostic criteria for Menière's disease. *J. Vestib. Res.* **2015**, *25*, 1–7. [CrossRef]
4. Frejo, L.; Soto-Varela, A.; Santos-Perez, S.; Aran, I.; Caletrio, A.B.; Perez-Guillen, V.; Perez-Garrigues, H.; Fraile, J.; Martin-Sanz, E.; Tapia, M.C.; et al. Clinical Subgroups in Bilateral Meniere Disease. *Front. Neurol.* **2016**, *7*, 182. [CrossRef] [PubMed]
5. Frejo, L.; Martin-Sanz, E.; Teggi, R.; Trinidad-Ruiz, G.; Soto-Varela, A.; Santos-Perez, S.; Manrique, R.; Perez, N.; Aran, I.; Almeida-Branco, M.S.; et al. Extended phenotype and clinical subgroups in unilateral Meniere disease: A cross-sectional study with cluster analysis. *Clin. Otolaryngol.* **2017**, *42*, 1172–1180. [CrossRef] [PubMed]
6. Requena, T.; Espinosa-Sanchez, J.M.; Cabrera, S.; Trinidad-Ruiz, G.; Soto-Varela, A.; Santos-Perez, S.; Teggi, R.; Perez, P.; Caletrio, A.B.; Fraile, J.; et al. Familial clustering and genetic heterogeneity in Meniere's disease. *Clin. Genet.* **2014**, *85*, 245–252. [CrossRef]
7. Lee, J.M.; Kim, M.J.; Jung, J.; Kim, H.J.; Seo, Y.J.; Kim, S.H. Genetic aspects and clinical characteristics of familial meniere's disease in a South Korean population. *Laryngoscope* **2015**, *125*, 2175–2180. [CrossRef]
8. Roman-Naranjo, P.; Gallego-Martinez, A.; Soto-Varela, A.; Aran, I.; Moleon, M.D.C.; Espinosa-Sanchez, J.M.; Amor-Dorado, J.C.; Batuecas-Caletrio, A.; Vázquez, P.P.; Lopez-Escamez, J.A. Burden of Rare Variants in the OTOG Gene in Familial Meniere's Disease. *Ear Hear.* **2020**, *41*, 1598–1605. [CrossRef]
9. Frejo, L.; Gallego-Martinez, A.; Requena, T.; Martin-Sanz, E.; Amor-Dorado, J.C.; Soto-Varela, A.; Santos-Perez, S.; Espinosa-Sanchez, J.M.; Batuecas-Caletrio, A.; Aran, I.; et al. Proinflammatory cytokines and response to molds in mononuclear cells of patients with Meniere disease. *Sci. Rep.* **2018**, *8*, 5974. [CrossRef] [PubMed]
10. Flook, M.; Frejo, L.; Gallego-Martinez, A.; Martin-Sanz, E.; Rossi-Izquierdo, M.; Amor-Dorado, J.C.; Soto-Varela, A.; Santos-Perez, S.; Batuecas-Caletrio, A.; Espinosa-Sanchez, J.M.; et al. Differential Proinflammatory Signature in Vestibular Migraine and Meniere Disease. *Front. Immunol.* **2019**, *10*, 1229. [CrossRef]
11. Flook, M.; Escamez, J.A.L. Meniere's Disease: Genetics and the Immune System. *Curr. Otorhinolaryngol. Rep.* **2018**, *6*, 24–31. [CrossRef]
12. Arnold, M. Headache Classification Committee of the International Headache Society (IHS) the International Classification of Headache Disorders. *Cephalalgia* **2018**, *38*, 1–211. [CrossRef]
13. Lempert, T.; Olesen, J.; Furman, J.; Waterston, J.; Seemungal, B.; Carey, J.; Bisdorff, A.; Versino, M.; Evers, S.; Newman-Toker, D. Vestibular migraine: Diagnostic criteria. *J. Vestib. Res.* **2012**, *22*, 167–172. [CrossRef]
14. Moore, D.S.; McCabe, G.P. *Introduction to the Practice of Statistics*, 5th ed.; W.H. Freeman & Company: New York, NY, USA, 2005.
15. Strupp, M.; Thurtell, M.; Shaikh, A.G.; Brandt, T.; Zee, D.S.; Leigh, R.J. Pharmacotherapy of vestibular and ocular motor disorders, including nystagmus. *J. Neurol.* **2011**, *258*, 1207–1222. [CrossRef] [PubMed]
16. Espinosa-Sanchez, J.M.; Lopez-Escamez, J. Menière's disease. In *The Human Hypothalamus—Neuroendocrine Disorders*; Elsevier BV: Amsterdam, The Netherlands, 2016; Volume 137, pp. 257–277.
17. Greco, A.; Gallo, A.; Fusconi, M.; Marinelli, C.; Macri, G.; de Vincentiis, M. Meniere's disease might be an autoimmune condition? *Autoimmun. Rev.* **2012**, *11*, 731–738. [CrossRef] [PubMed]
18. Bächinger, D.; Luu, N.-N.; Kempfle, J.S.; Barber, S.; Zürrer, D.; Lee, D.J.; Curtin, H.D.; Rauch, S.D.; Nadol, J.B.; Adams, J.C.; et al. Vestibular Aqueduct Morphology Correlates with Endolymphatic Sac Pathologies in Menière's Disease—A Correlative Histology and Computed Tomography Study. *Otol. Neurotol.* **2019**, *40*, e548–e555. [CrossRef]
19. Gallego-Martinez, A.; Requena, T.; Roman-Naranjo, P.; May, P.; A Lopez-Escamez, J. Enrichment of damaging missense variants in genes related with axonal guidance signalling in sporadic Meniere's disease. *J. Med. Genet.* **2019**, *57*, 82–88. [CrossRef] [PubMed]
20. Gallego-Martinez, A.; Requena, T.; Roman-Naranjo, P.; Lopez-Escamez, J.A. Excess of Rare Missense Variants in Hearing Loss Genes in Sporadic Meniere Disease. *Front. Genet.* **2019**, *10*, 76. [CrossRef]
21. Jin, L.; Batra, S.; Douda, D.N.; Palaniyar, N.; Jeyaseelan, S. CXCL1 Contributes to Host Defense in Polymicrobial Sepsis via Modulating T Cell and Neutrophil Functions. *J. Immunol.* **2014**, *193*, 3549–3558. [CrossRef]
22. Sawant, K.V.; Poluri, K.M.; Dutta, A.K.; Sepuru, K.M.; Troshkina, A.; Garofalo, R.P.; Rajarathnam, K. Chemokine CXCL1 mediated neutrophil recruitment: Role of glycosaminoglycan interactions. *Sci. Rep.* **2016**, *6*, 33123. [CrossRef]

23. Atri, C.; Guerfali, F.Z.; Laouini, D. Role of Human Macrophage Polarization in Inflammation during Infectious Diseases. *Int. J. Mol. Sci.* **2018**, *19*, 1801. [CrossRef]
24. Scheu, S.; Ali, S.; Ruland, C.; Arolt, V.; Alferink, J. The C-C Chemokines CCL17 and CCL22 and Their Receptor CCR4 in CNS Autoimmunity. *Int. J. Mol. Sci.* **2017**, *18*, 2306. [CrossRef]
25. Yamashita, U.; Kuroda, E. Regulation of Macrophage-Derived Chemokine (MDC/ CCL22) Production. *Crit. Rev. Immunol.* **2002**, *22*, 105–114. [CrossRef]
26. Tonndorf, J. Endolymphatic hydrops: Mechanical causes of hearing loss. *Eur. Arch. Oto-Rhino-Laryngol.* **1976**, *212*, 293–299. [CrossRef] [PubMed]
27. Vambutas, A.; Pathak, S. AAO: Autoimmune and Autoinflammatory (Disease) in Otology: What is New in Immune-Mediated Hearing Loss. *Laryngoscope* **2016**, *1*, 110–115. [CrossRef] [PubMed]
28. Empl, M.; Sostak, P.; Riedel, M.; Schwarz, M.; Müller, N.; Förderreuther, S.; Straube, A. Decreased Stnf-Ri in Migraine Patients? *Cephalalgia* **2003**, *23*, 55–58. [CrossRef] [PubMed]
29. Gurol, G.; Ciftci, I.H.; Harman, H.; Karakece, E.; Kamanli, A.; Tekeoglu, I. Roles of claudin-5 and von Willebrand factor in patients with rheumatoid arthritis. *Int. J. Clin. Exp. Pathol.* **2015**, *8*, 1979–1984.
30. Yücel, M.; Kotan, D.; Gurol Çiftçi, G.; Çiftçi, I.H.; Cikriklar, H.I. Serum levels of endocan, claudin-5 and cytokines in mi-graine. *Eur. Rev. Med. Pharmacol. Sci.* **2016**, *20*, 930–936.
31. Conti, P.; D'Ovidio, C.; Conti, C.; Gallenga, C.E.; Lauritano, D.; Caraffa, A.; Kritas, S.K.; Ronconi, G. Progression in migraine: Role of mast cells and pro-inflammatory and anti-inflammatory cytokines. *Eur. J. Pharmacol.* **2019**, *844*, 87–94. [CrossRef]
32. Fidan, I.; Yüksel, S.; Ýmir, T.; Irkeç, C.; Aksakal, F.N. The importance of cytokines, chemokines and nitric oxide in pathophysiology of migraine. *J. Neuroimmunol.* **2006**, *171*, 184–188. [CrossRef]
33. Oliveira, A.B.; Bachi, A.; Ribeiro, R.T.; de Mello, M.T.; Tufik, S.; Peres, M.F.P. Unbalanced plasma TNF-α and IL-12/IL-10 profile in women with migraine is associated with psychological and physiological outcomes. *J. Neuroimmunol.* **2017**, *313*, 138–144. [CrossRef] [PubMed]
34. Gallego-Martinez, A.; Lopez-Escamez, J.A. Genetic architecture of Meniere's disease. *Hear. Res.* **2020**, *397*, 107872. [CrossRef] [PubMed]

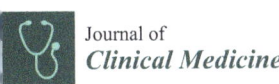

*Article*

# Hearing Benefits of Clinical Management for Meniere's Disease

Yi Zhang [1,2], Chenyi Wei [1,2], Zhengtao Sun [1,2], Yue Wu [1,2], Zhengli Chen [1,2] and Bo Liu [1,2,*]

1. Department of Otolaryngology Head and Neck Surgery, Beijing Tongren Hospital, Capital Medical University, Beijing 100730, China; zhangyi_trhos@mail.ccmu.edu.cn (Y.Z.); weichenyi_ent@163.com (C.W.); zhengtaosun@mail.ccmu.edu.cn (Z.S.); wuyue19940507@sina.com (Y.W.); chenzhengli@mail.ccmu.edu.cn (Z.C.)
2. Beijing Institute of Otolaryngology, Key Laboratory of Otolaryngology Head and Neck Surgery, Ministry of Education, Beijing 100730, China
* Correspondence: trliubo@xwh.ccmu.edu.cn; Tel.: +86-01-5826-5816

**Abstract:** Meniere's disease is a progressive hearing–disabling condition. Patients can benefit from strict clinical management, including lifestyle and dietary counseling, and medical treatment. A prospective cohort study was carried out with 154 patients with definite Meniere's disease, with an average age of 43.53 ± 11.40, and a male to female ratio of 0.97:1. The pure-tone thresholds of all 165 affected ears, over a one-year clinical management period, were analyzed. After one year, 87.27% of patients had improved or preserved their hearing at a low frequency, and 71.51% at a high frequency. The hearing threshold at frequencies from 250 Hz to 2000 Hz had improved significantly ($p < 0.001$, $p < 0.001$, $p < 0.001$, $p < 0.01$), and deteriorated slightly at 8000 Hz ($p < 0.05$). Of all the patients, 40.00% had a hearing average threshold that reached ≤25 dB HL after the clinical management period, among whom 27.27% were patients in stage 3. The restoration time was 2.5 (1.0, 4.125) months, with a range of 0.5–11.0 months, and the restoration time was longer for stage 3 than for stages 1 and 2 ($u = -2.542$, $p < 0.05$). The rising curves improved the most ($p < 0.05$), with most becoming peaks, whereas most peaks and flats remained the same. Patients who were initially in the earlier stages (95% CI 1.710~4.717, OR 2.840, $p < 0.001$), have an increased odds ratio of hearing by an average of ≤25 dB HL. Age (95% CI 1.003~1.074, OR 1.038, $p = 0.031$), peak curve (95% CI 1.038~5.945, OR = 2.484, $p = 0.041$), and flat curve (95% CI 1.056~19.590, OR = 4.549, $p = 0.042$), compared with the rising curve, increase the odds ratio of hearing on average by >25 dB HL. Most patients can have their hearing preserved or improved through strict clinical management, and sufficient follow-up is also essential. Stage 3 patients also have the potential for hearing improvement, although the restoration time is longer than in the early stages. The initial hearing stage, age, and audiogram pattern are related to the hearing benefits.

**Keywords:** Meniere's disease; sensorineural hearing loss; clinical management; pure-tone audiometry

**Citation:** Zhang, Y.; Wei, C.; Sun, Z.; Wu, Y.; Chen, Z.; Liu, B. Hearing Benefits of Clinical Management for Meniere's Disease. *J. Clin. Med.* **2022**, *11*, 3131. https://doi.org/10.3390/jcm11113131

Academic Editors: George Psillas and Eng Ooi

Received: 14 April 2022
Accepted: 28 May 2022
Published: 31 May 2022

**Publisher's Note:** MDPI stays neutral with regard to jurisdictional claims in published maps and institutional affiliations.

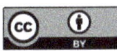

**Copyright:** © 2022 by the authors. Licensee MDPI, Basel, Switzerland. This article is an open access article distributed under the terms and conditions of the Creative Commons Attribution (CC BY) license (https://creativecommons.org/licenses/by/4.0/).

## 1. Introduction

Meniere's disease (MD) is a chronic unique inner ear disease associated with endolymphatic hydrops by histopathology, and is characterized by recurrent spontaneous vertigo, fluctuating sensorineural hearing loss (SNHL), tinnitus, and aural fullness [1]. Though not curable, patients with Meniere's disease can experience symptom relief and prevent permanent damage to their hearing through clinical management.

The Bárány society defines Meniere's disease as episodic vestibular syndrome in the International Classification of Vestibular Disorders (ICVD) [2]. The lesions of the auditory and vestibular system occur either simultaneously, or some precede others [3]. The effects of vertigo are always taken seriously; however, part of vertigo is the fluctuating and gradual decline in the hearing, which can potentially develop into a hearing disability. Hearing loss was included in the original description of this disease and is still considered a necessary criterion by the current international consensus. It is generally known that the audiogram has characteristic features and specific fluctuation patterns [4]. The hearing loss usually occurs at low frequencies and is accompanied by hearing fluctuations, which are characteristic of the early stages of Meniere's disease [5–7]. In this period, most patients' hearing loss is reversible; therefore, as the disease progresses, hearing tends to present full-frequency, moderate-to-severe hearing loss, and loss becomes permanent [8]. Those who have poor hearing often give up hopes of recovery. Nevertheless, residual hearing is vital. Progressive and occult hearing loss will often confuse patients and be ignored by doctors who have no complete knowledge system.

The treatment for Meniere's disease consists of reducing attacks, relieving symptoms, and preventing permanent damage to hearing. Lifestyle changes, diuretics, vasodilators, corticosteroids, intratympanic therapy, and surgical treatment methods are preferred. Although there is currently no complete cure for Meniere's disease, clinical management, which includes lifestyle and dietary changes, medical treatment, psychological counseling, or minimally invasive procedures, such as intratympanic steroid therapy, helps most patients [4,9,10]. Clinically, fluctuating and progressive sensorineural hearing loss is relatively refractory to treatment, whereas episodic vertigo is usually quite responsive [11]; however, the prevention of hearing disabilities is as important as the control of vertigo. The World Report on Hearing 2021 [12] revealed that nearly 1.5 billion people worldwide live with some degree of hearing loss, and nearly 430 million have moderate to severe hearing loss. Many studies have shown that more than half of Meniere's patients had hearing loss at an advanced stage, as they are either at stage 3 or 4 [13,14]. Control of the hearing lesion is the main aim of the management of Meniere's disease due to its great importance for the patients' quality of life, whether for symptom control, hearing disability prevention, functional rehabilitation, and even a reduction in the economic burden on patients and society.

The repeated attack, fluctuation, and progression of Meniere's disease are consistent with the modality of chronic disease; therefore, it also needs to be managed according to the clinical practice of chronic diseases. The importance of lifestyle adjustment is put forward in the guidelines for MD. We conducted a study with a small series of patients and found that the hearing restoration of MD patients takes months; however, that observation period was only three months. A more extended observation was needed. During this observation period, strict clinical management and close follow-ups were needed for practice. In this study, the term "clinical management", in its broadest sense, refers to the management of the core components of lifestyle adjustment and medical treatment.

Moreover, hearing features have rarely been studied and reported in recent years after the treatment and criteria were updated; there is no clear consensus among different studies regarding the characteristics and evolution of audiometric thresholds and the morphology of the audiogram of patients at different stages of Meniere's disease. In 1995, the American Academy of Otolaryngology-Head and Neck Surgery (AAO-HNS) devised a staging system based on the average hearing threshold of pure-tone audiometry (PTA) [15]. This staging system provides a relatively objective basis for the clinical classification of severity and emphasizes the importance of understanding the progression of hearing loss in this disease. According to previous studies, four main audiometric patterns have been described in patients with Meniere's disease: (1) the ascending type with low-frequency decline, (2) the descending type with high-frequency decline, (3) the peak type with low-frequency and high-frequency decline, and (4) the flat type with total frequency decline [16]. An audiogram and its changing regularity [17–19] provide the recognizable audiological features of the disease. Our study is based on the above practical staging system and audiometric patterns; therefore, we followed up with a group of patients with Meniere's disease, we analyzed and reported their hearing benefits after one year of strict clinical management, and investigated any hearing-related information that may be crucial for determining hearing prognosis in patients with Meniere's disease.

## 2. Materials and Methods

### 2.1. Study Participants

This is a prospective cohort study with pre- and post- intervention comparisons with the same group of patients. These patients were diagnosed with definite Meniere's disease for whom audiological data were collected in the Hearing and Vestibular Clinic of the Department of Otorhinolaryngology of the tertiary hospital from August 2017 to November 2020. All procedures carried out in studies involving human participants were consistent with the ethical standards of the Ethics Committee of the Hospital.

Inclusion criteria: (1) all patients were diagnosed with definite Meniere's disease according to the diagnostic criteria approved by the Classification Committee of the Bárány Society (2015) [1]: (a) two or more spontaneous episodes of vertigo, each lasting 20 min to 12 h; (b) audiometrically documented low-to-medium frequency sensorineural hearing loss in one ear, defining the affected ear on at least one occasion before, during, or after one of the episodes of vertigo; (c) fluctuating aural symptoms in the affected ear; and (d) symptoms not better accounted for by another vestibular diagnosis. (2) Subjects also met the following hearing loss criteria: low-frequency hearing of the affected ear is defined as greater increases in pure-tone thresholds (i.e., worse) than the contralateral ear by at least 30 dB HL at each of the two contiguous frequencies below 2000 Hz. In cases of bilateral hearing loss, the absolute low-frequency thresholds must be 35 dB HL or higher at each of the two contiguous frequencies below 2000 Hz. (3) All the patients consented to receive continuous follow-ups for one year or longer.

Exclusion criteria: (1) the specified conditions to be excluded include, including vestibular migraines, superior semicircular canal dehiscence syndrome, sudden hearing loss, labyrinthitis, drug-induced deafness, posterior circulation ischemia, schwannoma, definite autoimmune inner ear disease, delayed endolymphatic hydrops, and intracranial tumor. (2) Patients with Meniere's disease who had received an intratympanic gentamicin injection, endolymphatic sac surgery, semicircular canal occlusion, vestibular neurectomy, or cochlear implant surgery were excluded.

Ultimately, a total of 156 patients were enrolled in the study, for two of whom follow-up data were lost for not coming back on time. Finally, the hearing of 165 ears in 154 patients was analyzed. There was unilateral Meniere's disease in 143 ears and bilateral Meniere's disease in 22 ears, with an average age of 43.53 ± 11.40 (19–70 years old), consisting of 76 males (49.35%) and 78 females (50.65%), with a male-to-female ratio of 0.97:1 (Table 1).

Table 1. Overview of the patients with definite Meniere's disease.

| Clinical Features | Unilateral MD | Bilateral MD | p-Value |
|---|---|---|---|
| Age (year) (mean ± SD) | 43.24 ± 11.56 | 47.27 ± 8.60 | 0.260 • |
| Sex (n) | | | |
| Male | 70 | 6 | 0.764 † |
| Female | 73 | 5 | |
| Sides (n) | | | |
| Right | 67 | 11 | 0.822 † |
| Left | 76 | 11 | |
| Comorbidities (n) | | | |
| Migraine | 36 | 1 | 0.403 ° |
| Familial Meniere's history | 2 | 0 | 1.000 * |
| Autoimmune disease | 6 | 2 | 0.190 ° |
| Duration of the disease (months) (Median, IQR) | 16 (6, 27) | 36 (6, 48) | 0.293 # |
| Initial hearing average (dB HL) | 41.84 ± 15.76 | 40.15 ± 12.90 | 0.632 • |
| Initial stage (n) | | | |
| 1 | 24 | 4 | |
| 2 | 46 | 7 | 1.000 * |
| 3 | 69 | 11 | |
| 4 | 4 | 0 | |

• Student's t-test; † Chi-square test; * Fisher's test; ° Continuity Correction; # Mann–Whitney U test.

*2.2. Procedures*

All the patients registered clinical information in detail, including sex and age. Medical histories were recorded in detail. Examination of otology was routinely performed. Pure tone audiometry was taken routinely. MRI of the internal auditory canal and posterior fossa was taken to exclude other diseases which can present vertigo and audiometrically verified asymmetric sensorineural hearing loss. Caloric and head impulse tests were used for the evaluation of the vestibular system's status. The audiograms were analyzed as evidence.

Regarding clinical management, when they received the diagnosis, all patients received education regarding a low-sodium diet, avoidance of particular foods and products, such as alcohol, caffeine, monosodium glutamate, excessive tea, and so on. Healthy lifestyle modifications and psychological counseling are needed, such as quitting smoking, avoiding allergy triggers, getting plenty of sleep, maintaining a good mood, taking part in appropriate physical activities, and so on. Patients were encouraged to make notes relating to their health. During the treatment course, patients were provided pharmacologic treatment with necessary steroids, betahistine, diuretics, or ginkgo preparation for the days or months of the trial, in order to control symptoms and maintain a stable state. When patients experienced an acute attack, systemic steroid therapy or local steroid injection were options for treating patients' hearing loss. The systemic steroid was given prednisone 5 mg/kg/d as an initial dosage, for approximately 10–14 days with a slow tapering dose, and a local steroid injection was performed instead if there were contraindications with the systemic use of the steroid or when used as a supplementary treatment. Moreover, the patients temporarily used vestibular inhibitors during acute vertigo attacks and used betahistine with other medications for vertigo control at other times. We used betahistine 36 mg/d, for the attack and interval therapy. The treatment duration depends on patients' symptoms, including vertigo and hearing loss. Hence, some patients used betahistine for several months, usually 3 to 6. Hydrochlorothiazide 25 mg/d as diuretics were used when patients were refractory to steroids and betahistine. Ginkgo biloba preparations at 57.6 mg/d, were not opposed to if needed. Vestibular rehabilitation exercise was performed during the non-acute period if needed. Patients were encouraged to keep a health diary. In addition, a one-year clinical follow-up was conducted.

*2.3. Audiometric Measurement*

The pure-tone audiometric data were collected by professionals with a GSI 61 audiometer in a standard soundproof room, which limited the background noise to below 18 dB A. The audiometric thresholds for 250, 500, 1000, 2000, 4000, and 8000 Hz were determined by air and bone conduction, and narrow-band noise was used for masking.

The poorest audiogram within six months of the interval before entering the study determined the patients' onset hearing level, and their poorest audiogram at the one-year point (12 months ± 0.5 months) was taken as the hearing level after the one-year follow-up. For the criterion of clinical hearing improvement or deterioration, a greater than 5 dB change was used as an outcome measure [5,20]. The pure-tone threshold results were analyzed using two groups of frequencies: (1) low frequency (the average threshold value of 250, 500, and 1000 Hz) and (2) high frequency (the average threshold value of 4000 and 8000 Hz). As the Bárány Society (2015) [1] and the AAO-HNS Committee on Hearing and Equilibrium criteria for Meniere's disease (1995) [15] have recommended, we finally staged the hearing from stage 1 to stage 4 using the average threshold corresponding to ≤25 dB HL, 26–40 dB HL, 41–70 dB HL, and >70 dB HL, respectively. In this study, staging was applied to evaluate the status of patients before treatment. During the one year of follow-up, the patients' hearing was re-evaluated in order to draw comparisons.

To classify different types of the audiometric curve objectively, we referred to the function that Mateijsen and his colleagues [16] used to classify the curves, and made fine-tuning corrections according to the methods of other studies found in the literature [21,22]. Two professionals performed the fine-tuning. If the advice reached an agreement, the correction was made; however, if there was no consensus, the final result was based on the formula.

## 2.4. Statistical Analysis

The database was established using Excel 2016, and statistical analysis was conducted using IBM SPSS Statistics for Windows, Version 24.0 (IBM Corp., Armonk, NY, USA). MATLAB was used for visualization. The data presented a normal distribution using the Kolmogorov–Smirnov test and are expressed as the mean and standard deviation; Student's *t*-test and a chi-square test were used for comparisons between groups. Nonnormally distributed data were represented by quartile spacing and the Wilcoxon signed-rank test, whereas Spearman's rank–order correlation test was used for comparisons between groups. Binary logistic regression was used to analyze risk factors. $p < 0.05$ was considered statistically significant.

## 3. Results

### 3.1. Initial Hearing

Affected ears at stage 3, and with a peak curve, represented the greatest proportion of all the collected hearing data. Table 2 showed the distribution of different stages and audiometric curves of these patients. The proportion of patients at stage 3 reached their highest at 49% (80/165); the rest were 17% (28/165) at stage 1, 32% (53/165) at stage 2, and 2% (4/165) at stage 4, respectively. The peak curves accounted for the greatest proportion in each stage. Moreover, the proportion of flat curves rose from stage 1 to stage 4. There was no difference in the composition of the curve type of each stage ($\chi^2 = 14.064$, $p = 0.08$). There was a significant correlation between the average threshold of low and high frequencies ($r = 0.433$, $p < 0.001$), and the coefficient of high frequency:low frequency was 0.676:1.

**Table 2.** The number and proportion of each stage and curve type (n (%)).

|         | Rising  | Falling | Peak    | Flat    | Total     |
|---------|---------|---------|---------|---------|-----------|
| Stage 1 | 10 (36) | 2 (7)   | 16 (57) | 0 (0)   | 28 (100)  |
| Stage 2 | 14 (26) | 11 (21) | 25 (47) | 3 (6)   | 53 (100)  |
| Stage 3 | 23 (29) | 16 (20) | 28 (35) | 13 (16) | 80 (100)  |
| Stage 4 | 1 (25)  | 0 (0)   | 2 (50)  | 1 (25)  | 4 (100)   |
| Total   | 48 (29) | 29 (18) | 71 (43) | 17 (10) | 165 (100) |

### 3.2. Hearing Benefits after Clinical Management

#### 3.2.1. Hearing Benefits and Hearing Restoration

Of the affected ears, 87.27% had improved or preserved hearing at a low frequency (66.06% improved and 21.21% preserved), and 71.51% at a high frequency (24.24% improved and 47.27% preserved). In Figure 1, a clear, steady hearing improvement can be seen at 250 Hz ($z = -8.330$, $p < 0.001$), 500 Hz ($z = -7.391$, $p < 0.001$), 1000 Hz ($z = -5.856$, $p < 0.001$), and 2000 Hz ($z = -2.845$, $p = 0.004$). Notably, at 4000 Hz, there is no significant difference ($z = -0.263$, $p = 0.792$). In contrast, the 8000 Hz threshold showed a slight deterioration ($z = -2.001$, $p = 0.045$).

The most striking result that emerged from the data is that 66 affected ears (40.00%) were restored to, or preserved at, a normal hearing level (average threshold $\leq 25$ dB HL). The restoration time was 2.5 (1.0, 4.125) months, with a range of 0.5–11.0 months. The restoration time of the advanced stages (stages 3 and 4) (3.0 (1.75, 6.25 months)) was longer than that of the early stages (stages 1 and 2) (2.0 (0.56, 3.00 months)), and the differences were statistically significant ($u = -2.542$, $p = 0.011$). The patients with hearing thresholds that reached $\leq 25$ dB HL were younger than those with a hearing average >25 dB HL. Whether the hearing reached $\leq 25$ dB HL or not had no relationship to sex, but there was a significant difference with regard to the initial audiometric curve patterns (Table 3).

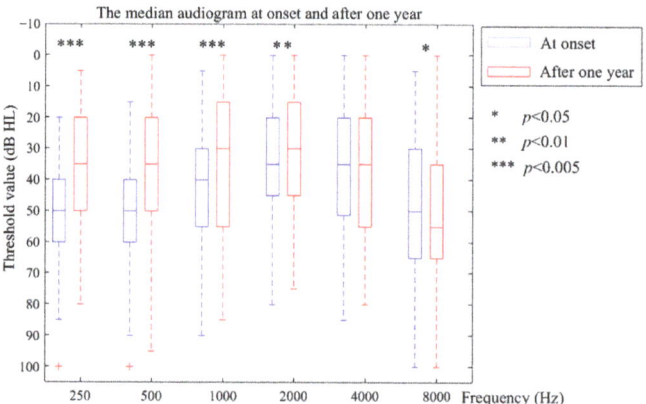

**Figure 1.** The medium audiogram at onset and after one year.

**Table 3.** The comparison between different hearing results of the patients after clinical management.

| | Group | Restored Average Thresholds ≤ 25 dB HL | Restored Average Thresholds > 25 dB HL | p-Value |
|---|---|---|---|---|
| N | | 66 | 99 | |
| Age (year) | | 40.05 ± 10.70 | 46.26 ± 11.01 | <0.001 • |
| Sex (n) | | | | |
| | male | 30 | 52 | |
| | female | 36 | 47 | 0.428 † |
| Initial stage (n) | | | | |
| | 1 | 19 | 9 | |
| | 2 | 29 | 24 | |
| | 3 | 18 | 62 | <0.001 * |
| | 4 | 0 | 4 | |
| Initial curve (n) | | | | |
| | rising | 28 | 20 | |
| | falling | 8 | 21 | |
| | peak | 27 | 44 | 0.007 † |
| | flat | 3 | 14 | |

• Student's *t*-test; † Chi-square test; * Fisher's test.

### 3.2.2. Hearing Benefits for Different Stages

The advanced stages still have potential for improvement. Figure 2 reveals that there were steady hearing benefits in the most affected ears after the one-year clinical management period. At the low frequency, the hearing at stage 2 (t = 4.945, $p < 0.001$) and stage 3 (t = 8.349, $p < 0.001$) improved significantly, whereas at stage 1 (t = 1.166, $p > 0.05$) and stage 4 (t = 2.818, $p = 0.067$), it did not show a significant difference. At 2000 Hz, at stage 1 (t = −2.228, $p = 0.034$), hearing deteriorated, and at stage 3 (t = 4.518, $p < 0.001$), it improved, whereas the changes in the other two stages did not show a significant difference ($p > 0.05$). At the high frequency, at stage 1 (t = −2.273, $p = 0.031$), hearing deteriorated, and at stage 4 (t = 4.371, $p = 0.022$), it improved significantly, whereas the change in the other two stages did not show a significant difference ($p > 0.05$). In terms of average hearing threshold value, at stage 2 (t = 3.283, $p = 0.002$), hearing deteriorated slightly, and at stage 3 (t = 7.436, $p < 0.001$), it improved slightly. The hearing of patients at advanced stages (stages 3 and 4) improved more both at low (t = 3.409, $p = 0.001$) and high (t = 2.333, $p = 0.021$) frequencies than that of patients at an early stage (stages 1 and 2).

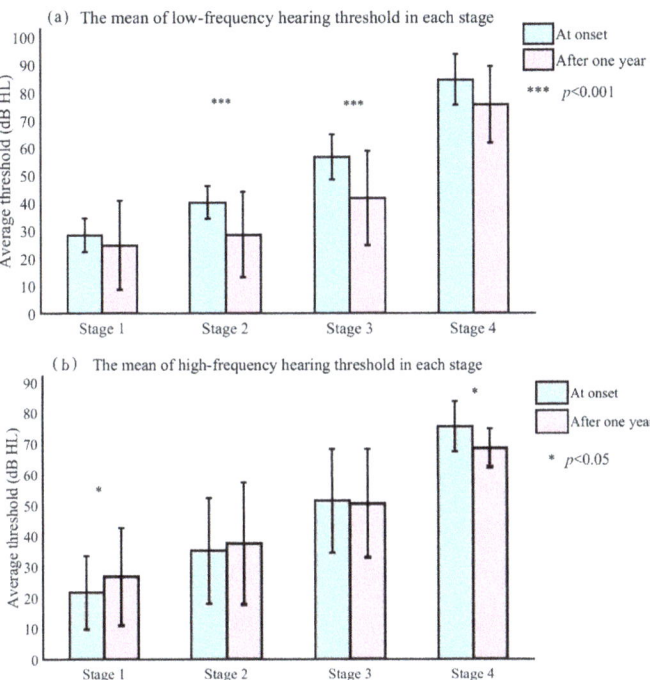

**Figure 2.** The mean low-frequency and high-frequency hearing thresholds at onset and after one year for each stage.

What stands out in Figure 3 is that the majority of the affected ears had an improved or preserved hearing level. For the individuals, the hearing of the majority (67.86%) at stage 1 was still ≤25 dB HL, whereas a small proportion had progressed to stage 2 (21.43%) or stage 3 (10.71%); nearly half (54.72%) of the affected ears at stage 2 improved their hearing to ≤25 dB HL, 26.42% remained at 26–40 dB HL, and 18.87% progressed to 41–70 dB HL; half (50.00%) of the stage 3 patients remained at 41–70 dB HL, 22.50% improved to <25 dB HL, 26.25% improved to 26–40 dB HL, and 1.25% progressed to >70 dB HL. Of the four affected ears at stage 4, two improved to 41–70 dB HL, and the other two remained at >70 dB HL.

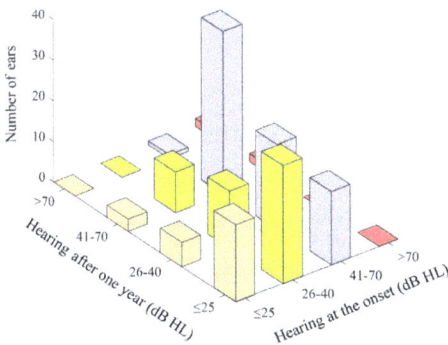

**Figure 3.** The changes in patients' average hearing thresholds over one year.

### 3.2.3. Hearing Benefits for Different Audiometric Curves

Figure 4 shows that there were steady hearing benefits in most patients with different audiometric curves. At the low frequency, all types improved significantly (i.e., from 50.49 dB HL to 30.63 dB HL (t = 9.688, $p < 0.001$), 42.41 dB HL to 35.29 dB HL (t = 2.390, $p = 0.024$), 44.79 dB HL to 35.49 dB HL (t = 4.555, $p < 0.001$), and 56.67 dB HL to 47.35 dB HL (t = 2.336, $p = 0.033$)) by means of rising, falling, peak, and flat curves, respectively. At the high frequency, there was a slight deterioration in the rising (t = −2.032, $p = 0.048$) and peak curves (t = −1.215, $p > 0.05$), and a slight improvement in the falling (t = 1.333, $p = 0.193$) and flat curves (t = 1.065, $p = 0.303$), but there was no significant difference between various types (F = 2.539, $p = 0.058$).

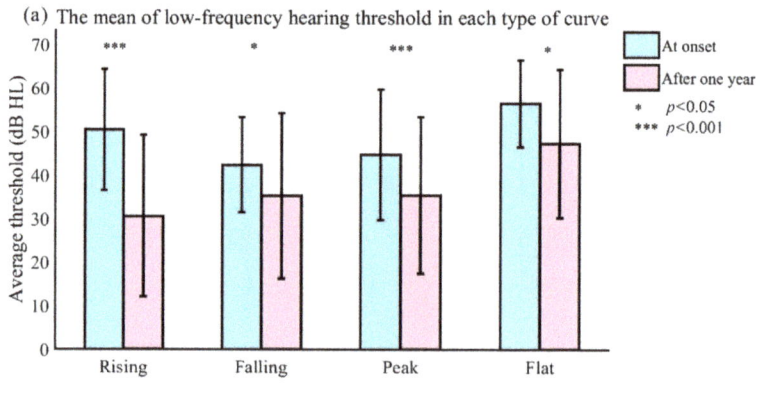

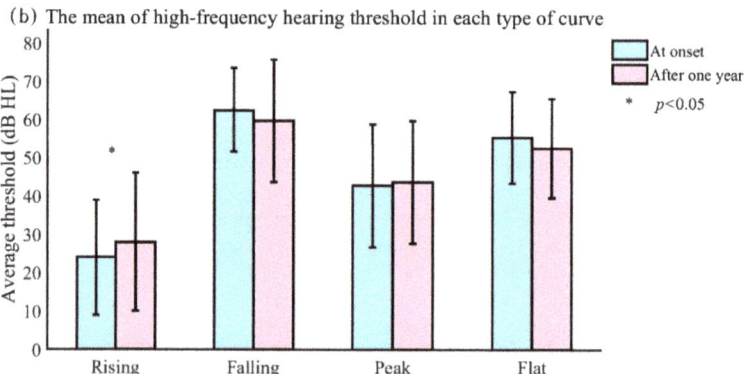

**Figure 4.** The mean of the low- and high-frequency hearing thresholds at onset and after one year of each type of curve.

What can be clearly seen in Figure 5 is the general pattern of the changes in the audiometric curves. For 46.48% of individuals, the rising curves at onset were likely to turn to peak curves after one year; for 14.58%, rising curves were maintained as rising curves; 14.58% showed a change to falling curves; and 29.17% showed a change to flat curves. The majority (89.66%) of the falling curves maintained the same type of curve. Nearly half (46.48%) of the peak curves were maintained as peak curves, 30.99% became falling curves, 18.31% became flat curves, and 4.23% became rising curves. Nearly half (47.06%) of the flat curves remained flat, whereas 29.41% became falling curves, 17.65% became peak curves, and 5.88% became rising curves.

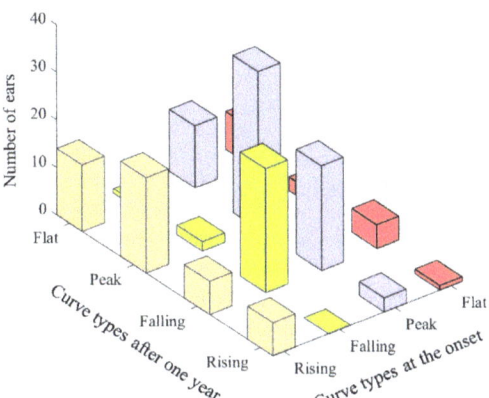

**Figure 5.** Changes in patients' curve types over one year.

3.2.4. Multiple Factors Analysis of Hearing Benefits Based on Pure-Tone Audiometry

The dependent variable was defined as whether the average thresholds reached ≤25 dB HL after clinical management, and the independent variables and covariates included sex (male, female), age, audiometric curve (four types), and the initial stage (stage 1, 2, 3, and 4). Patients at an earlier stage initially (95% CI 1.710~4.717, OR 2.840, $p < 0.001$) had an increased odds ratio of hearing, on average, ≤ 25 dB HL. Age (95% CI 1.003~1.074, OR 1.038, $p = 0.031$) increased the odds ratio of hearing to an average of > 25 dB HL. Compared with the rising curve, the peak curve (95% CI 1.038~5.945, OR = 2.484, $p = 0.041$) and flat curve (95% CI 1.056~19.590, OR = 4.549, $p = 0.042$) increased the odds ratio of hearing to an average threshold of >25 dB HL. There was no relationship between sex and hearing restoration.

## 4. Discussion

In this study, we proposed a practical clinical management plan. Clinical and laboratory studies have indicated that Meniere's disease is the clinical expression of inner ear changes caused by the progressive dysfunction of the accumulated endolymph and can progress to hearing disability. Although initial treatment includes lifestyle changes and pharmacologic therapy, many individuals eventually progress to hearing loss, but few lose hearing entirely, even in the later stages [23]; therefore, it is necessary to preserve the patient's hearing as early as possible. The treatment is complicated since hearing, vertigo control, tinnitus, and suppression are all intertwined, and thus, are tricky to treat separately. Both pharmacologic and surgical treatment may be effective for some patients and ineffective for others [24,25]; however, there is no current cure for Meniere's disease, which is especially crucial for sensorineural hearing loss. For surgical therapy, patients and doctors sometimes find a clinical course difficult to decide on. This does not mean an opposition to surgery, but we need to determine when and how to choose. Preserving the structure appropriately is of the same importance. Nevertheless, most patients will benefit from criterial clinical management.

In this study, pure-tone audiometry is used for data collection and deep analysis. The treatment of hearing in Meniere's disease consists of a series of practical methods, which needs efficient management. High-efficiency diagnosis and evaluation are the key points; however, high-efficiency diagnosis and management remain challenging for clinicians. During the past decade, magnetic resonance imaging, electrocochleography, and many other techniques have been developed for the inner ear, leading to advancements in diagnosing Meniere's disease; however, we still require a non-invasive, cost-effective, and universally available test with high sensitivity and specificity for Meniere's disease. Pure-tone audiometry meets these requirements. The hearing loss pattern can provide information for future efforts to slow down its progress [26].

In our series of patients with definite Meniere's disease, nearly half of the patients had moderate to severe hearing loss, and their average hearing thresholds displayed a predominance of stage 3 and stage 4. This observation was similar to that of others, which is noted in the literature [8]. The proportion of patients with moderate to severe hearing loss in this study was less than that previously published [14]. This may be due partly to the increased attention and improvement of the early diagnosis of Meniere's disease. Furthermore, a focus on patient education could enable more patients to be aware of their symptoms and to see a doctor at an earlier stage.

Encouragingly, after one year of strict clinical management, most patients improved their hearing at a low frequency and/or maintained their hearing at a high frequency. Only a few had their hearing deteriorate at low and high frequencies. Thus, most patients benefitted from criterial clinical management and sufficient observation. This result is better than that of a former study, which suggested that the percentage of patients who experienced fluctuations resulting in hearing deterioration ranged from 58% to 67% [5]. Additionally, a slightly higher value than Molnár A's result of intratympanic steroid therapy of 68.6% [27] was achieved. The different length of the follow-up period and the development of the criteria of the disease are possible reasons for the different results.

What is surprising, is that 40% of patients had their hearing thresholds reach $\leq$25 dB HL, even the 18 patients in stage 3. A long period, comprising months, was required for patients to restore their hearing. Their hearing did not always improve rapidly after the treatment, but it was gradually restored after months of waiting. This has not been reported before, and it subverts our inherent understanding of this issue; however, it provides essential data on the timing of hearing restoration. The restoration time of the advanced stage was longer than that of the earlier stages. The longest time was 11 months, the middle time for advanced stages was 3 months, and for the early stages, it was 2 months. According to this result, we recommend a hearing observation period for patients of Meniere's disease of at least one year. Furthermore, compared with early stages (stages 1 and 2), patients' hearing in advanced stages (stages 3 and 4) improved more at low and high frequencies. Patients in advanced stages should not be neglected, nor should they give up on rescuing their hearing. Instead, we emphasize that more attention should be paid to their symptoms, and they should attend follow-up appointments with their clinician to maintain their residual hearing. The hearing changes associated with Meniere's disease need further observation to determine when to carry out an artificial hearing intervention or surgery, as irreversible hearing loss may occur.

The importance of examining individual frequency thresholds is emphasized as one evaluates and monitors patients with Meniere's disease over time [28]. The proportion of patients with low-frequency hearing improvements was the highest. Low-frequency hearing in stages 1 to 4 improved, and the improvements in stages 2 and 3 were significantly different; however, few studies have focused on high-frequency hearing loss. Some studies [17] have suggested that high-frequency hearing is related to presbycusis and that the effect of age is greater than the effect of the duration of the disease, which means that an audiogram shows an ascending curve when age correction is carried out; however, we report here that the decline in the high-frequency hearing was not due to age. We found a correlation between the average threshold of low- and high-frequency hearing. As the low frequencies declined, the high frequencies also declined relatively slowly. After one year, the high frequency deteriorated at stages 1 and 2, especially in stage 1, with a significant difference; it improved at stages 3 and 4, especially at stage 4. This outcome indicates that the decline in high frequency is somewhat associated with changes in the pathological progress of the disease itself, instead of aging. This argument is similar to that of Albre [29] and colleagues, who concluded that age does not influence the course of hearing loss of a pure-tone average threshold in patients with Meniere's disease.

The proportion of the peak curve was the greatest, which is similar to the findings of Paparella [18] and Lee [19], who reported a significant prevalence of the peak curve of 42.9% and 50.26%, respectively. The ascending-type curve is generally considered to be characteristic of Meniere's disease; however, it is usually not the most common type of curve in practice. Some studies observed a predominantly flat audiometric curve [13,22,30], even in very early times [22]. Enander [22] and colleagues observed that flat curves accounted for 60% of all patients. Thomas [30] and colleagues found that flat curves accounted for 44.5–45.9%. Other studies observed that the peak curve is the most common, represented by hearing loss at low and high frequencies and an audiogram peak at approximately 2 kHz [18,19]. There is no consensus regarding the standard of curve type in previous studies. In our research, we referred to the classification and calculation method in the literature when judging the curve type to make the decision objectively. Moreover, we manually reviewed and corrected the calculation results, which made the judgment of the audiogram curve more unified and standardized to reduce bias. This is the virtue of this essay when studying the audiometric curve. All four types improved significantly for different curves, utilizing rising, falling, peak, and flat types for the low frequency. Although there was no significant difference for the high frequency, it still surprisingly showed a slight deterioration in the rising and peak curves, and showed a slight improvement in the falling and flat curves. Patients who had rising curves at onset were most likely to have a peak after one year. This may have contributed to the percentage of the rising curve being the highest, and the decrease in the hearing of high-frequency patients at stage 1. Most patients with the falling curve still had this type (89.66%). Approximately half of the patients with a peak curve maintained a peak curve (46.48%). Most patients with flat curves remained flat (47.06%). Savastano [21] and colleagues reported that with disease development, an audiometric pattern tends to develop from the peak shape to the flat shape in a long-term follow-up (i.e., for ten years). After 15 years of follow-ups, the rate of the appearance of the flat type of audiogram increased from 21% to 75% [13].

We speculate that hearing loss appears in the low frequency initially, then in the high frequency, and then in the entire frequency, gradually deteriorating in this way. New studies report that the hearing loss profile does not only affect the low frequency in the early stages; however, a flat sensorineural hearing loss was observed in patients with familial Meniere's disease and mutations in OTOG and MYO7A [31]. In our group only three patients exhibited a flat pattern in stages 1 and 2, potentially related to the fact that there were only two patients with familial histories of Meniere's disease. More specifically, although our results show that patients had satisfactory hearing improvement, in the long term, the hearing improvement might not necessarily be the result of any treatment but rather the result of fluctuation in Meniere's disease itself. The allelic variant may associate with the progression of hearing loss in patients with MD, such as major histocompatibility complex class I chain-related A (MICA) [32] and Toll Like Receptor 10 (TLR10) [33]. The beginning of high-frequency hearing loss often occurs in the early stage, which is also part of the hearing fluctuation and the process of Meniere's disease. Changes in different frequencies may provide suggestive information regarding the prognosis. High-frequency hearing loss in the first audiogram, age of onset, and migraine can help to assess the risk of bilateral SNHL in MD [34]. In our group, there were a few bilateral MD cases with no familial histories, and with an increasing number of patients, further investigations will be conducted. The improvement of sensorineural hearing loss is strongly associated with the prognosis of tinnitus [35], which argues for future research on aural symptoms in patients. The characterization of the manifestation of hearing loss is essential for appropriate counseling and an improved understanding of the disease. Sufficient longitudinal follow-up and hearing evaluation are cardinal when making clinical practice decisions.

More long-term follow-up studies are needed to investigate the progressive patterns of different patients and different treatment outcomes with Meniere's disease. The hearing of the patients fluctuates alternatively between improvement and deterioration. The results of a five- or ten-year follow-up are expected in the future for more clinical information. Although vestibular migraines are excluded from the study, migraine symptoms are usually complex, and the influencing factors should be strictly limited when observing Meniere's disease hearing changes. In the future, research needs to include more details. The influencing factors should be more strictly limited. Further in-depth comparative analysis should be conducted when the case numbers increase. Future research directions may also be highlighted in terms of predictive factors of listening outcomes.

## 5. Conclusions

Most patients can have their hearing preserved or improved through strict clinical management, and sufficient follow-up time is also essential. Stage 3 patients also have potential for improvement, and their restoration time is longer than in the early stages. Initial hearing stage, age, and audiogram pattern are related to the hearing benefits.

**Author Contributions:** Conceptualization, B.L.; original draft, Y.Z.; formal analysis, Y.Z., Z.S. and C.W.; software, Z.S.; data curation, Y.Z.; review, B.L.; visualization, Z.S.; resources, Y.W. and Z.C.; funding acquisition, B.L. and Y.Z. All authors have read and agreed to the published version of the manuscript.

**Funding:** This work was supported by the National Key Research and Development Program (2020YFC2005200) and the Priority Medical Science Program of Tongren Hospital (trzdyxzy201802).

**Institutional Review Board Statement:** The study was conducted in accordance with the Declaration of Helsinki and approved by the Institutional Ethics Committee of Beijing Tongren Hospital (TRECKY2019-045).

**Informed Consent Statement:** Informed consent was obtained from all subjects involved in the study.

**Data Availability Statement:** The data presented in this study are available on request from the corresponding author. The data are not publicly available because the health examination data of a private hospital were used.

**Conflicts of Interest:** The authors declare no conflict of interest.

## References

1. Lopez-Escamez, J.A.; Carey, J.; Chung, W.-H.; Goebel, J.A.; Magnusson, M.; Mandalà, M.; Newman-Toker, D.E.; Strupp, M.; Suzuki, M.; Trabalzini, F.; et al. Diagnostic criteria for Menière's disease. *J. Vestib. Res.* **2015**, *25*, 1–7. [CrossRef]
2. Bisdorff, A.R.; Staab, J.P.; Newman-Toker, D.E. Overview of the International Classification of Vestibular Disorders. *Neurol. Clin.* **2015**, *33*, 541–550. [CrossRef]
3. Belinchon, A.; Perez-Garrigues, H.; Tenias, J.M. Evolution of symptoms in Ménière's disease. *Audiol. Neurootol.* **2012**, *17*, 126–132. [CrossRef]
4. Sajjadi, H.; Paparella, M.M. Meniere's disease. *Lancet* **2008**, *372*, 406–414. [CrossRef]
5. Havia, M.; Kentala, E.; Pyykkö, I. Hearing loss and tinnitus in Meniere's disease. *Auris Nasus Larynx* **2002**, *29*, 115–119. [CrossRef]
6. Hoa, M.; Friedman, R.A.; Fisher, L.M.; Derebery, M.J. Prognostic implications of and audiometric evidence for hearing fluctuation in Meniere's disease. *Laryngoscope* **2015**, *125* (Suppl. S12), S1–S12. [CrossRef]
7. McNeill, C.; Freeman, S.R.M.; McMahon, C. Short-term hearing fluctuation in Meniere's disease. *Int. J. Audiol.* **2009**, *48*, 594–600. [CrossRef]
8. Huppert, D.; Strupp, M.; Brandt, T. Long-term course of Menière's disease revisited. *Acta Otolaryngol.* **2010**, *130*, 644–651. [CrossRef]
9. Hussain, K.; Murdin, L.; Schilder, A.G. Restriction of salt, caffeine and alcohol intake for the treatment of Ménière's disease or syndrome. *Cochrane. Database Syst. Rev.* **2018**, *12*, CD012173. [CrossRef]
10. Oğuz, E.; Cebeci, A.; Geçici, C.R. The relationship between nutrition and Ménière's disease. *Auris Nasus Larynx* **2021**, *48*, 803–808. [CrossRef]
11. Rauch, S.D. Ménière's disease: Damaged hearing but reduced vertigo. *Lancet* **2016**, *388*, 2716–2717. [CrossRef]
12. Chadha, S.; Kamenov, K.; Cieza, A. The world report on hearing, 2021. *Bull. World Health Organ.* **2021**, *99*, 242. [CrossRef] [PubMed]
13. Stahle, J.; Friberg, U.; Svedberg, A. Long-term progression of Meniére's disease. *Acta Oto-Laryngol. Suppl.* **1991**, *485*, 78–83. [CrossRef] [PubMed]

14. Zhang, Y.; Liu, B.; Wang, R.; Jia, R.; Gu, X. Characteristics of the Cochlear Symptoms and Functions in Meniere's Disease. *Chin. Med. J.* **2016**, *129*, 2445–2450. [CrossRef]
15. Committee on Hearing and Equilibrium. Committee on Hearing and Equilibrium guidelines for the evaluation of results of treatment of conductive hearing loss. In *Otolaryngology-Head and Neck Surgery: Official Journal of American Academy of Otolaryngology-Head and Neck Surgery*; American Academy of Otolaryngology-Head and Neck Surgery Ffoundation, Inc.: Alexandria, VA, USA, 1995; Volume 113, pp. 181–185.
16. Mateijsen, D.J.; Van Hengel, P.W.; Van Huffelen, W.M.; Wit, H.P.; Albers, F.W. Pure-tone and speech audiometry in patients with Menière's disease. *Clin. Otolaryngol. Allied Sci.* **2001**, *26*, 379–387. [CrossRef] [PubMed]
17. Belinchon, A.; Perez-Garrigues, H.; Tenias, J.M.; Lopez, A. Hearing assessment in Menière's disease. *Laryngoscope* **2011**, *121*, 622–626. [CrossRef]
18. Paparella, M.M.; McDermott, J.C.; de Sousa, L.C. Meniere's disease and the peak audiogram. *Arch. Otolaryngol.* **1982**, *108*, 555–559. [CrossRef]
19. Lee, C.S.; Paparella, M.M.; Margolis, R.H.; Le, C. Audiological profiles and Menière's disease. *Ear Nose Throat J.* **1995**, *74*, 527–532. [CrossRef]
20. Harris, J.P.; Weisman, M.H.; Derebery, J.M.; Espeland, M.A.; Gantz, B.J.; Gulya, A.J.; Hammerschlag, P.E.; Hannley, M.; Hughes, G.B.; Moscicki, R.; et al. Treatment of corticosteroid-responsive autoimmune inner ear disease with methotrexate: A randomized controlled trial. *JAMA* **2003**, *290*, 1875–1883. [CrossRef]
21. Savastano, M.; Guerrieri, V.; Marioni, G. Evolution of audiometric pattern in Meniere's disease: Long-term survey of 380 cases evaluated according to the 1995 guidelines of the American Academy of Otolaryngology-Head and Neck Surgery. *J. Otolaryngol.* **2006**, *35*, 26–29. [CrossRef]
22. Enander, A.; Stahle, J. Hearing in Menière's disease. A study of pure-tone audiograms in 334 patients. *Acta Otolaryngol.* **1967**, *64*, 543–556. [CrossRef] [PubMed]
23. Rauch, S.D. Clinical hints and precipitating factors in patients suffering from Meniere's disease. *Otolaryngol. Clin. N. Am.* **2010**, *43*, 1011–1017. [CrossRef] [PubMed]
24. Lee, S.-Y.; Kim, Y.S.; Jeong, B.; Carandang, M.; Koo, J.-W.; Oh, S.H.; Lee, J.H. Intratympanic steroid versus gentamicin for treatment of refractory Meniere's disease: A meta-analysis. *Am. J. Otolaryngol.* **2021**, *42*, 103086. [CrossRef] [PubMed]
25. Kersbergen, C.J.; Ward, B.K. A Historical Perspective on Surgical Manipulation of the Membranous Labyrinth for Treatment of Meniere's Disease. *Front. Neurol.* **2021**, *12*, 794741. [CrossRef] [PubMed]
26. Ruckenstein, M.J. *Meniere's Disease: Evidence and Outcomes*; Plural Publishing: Abingdon, UK, 2010; pp. 69–71.
27. Molnár, A.; Maihoub, S.; Tamás, L.; Szirmai, Á. Intratympanically administered steroid for progressive sensorineural hearing loss in Ménière's disease. *Acta Otolaryngol.* **2019**, *139*, 982–986. [CrossRef]
28. Pfaltz, C.R.; Alford, B.R. *Controversial Aspects of Ménière's Disease*; Thieme: New York, NY, USA, 1986.
29. Albera, R.; Canale, A.; Cassandro, C.; Albera, A.; Sammartano, A.M.; Dagna, F. Relationship between hearing threshold at the affected and unaffected ear in unilateral Meniere's disease. *Eur. Arch. Otorhinolaryngol.* **2016**, *273*, 51–56. [CrossRef]
30. Thomas, K.; Harrison, M.S. Long-term follow up of 610 cases of Ménière's disease. *Proc. R Soc. Med.* **1971**, *64*, 853–857. [CrossRef]
31. Roman-Naranjo, P.; Gallego-Martinez, A.; Soto-Varela, A.; Aran, I.; Moleon, M.D.C.; Espinosa-Sanchez, J.M.; Amor-Dorado, J.C.; Batuecas-Caletrio, A.; Perez-Vazquez, P.; Lopez-Escamez, J.A. Burden of Rare Variants in the OTOG Gene in Familial Meniere's Disease. *Ear Hear.* **2020**, *41*, 1598–1605. [CrossRef]
32. Gazquez, I.; Moreno, A.; Aran, I.; Soto-Varela, A.; Santos, S.; Perez-Garrigues, H.; Lopez-Nevot, A.; Requena, T.; Lopez-Nevot, M.A.; Lopez-Escamez, J.A. MICA-STR A.4 is associated with slower hearing loss progression in patients with Ménière's disease. *Otol. Neurotol.* **2012**, *33*, 223–229. [CrossRef]
33. Requena, T.; Gazquez, I.; Moreno, A.; Batuecas, A.; Aran, I.; Soto-Varela, A.; Santos-Perez, S.; Perez, N.; Perez-Garrigues, H.; Lopez-Nevot, A.; et al. Allelic variants in TLR10 gene may influence bilateral affectation and clinical course of Meniere's disease. *Immunogenetics* **2013**, *65*, 345–355. [CrossRef]
34. Moleon, M.D.C.; Torres-Garcia, L.; Batuecas-Caletrio, A.; Castillo-Ledesma, N.; Gonzalez-Aguado, R.; Magnoni, L.; Rossi, M.; Di Berardino, F.; Perez-Guillen, V.; Trinidad-Ruiz, G.; et al. A Predictive Model of Bilateral Sensorineural Hearing Loss in Meniere Disease Using Clinical Data. *Ear Hear.* **2022**, *43*, 1079–1085. [CrossRef] [PubMed]
35. Ding, X.; Zhang, X.; Huang, Z.; Feng, X. The Characteristic and Short-Term Prognosis of Tinnitus Associated with Sudden Sensorineural Hearing Loss. *Neural Plast.* **2018**, *2018*, 6059697. [CrossRef] [PubMed]

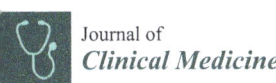 

*Review*

# Risk Factors for Recurrence of Benign Paroxysmal Positional Vertigo. A Clinical Review

Ioanna Sfakianaki [1], Paris Binos [2], Petros Karkos [1], Grigorios G. Dimas [3] and George Psillas [1,*]

[1] 1st Academic ENT Department, AHEPA Hospital, Aristotle University of Thessaloniki, 1, Stilponos Kyriakidi St., 546 36 Thessaloniki, Greece; g_sfakianaki@yahoo.com (I.S.); pkarkos@aol.com (P.K.)

[2] Department of Rehabilitation Sciences, Cyprus University of Technology, Limassol 3036, Cyprus; paris.binos@cut.ac.cy

[3] 1st Propaedeutic Department of Internal Medicine, AHEPA Hospital, Aristotle University of Thessaloniki, 1, Stilponos Kyriakidi St., 546 36 Thessaloniki, Greece; gregorydimas@yahoo.gr

* Correspondence: psill@otenet.gr; Tel.: +30-2310-994-762; Fax: +30-2310-994-916

**Abstract:** Benign paroxysmal positional vertigo (BPPV) is one of the most common peripheral vestibular dysfunctions encountered in clinical practice. Although the treatment of BPPV is relatively successful, many patients develop recurrence after treatment. Our purpose is to evaluate the mean recurrence rate and risk factors of BPPV after treatment. A review of the literature on the risk factors of BPPV recurrence was performed. A thorough search was conducted using electronic databases, namely Pubmed, CINAHL, Academic Search Complete and Scopus for studies published from 2000 to 2020. Thirty studies were included in this review with 13,358 participants. The recurrence rate of BPPV ranged from 13.7% to 48% for studies with follow-up <1 year, and from 13.3% to 65% for studies with follow-up ≥2 years. Pathophysiologic mechanisms and implication of each of the following risk factors in the recurrence of BPPV were described: advanced age, female gender, Meniere's disease, trauma, osteopenia or osteoporosis, vitamin D deficiency, diabetes mellitus, hypertension, hyperlipidemia, cardiovascular disease, migraine, bilateral/multicanal BPPV, cervical osteoarthrosis and sleep disorders. Patients with hyperlipidemia and hypertension had the highest recurrence rates of BPPV, 67.80% and 55.89%, respectively, indicating that vascular comorbidities increase the risk of BPPV recurrence. In addition, more than half of patients (53.48%) with diabetes mellitus and BPPV experienced recurrence of BPPV. Knowledge and awareness of risk factors for recurrence of BPPV are essential for the assessment and long-term prognosis of patients. Identification of these relapse risk factors may enhance the ability of clinicians to accurately counsel patients regarding BPPV and associated comorbidities.

**Keywords:** BPPV; BPPV recurrence; risk factors

## 1. Introduction

Benign paroxysmal positional vertigo (BPPV) is the commonest peripheral vestibular condition encountered in a neurotology clinic and it accounts for about 20% to 30% of all the vestibular complaints [1–3]. The mechanism of BPPV has been based on dislodged otoliths that leave the utricle and freely float in the semicircular canals or attach to the cupula, making the labyrinth sensitive to gravitational forces. BPPV is characterized by recurrent and brief vertigo with corresponding nystagmus when extending or turning the neck, getting up or lying down, or rolling over in bed. In most cases, BPPV is idiopathic, but also can be secondary (following head trauma, viral infection, Meniere's disease, migraine, otologic and non-otologic surgery, prolonged bed rest [4,5].

It was reported that using canalith repositioning therapy (CRT), such as Epley's maneuver, otoliths are moved from the semicircular canal to the vestibule where they are absorbed. Complete recovery with resolution of symptoms and disappearance of positional nystagmus after a single maneuver is achieved in about 50–60% of the patients, and after repetitive maneuvers in more than 90% [6]. Posterior semicircular canal involvement is the most common form in BPPV (90–91%), but lateral and anterior canals can also be involved [7].

The BPPV recurrence has been defined as the reappearance of positional vertigo and nystagmus after at least one month from the execution of an effective CRT [8]. The frequent recurrence of BPPV may cause great inconvenience in the daily life of patients with reoccurring BPPV. Many recent studies found that BPPV can be associated with other comorbidity diseases, including hypertension, diabetes, thyroid disorders, hyperlipidemia, and osteoporosis and may be responsible for increased frequency of recurrence of BPPV following treatment [2]. If such a correlation between common comorbidities and BPPV exists, appropriate treatment of these conditions may be useful in limiting chronicity and reducing the frequency of recurrence.

The purpose of this review is to assess the recurrence rate and the time interval, as well as to identify the etiologic factors that may contribute to the recurrence of BPPV. Thus, our aim is to provide an overview of the literature in an area that is still unclear, direct physician's attention to what factors should assess when encountering patients with BPPV as well as contribute to the knowledge on the mechanisms of the risk factors implicated.

## 2. Materials and Methods

### 2.1. Literature Search

A review of the literature on the risk factors of BPPV recurrence was performed. The articles were identified using MeSH descriptors in the Pubmed database, for studies published until December 2020 (Figure 1); the electronic databases of CINAHL, Academic Search Complete and Scopus were also used for the same period. After combining specific keywords, "BPPV", "Benign paroxysmal positional vertigo", "Recurrence", "Recurrent", 410 articles were identified. Each title was screened for eligibility according to the predetermined requirements by first author (IS), followed by an independent screening of the abstract and full text by all authors (PB, PK, GGD, GP). All the full texts were verified by the assigned authors. Any discrepancies between the authors' decisions were addressed through dialogue until a decision was reached.

### 2.2. Eligibility and Exclusion Criteria for Study Selection

The eligibility criteria for inclusion in the analysis were the following:
- Retrospective or prospective studies on the recurrence of BPPV.
- BPPV diagnosis according to clinical practice guideline [9]
- Assessment of the demographics (sex, age) of recurrent BPPV patients and the potential risk factors of BPPV recurrence.
- Articles published in English.

The exclusion criteria in the analysis were the following:
- Systematic reviews, case reports, book chapters.
- Experimental studies.
- Studies not based on outcomes of canalith repositioning procedure (CRP).
- Studies with insufficient data for analysis.
- Diagnosis, treatment, or definition of recurrence of BPPV was not clear.
- Follow-up time less than 6 months or unstated.

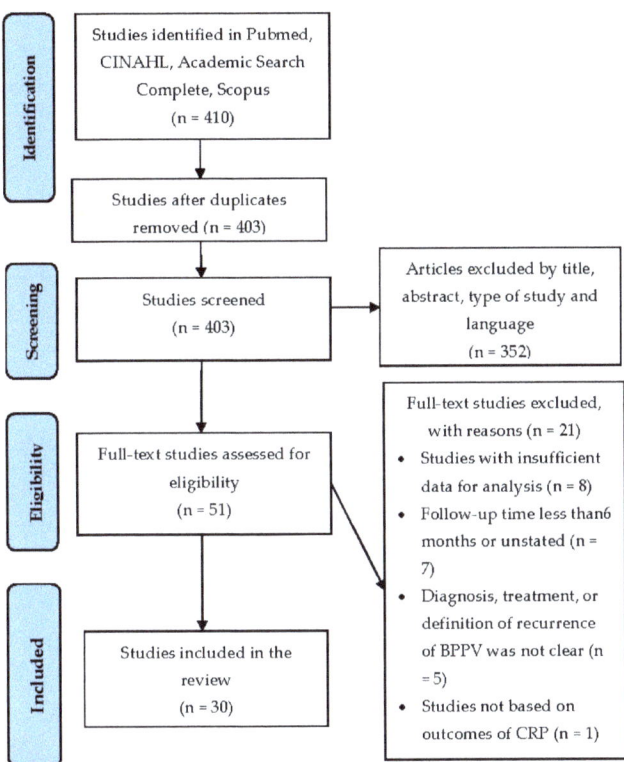

**Figure 1.** Flowchart of data search and studies selection.

*2.3. Data Extraction*

Studies were initially identified on the basis of title and abstract and then assessed for eligibility by full text, in order to establish the final set of studies included. The following data were extracted and evaluated: First author, year of publication, type of study design, population size, mean age, gender, location of BPPV, follow-up time, recurrence rate, time to recurrence, location of recurrence, risk factors assessed.

## 3. Results

*3.1. Study Selection*

A total of 403 articles were initially retrieved from databases (Figure 1). Of these, 352 articles were excluded by title, abstract, type of study and language. Of the remaining 51 articles, after further, full-text evaluation, 21 were excluded according to the abovementioned criteria. Finally, 30 articles met the eligibility criteria for the study (Table 1).

Table 1. Assessed characteristics of the included studies.

| Authors | Year | Study | Patients (M/F) | Mean Age | Location of BPPV | Follow up | Recurrence Rate | Time to Recurrence | Location of Recurrence | Risk Factors Assessed |
|---|---|---|---|---|---|---|---|---|---|---|
| Del Rio et al. [10] | 2004 | R | 104 (35/69) | 64.3 y | PSC | 6–15 mo | 22.6% (21/93) | 118 d | N/A | RF3 *:7/16 ** RF4:1/12 |
| Korres et al. [11] | 2006 | R | 143 (62/81) | 59.9 y | 3SC bilateral multicanal | 24 mo | 13.3 % (19/143) | N/A | PSC HSC bilateral 2-canals | RF1 *:19/124 RF2: 11/81 RF4: 1/4 RF12 *:5/8 |
| Kansu et al. [7] | 2010 | R | 118 (44/74) | 51.8 y | PSC | 53–78 mo | 33.1% (39/118) | 53.8% within 2 y 33.1% within 5 y | PSC bilateral | RF1: 39/79 RF2: 25/74 RF3 *: 3/8 RF4 *:12/25 RF11:5/16 RF12: 2/5 |
| Choi et al. [12] | 2012 | R | 120 (43/77) | 50.4 y | PSC HSC | 6–29 mo | 10% (12/120) | N/A | PSC HSC | RF3 *: 2/2 RF4 *: 2/8 |
| Yamanaka et al. [13] | 2013 | R | 61 (0/61) | 63.7 y | N/A | 12 mo | 56% (9/16) | N/A | N/A | RF5 *: 9/16 |
| Webster et al. [14] | 2014 | P | 72 (N/A) | N/A | N/A | 41 mo | 36.1% (26/72) | N/A | N/A | RF7 * |
| De Stefano et al. [1] | 2013 | R | 1092 (407/685) | 72.9 y | 3SC multicanal | 6–24 mo | 50.5% (551/1092) | N/A | PSC (36.8%) | RF5: 1/13 RF7 *: 10/16 RF8 *: 100/163 RF13 *: 8/13 |
| Babac et al. [15] | 2014 | P | 400 (119/281) | 58.7 y | 3SC bilateral multicanal | 12 mo | 15.5% (62/400) | 48.4% within 3 mo | ipsilateral PSC (61.29%) contralateral PSC (30.65%) multicanal ipsilateral (1 case) | RF1(>50 y): 51/254 RF2: 48/281 RF4: 4/18 RF5: 12/65 RF11: 6/55 RF10: 36/224 RF12: 0/5 |

Table 1. Cont.

| Authors | Year | Study | Patients (M/F) | Mean Age | Location of BPPV | Follow up | Recurrence Rate | Time to Recurrence | Location of Recurrence | Risk Factors Assessed |
|---|---|---|---|---|---|---|---|---|---|---|
| Su et al. [3] | 2016 | R | 243 (47/19) | 57.5 y | PSC | 24 mo | 18.9% (46/243) | | | RF1(>65 y): 15/58 RF2 *: 42/196 RF4: 2/11 RF10: 20/80 RF14 *: 14/40 |
| Kim et al. [8] | 2017 | R | 198 (59/139) | 62.9 y | 3SC | ≥12 mo | 33.8% (67/198) | mean period of 11.6 mo | 16% in different SC | RF1: 67/131 RF2: 49/139 RF5: 7/14 RF7 *:14/17 RF8 *:27/32 |
| Luryi et al. [16] | 2018 | R | 1105 (315/790) | 64.8 y | 3SC bilateral | 602 d | 37% | 76% within 2 y | 28% in the same ear | RF1(>60 y):267/700 RF2 *: 319/790 RF3: 31/103 RF4: 27/82 RF7: 47/134 |
| Nunez et al. [17] | 2000 | P | 151 (44/107) | 63.0 y | PSC | 15.9 mo | 26.8% (37/138) | 15% per year 40% within 40 mo | PSC | RF4: 10/27 |
| Brandt et al. [6] | 2009 | R | 125 (49/76) | 55.1 y | PSC | 10.3 y | 50% | 80% within 1 y 94% within 5 y | | RF1: 37/54 * RF2 *: 44/76 RF4: 7/17 RF11: 8/15 |
| Perez et al. [5] | 2012 | P | 69 (25/44) | 62.0 y | 3SC bilateral multicanal | 47 mo | 27% (19/69) | 50% within 6 mo | 7/19 contralateral ear 5/7 other canal 6/12 other canal | RF1: 19/69 RF2 RF4 *: 3/6 RF12 *: 8/17 |

Table 1. Cont.

| Authors | Year | Study | Patients (M/F) | Mean Age | Location of BPPV | Follow up | Recurrence Rate | Time to Recurrence | Location of Recurrence | Risk Factors Assessed |
|---|---|---|---|---|---|---|---|---|---|---|
| Zhu et al. [18] | 2019 | R | 1012 (316/696) | 54.6 y | PSC HSC multicanal | 12 mo | 33,7% (255/757) | 12 mo | | RF1(>60 y): 91/315 RF2*: 187/696 RF3*: 16/24 RF7: 24/87 RF8*: 89/276 RF9*: 84/266 RF10: 77/258 RF11*: 14/29 |
| Messina et al. [19] | 2017 | R | 2682 (1008/1571) | 59.3 y | 3SC | ≥6 mo | 52.5% (1386/2638) | 1–5 episodes per year (84.3%) | 49.2% same canal | RF7*: 261/413 RF8*: 844/1401 RF9*: 1401/1906 RF10*: 82/265 |
| Sreenivas et al. [2] | 2019 | R | 71 (31/40) | 49.0 y | N/A | 6–12 mo | 22.5% (16/71) | | | RF1(>60 y)*: 5/11 RF6: 12/56 RF7*: 5/8 RF8: 8/21 RF9: 10/33 |
| Rhim et al. [20] | 2016 | R | 232 (63/169) | 50.35 y | 3SC bilateral multicanal | 10.2 mo | 17.7% (41/232) | N/A | N/A | RF1:41/191 RF2: 31/169 RF6*:41/191 RF12: 6/28 |
| Balatsouras [21] | 2012 | R | 262 (97/165) 233 iBPPV 29 mBPPV | 53.4 y | 3SC bilateral multicanal | 12 mo | 44.4% (iBPPV) 13.3% (mBPPV) | N/A | N/A | RF3*: 12/27 |
| Talaat et al. [22] | 2014 | P | 80 (28/52) | 47.6 y | 3SC | ≥12 mo | 45% (36/80) | N/A | N/A | RF1: 36/44 RF2: 27/52 RF5*: 22/48 RF6*: 34/72 |

Table 1. Cont.

| Authors | Year | Study | Patients (M/F) | Mean Age | Location of BPPV | Follow up | Recurrence Rate | Time to Recurrence | Location of Recurrence | Risk Factors Assessed |
|---|---|---|---|---|---|---|---|---|---|---|
| Yang CJ et al. [23] | 2017 | R | 130 (30/100) | 54.9 y | 3SC | 12 mo | 48% (63/130) | N/A | N/A | RF1 *: 63/67<br>RF2: 50/100<br>RF5: 39/68<br>RF6: 63/67 |
| Wei et al. [24] | 2018 | R | 127 (46/81) | 53.9 y | 3SC | 6 mo | 14.17% | 6 mo | N/A | RF1(>60y)<br>RF2<br>RF7<br>RF8<br>RF9<br>RF11<br>RF13 |
| Faralli et al. [25] | 2006 | R | 566 (204/362) | 56.8 y | 3SC | 6 mo | 13.7% (77/560) | N/A | N/A | RF1(>50 y):<br>64/396<br>RF10 *: 22/111 |
| Piccioti et al. [4] | 2016 | R | 475 (188/287) | 61.9 y | PSC HSC | 30 mo | 23.4% (139/475) | N/A | N/A | RF1 *: 139/475<br>RF2 *: 95/287<br>RF4: 13/42<br>RF7 *<br>RF8 *<br>RF9 *<br>RF10 * |
| Tan et al. [26] | 2016 | R | 88 (33/55) 47 i-BPPV 41 h-BPPV | 53.44 y (h-BPPV) 51.64 y (i-BPPV) | 3SC | ≥12 mo | 12.7% (6/47, i-BPPV) 31.7% (13/41, h-BPPV) | N/A | N/A | RF8 *: 13/41 |
| Prokopakis et al. [27] | 2012 | P | 965 (481/484) | N/A | 3SC | 74 mo | 15.5% (139/895) | N/A | N/A | RF1(>70 y) *<br>RF4 * |

Table 1. Cont.

| Authors | Year | Study | Patients (M/F) | Mean Age | Location of BPPV | Follow up | Recurrence Rate | Time to Recurrence | Location of Recurrence | Risk Factors Assessed |
|---|---|---|---|---|---|---|---|---|---|---|
| Rashad et al. [28] | 2009 | P | 103 (45/58) | 48.2 y | PSC | 5 y | 65% (67/103) | 46.3 mo | N/A | RF1(≥40 y) *: 49/82 RF2: 34/58 |
| Hilton et al. [29] | 2020 | R | 1481 (389/1092) | 63.3 y | N/A | ≥6 mo | 33.8% (267/791) | N/A | N/A | RF11: 80/209 |
| Ishiyama et al. [30] | 2000 | R | 247 (93/154) | N/A | PSC | ≥6 mo | 68.4% (169/247) | N/A | N/A | RF11 *: 48/62 |
| Gordon et al. [31] | 2004 | R | 21 t-BPPV (10/11) 42 i-BPPV (10/32) | 56.3 y (t-BPPV) 61.1 y (i-BPPV) | PSC HSC bilateral | 6–42 mo | 57% (12/21, t-BPPV) 19% (8/42, i-BPPV) | N/A | N/A | RF4 *: 12/21 |

* Statistically significant Risk Factors. RF1: Advanced age, RF2: Female gender, RF3: Meniere's disease/Hydrops, RF4: Head trauma, RF5: Osteopenia/Osteoporosis, RF6: Vitamin D deficiency RF7: Diabetes mellitus/Hyperinsulinism/Hyperglycemia, RF8: Hypertension, RF9: Hyperlipidemia, RF10: Cardiovascular disease, RF11: Migraine, RF12: Bilateral/Multicanal BPPV, RF13: Cervical osteoarthrosis, RF14: Sleep disorders. N/A: Not available, R: Retrospective study, P: Prospective study, PSC, HSC: posterior, horizontal semicircular canal, SC: semicircular canals, y: years, mo: months, d: days, t-BPPV, i-BPPV: traumatic, idiopathic benign paroxysmal positional vertigo. ** In the last column, the number of patients with reoccurring BPPV is shown among the total number of patients having the corresponding risk factor.

*3.2. Findings*

Thirty articles examined 14 risk factors for recurrence of BPPV and they included 12,585 participants (Table 2). Twenty-three were retrospective studies [1–4,6–8,10–13,16,18–21,23–26,29–31] and seven were prospective cohort studies [5,14,15,17,22,27,28]. In all studies, the diagnosis of BPPV was established by positive positional tests (Dix-Hallpike, roll tests). Twenty-nine of the thirty studies provided data on gender of which 7912 of the 12,513 patients were female (62.9%). In one study [14] the proportion of gender was not stated. The mean age of the participants in twenty-seven of the thirty studies was 57.5 years; three studies did not provide sufficient information on the mean age of their participants [14,27,30].

**Table 2.** Analysis of each included risk factor for BPPV recurrence in this review.

| | N of Studies Assessed | N of Studies with Statistical Significance | Recurrence/ Non-Recurrence (Cases) | Recurrence (%) |
|---|---|---|---|---|
| Advanced Age | 18 | 6 | 976/2069 | 32.05% |
| Female gender | 15 | 5 | 962/2037 | 32.08% |
| Meniere's disease | 6 | 5 | 71/109 | 39.44% |
| Trauma | 12 | 4 | 94/176 | 34.81% |
| Osteopenia/Osteoporosis | 6 | 2 | 90/134 | 40.18% |
| Vitamin D deficiency | 4 | 2 | 150/236 | 38.86% |
| Diabetesmellitus/Hyperisulinism/Hyperglycemia | 9 | 6 | 361/314 | 53.48% |
| Hypertension | 8 | 6 | 1081/853 | 55.89% |
| Hyperlipidemia | 5 | 3 | 1495/710 | 67.80% |
| Cardiovascular disease | 6 | 3 | 237/701 | 25.27% |
| Migraine | 7 | 2 | 161/225 | 41.71% |
| Bilateral/multicanal BPPV | 5 | 2 | 21/42 | 33.33% |
| Cervical osteoarthrosis | 2 | 1 | 8/5 | 61.54% |
| Sleep disorders | 1 | 1 | 14/26 | 35.00% |

N: Number.

*Initial semicircular canal involvement.* Seven studies [3,6,7,10,17,28,30] examined cases of unilateral posterior canal BPPV; eight studies [8,19,22–27] analyzed unilateral BPPV cases involving the three semicircular canals (posterior, horizontal, anterior) and nine studies [1,5,11,15,16,18,20,21,31] reported cases of bilateral or multiple-canal BPPV.

*Follow-up time.* Nine studies [2,13,15,18,20,21,23–25] had a follow-up duration greater than 6 months to less than a year, reporting a recurrence rate (RR) in the range of 13.7% [25] to 48% [23]. Furthermore, ten studies [3–7,11,14,27,28,31] had a follow-up time ≥2 years with a recurrence rate varying from 13.3% [11] to 65% [28].

*Time to recurrence.* The majority of the studies -nine out of twelve- found that most of the recurrent episodes developed within the first year [5,6,8,10,15,16,18,19,24]. In particular, Perez et al. [5] reported that 50% of the recurrent episodes occurred within the first 6 months. Luryi et al. [16] and Brandt et al. found [6] that 56% and 80% of recurrences, respectively, developed within the first year and Kim et al. [8] reported that the mean period of recurrence was 11.6 months. On the contrary, Kansu et al. [7] found that most of the patients (53%) experienced recurrence within the first two years whereas two studies [17,28] found that the majority of the recurrent episodes occurred within 4 years after the initial treatment. Specifically, Nunez et al. [17] reported that by 40 months the overall incidence of recurrent episodes approached 50% and Rashad et al. [28] found that the overall mean time to recurrence was 46.3 months.

*Location of recurrence.* Compared to the initial location of BPPV, ipsilateral side was the most affected side in the range of 63% [5] to 76% [16] of the recurrences, while Messina et al. [19] found that 49.2 % of the recurrent episodes developed in the same canal. In addition, Babac et al. [15] reported that 30.65% of the recurrences affected the posterior canal of the contralateral side and Kim et al. [8] found that 16% of the patients suffered recurrence in a different semicircular canal from the one initially involved.

*Analysis of each included risk factor for BPPV recurrence* (Table 2). Patients with hyperlipidemia and hypertension had the highest recurrence rates of BPPV, 67.80% and 55.89%, respectively. Moreover, it seems that more than half of patients (53.48%) with diabetes mellitus and BPPV experienced recurrence of BPPV. In addition, it appears that migraine is also a contributor to the recurrence of BPPV as BPPV recurs in 41.71% of the cases. The rate of BPPV recurrence among the patients who also suffer from osteopenia/osteoporosis and vitamin D deficiency is 40.18% and 38.86%, respectively. Furthermore, our study showed that BPPV recurs in 39.44% of the cases that are comorbid with Meniere's disease and in 34.81% of the posttraumatic cases of BPPV. Lower recurrence rates have been observed in cases of bilateral/multicanal BPPV (33.33%), in cases of patients with advanced age (32.05%) and in the female patients (32.08%). Sleep disorders and cervical osteoarthrosis had been studied in a small sample size of patients suffering from BPPV recurrence, therefore the conclusions are ambiguous.

## 4. Discussion

*4.1. Age*

Progressive demineralization with advancing age leads to degradation, fragmentation and detachment of utricular otoconia, resulting in BPPV [32]. Additionally, the higher number of recurrences in the elderly patients might be explained by the reduction in daily activities, limited mobility, fatigue and increase in falls [11,15,18]. Whether age represents an independent prognostic factor is controversial. Contrary to studies [7,25] the recurrence rate was demonstrated to be increased with advancing age [4,11]. In studies with large samples, it has been shown that patients older than 40 years [28], or 50 years [15], or 65 years [6] or in the sixth [6] or mainly seventh decade of age [2] were more likely to relapse. Piccioti et al. [4] supported that the risk for recurrence of BPPV was found to be 1.6 times more in patients older than 65 years compared to younger than 65 years; they also noted that the presence of comorbidity (hypertension, diabetes, vascular diseases) might increase the rate of recurrence in aged patients.

*4.2. Gender*

BPPV is frequent in females older than 50 years old [13]. This trend could be attributed to the increased prevalence of osteoporosis and osteopenia in postmenopausal women [33,34], due to the decrease in estrogen secretion (as discussed below). In contrast to age, fewer studies [3,18] have supported that females were more likely to exhibit recurrences of BPPV compared to studies in which the recurrence was shown to not significantly relate to gender [11,28]. However, according to a very recent meta-analysis [33], females were more prone to relapse. Brandt et al. [6] reported higher rate of recurrence in women with a quoted female-to-male ratio 3:2.

*4.3. Meniere's Disease*

Meniere's disease is commonly associated with BPPV. However, this association is still ambiguous and could be attributed to the repeated distention of the membranous labyrinth due to hydrops, which may lead to otoconia detachment, loss of resilience and partial collapse of the semicircular canal; the resulted partial obstruction prevents the otoliths from returning to vestibule during the repositioning maneuvers, increasing the rate of treatment failure [35]. Partial obstruction may also be due to a dilated saccule or adhesion of otoliths to the membranous labyrinth [21]. It has been reported that BPPV patients with Meniere's disease have a 6.009-fold higher risk of recurrence compared to those without Meniere's disease [18], or a 35% recurrence rate when endolymphatic hydrops and BPPV were associated [10]. However, Luryi et al. [16] did not support the association between BPPV recurrence with pre-existing Meniere's disease, reporting that signs and symptoms of Meniere's disease may be conflated with symptoms of concurrent BPPV. Patients with

BPPV and Meniere's disease required more canal repositioning maneuvers than those with idiopathic BPPV without Meniere's disease [10].

*4.4. Trauma*

Trauma is considered one of the most common causes of secondary BPPV [31,36]. The nature and severity of traumas are diverse and include head trauma, whiplash injury, head and neck surgery. Traumatic BPPV (t-BPPV) has certain distinctive clinical characteristics. In particular, it is associated with a higher incidence of bilateral or multicanal involvement, a greater number of repositioning maneuvers for resolution and a higher recurrence rate [5,12,31,36]. Regarding the persistence of t-BPPV, there is a general consensus that posttraumatic BPPV is more difficult to cure than the idiopathic type (i-BPPV) [4,5,10,12,15,31]. However, there has been a lot of controversy over the recurrence of t-BPPV. Gordon et al. [31] reviewed the clinical records of 21 patients with t-BPPV and compared the outcome with the results of 42 patients with i-BPPV. They found that, during a mean follow-up of 22 months, recurrence was significantly more common in t-BPPV patients (57%) than in idiopathic cases (19%). They also suggested a possible pathogenetic mechanism according to which posttraumatic otoconial detachment and associated microscopic hemorrhage or tissue impairment, resulting in biochemical changes that enhance the reformation of otoconial clots. Kansu et al. [7] in a retrospective study with a long-term follow-up period, found that patients with BPPV caused by head traumas are more likely to relapse compared to i-BPPV patients. In the same line, Choi et al. [12] found that persistent and recurrent BPPV had a higher incidence rate in patients with secondary BPPV including BPPV caused by trauma. Prokopakis et al. [27] in a large prospective study with a mean follow-up of 74 months, also indicated that head trauma, among other causes, increases the risk of recurrence significantly ($p < 0.001$). Perez et al. [5] suggested that cases of traumatic BPPV are considered complex and therefore tend to relapse more often, but found no significant difference in the rate of recurrence. They also suggested that it is the BPPV syndrome that relapses rather than BPPV affecting a particular side or canal. On the other hand, most of the studies in our review did not find a significant correlation between trauma and BPPV recurrence [3,4,6,10,15–17].

There are certain difficulties in assessing trauma as a risk factor of recurrence. Firstly, there is high heterogeneity in the type and the severity of trauma, as well as on the intervals between the traumatic event and the diagnosis of BPPV due to other possible medical issues that patients experience after the event. In addition, the repositioning maneuvers in patients with severe traumas could cause pain and discomfort; therefore, in some cases, they are avoided. In most studies of our review, the cohort size was small, and the information provided about the nature of trauma was insufficient. Thus, more prospective studies with more precise data about the history and the clinical characteristics of traumatic BPPV are necessary, in order to clarify the role of trauma in BPPV.

*4.5. Osteoporosis*

Otoconia are a result of inorganic calcium carbonate deposited onto an organic matrix core composed of glycoproteins, mainly otoconin 90 [22,23,37]. Otoconia are in a dynamic state and calcium is required for their mineralization and turnover [38,39]. Calcium and carbonate levels in the endolymph should be kept at a critical level to initiate and maintain the mineralization of the otoconia protein matrix but also avoid unnecessary mineralization [40,41]. This critical balance is achieved by pore-like openings located on the crystalline surface of otoconia, playing an important role in the control of homeostasis [41]. It is speculated that disturbance of calcium metabolism induced by osteoporosis/osteopenia can lead to BPPV by different mechanisms. Vibert et al. [40] found that in ovariectomized osteopenic/osteoporotic female adult rats, otoconia were modified, regarding size and density, suggesting two possible mechanisms. Firstly, they assumed that the reduction in estrogen level can decrease fixation of calcium and subsequently, generate failures in the remodeling of the internal structure of the otoconia as well as in their attachment on the gelatinous matrix. Secondly, an increased concentration of free calcium in the endolymph might induce a reduction in its capacity to dissolve dislodged otoconia and also disturb electromechanical transduction of the sensory epithelium [40,42]. Furthermore, it has been suggested that osteopontin, a bone matrix protein that is considered to form a complex with calcium carbonate crystals at the otolith margin, is reduced in patients with osteoporosis, leading to an impaired otolith formation [43]. Thus, in patients with BPPV and osteoporosis, calcium metabolism failure may be present as a common pathogenesis, leading to the synthesis of atrophic fragile otoliths [13].

There has been controversy about the implication of osteoporosis on the recurrence of BPPV. Babac et al. [15] found that osteoporosis is a potential risk factor for poor treatment results but not for recurrence. Kim et al. found [8] that decreased mineral density (BMD) did not show significant association with BPPV recurrence but showed a significant relation with BPPV occurrence. As a study result similar to Kim et al., Yang et al. [23] found BMD in women is associated with the occurrence of BPPV, though a low BMD and age correlate with the recurrence of BPPV. De Stefano et al. [1], in a multicenter observational study, found that osteoporosis was related to an increased risk of relapse when it was in combination with other comorbidities and defined "groups of risk". Contrary to the above, a few studies have demonstrated an apparent association between BPPV recurrence and BMD score. Yamanaka et al. [13] did not find a clinical association between BPPV and osteoporosis but the results of his study suggest that osteoporosis is a risk factor for BPPV recurrence and that the prognosis of the BPPV might be clinically predicted by BMD reduction. Talaat et al. [22] in their study found that there was an association between reduced BMD and development/recurrence of BPPV. In a retrospective chart review, Mikulec et al. [44] found a significant negative association between BPPV and treated osteoporosis in women aged 51 to 60 years suggesting the possibility that anti-osteoporotic medication may provide protection against BPPV.

These controversies may be explained by different methodologies to measure osteoporotic changes (location for measuring BMD, bone turnover markers), different definitions of BPPV recurrence and follow- up and various distributions of age or gender in study populations. In particular, most of the studies included women, especially older women because BPPV is more common in women between 41 to 61 years old. In addition, most of the studies are retrospective studies where it is difficult to elucidate causal relationships between the recurrence of BPPV and variables including BMD.

### 4.6. Vitamin D

Vitamin D plays a crucial role in the homeostasis of calcium and phosphorus. Normal serum level of vitamin D is essential for the development of normal otoconia through keeping the calcium concentration in the vestibular endolymph at a normal critical level [45,46]. The epithelial $Ca^{2+}$ channel transport system, $Na^+/Ca^{2+}$ exchangers, and plasma membrane $Ca^{2+}$ pumps expressed in the inner ear contribute to this critical balance of calcium levels by transepithelial absorption of $Ca^{2+}$ from the endolymph of the inner ear [47]. Vitamin D receptors in the epithelial cells of the inner ear regulate the expression of some $Ca^{2+}$ binding proteins [20,22,23]. Therefore, it has been suggested that vitamin D deficiency also contributes to the development and recurrence of BPPV by abnormal calcium metabolism in the inner ear [23]. Rhim et al. [20] found that vitamin D affects BPPV as a recurrence factor independent of age, gender, follow-up period and type of BPPV. Talaat et al. [22] found that low levels of Vitamin D were related to the development of BPPV while very low levels were associated with recurrence of BPPV. Hence, in the following study, Talaat et al. [48] analyzed the effect of treatment of severe vitamin D deficiency on the recurrence rate of BPPV and found that improvement of serum 25-hydroxyvitamin D3 levels is associated with a substantial decrease in recurrence of BPPV. On the contrary, Yang et al. [23] found that the levels of vitamin D are significantly decreased in men with idiopathic BPPV but they are not associated with the recurrence of BPPV. Similarly, Sreenivas et al. [2] found that the recurrence among patients with vitamin D deficiency was not statistically significant.

They assumed that there are significant differences between bone and otoconia formation and this could be partially explained by the fact that the calcium for otoconia formation comes from the endolymph; therefore they speculated that serum markers of turnover are not directly involved in the pathogenesis of BPPV [2].

In most of the studies, blood samples were not obtained at a constant time. Given that there is seasonality of vitamin D, it is critical that future studies should take more parameters into account that affect vitamin D levels such as season, country's climate, lifestyle and skin color.

*4.7. Diabetes Mellitus/Hyperinsulinism/Hyperglycemia*

Changes in glucose metabolism have been associated with a high prevalence of inner ear disorders, hence with BPPV occurrence and recurrence [14,49,50]. These metabolic disorders can act as a principal etiologic factor in vestibular dysfunction, as well as an aggravating factor of a pre-existing vestibular disorder [51]. Yoda et al. [50] reviewed temporal bones of patients with type 1 diabetes and found that they exhibit a much higher prevalence of migration of otocone debris coming from the utricle, compared to healthy patients. In addition, they found that this difference was associated with the duration of the disease. D'Silva et al. [52] reported a higher prevalence of BPPV in patients with type 2 diabetes and found that this association was mediated by hypertension. The pathophysiologic mechanism for this correlation is still elusive. Hyperglycemia increases vascular resistance by inhibiting nitric oxide-related vasodilation, thus a combination of hypertension and diabetes may lead to tissue hypoxia and cochleovestibular degeneration [52]. In diabetes the histopathological changes of microangiopathy and vestibular neuropathy are present. Therefore, diabetes-associated neuropathy and vasculopathy as well as microvascular damage, including atherosclerosis, contribute to otoconial degeneration and thus precipitate BPPV [2,19]. In addition, diabetic patients have a poorer capacity for recovery from mild insults, such as viral infections or mild trauma, making these insults more severe [2]. Furthermore, these patients present mutations in the BETA2/NeuroD1 gene which is essential for the normal development of the sensory epithelia of the cochlea, utricle, saccule, and crista ampullaris [53]. On the other hand, hyperinsulinism may disrupt inner ear homeostasis and alter the ionic and metabolic characteristics of the stria vascularis, which is responsible for maintaining endocochlear potential through potassium secretion in the endolymphatic space [49,51]. The inner ear is also affected by hyperinsulinism due to a large number of the insulin receptors present in the endolymphatic sac [14].

In our review, Webster et al. [14] in a prospective study, found that both hyperinsulinism and hyperglycemia behaved as a risk factor for recurrence of idiopathic BPPV and also that a normal glucose tolerance test acted as a protective factor. De Stefano et al. [1] and Messina et al. [19] conducted multicenter observational studies with a large number of subjects. They evaluated the correlation between comorbidities and recurrent episodes of BPPV and found, among other things, that the presence of diabetes is associated with a statistically significant increased risk of recurrence. Piccioti et al. [4] also found that diabetes was associated with the recurrence of BPPV and that in the recurrent group, patients with more than one comorbidity were significantly more numerous compared with patients with one comorbidity. In line with the abovementioned studies, Kim et al. [8] in a smaller study group, found that comorbidities of diabetes and hypertension were associated with recurrence of BPPV. On the other hand, Sreenivas et al. [2] found a significant association between recurrence of BPPV and diabetes mellitus but not hypertension. However, there are few recent studies that found no significant rate of recurrence among diabetic patients. Specifically, Luryi et al. [16] and Zhu et al. [18] in two large single-institution studies of recurrence of BPPV, found no association between recurrence and diabetes mellitus. Wei et al. [24] in a smaller retrospective study, also did not find a correlation between the presence of comorbidities in general and diabetes mellitus in particular and increased recurrence rates of BPPV.

It seems that diabetes mellitus, as with other comorbidities, plays an important role in BPPV occurrence and recurrence. However, most studies were observational studies that did not investigate whether the patients had a good glucose control (hemoglobin A1C levels), or provide information about subcategories of diabetes (Type 1 versus Type 2), resulting in a limitation of potential therapeutic guidance. Therefore, further studies should be conducted in order to evaluate the possibility that proper treatment may reduce the prevalence and recurrence of BPPV.

*4.8. Vascular Comorbidities (Hypertension, Hyperlipidemia, Cardiovascular Disease)*

Numerous epidemiological studies have shown a possible association between BPPV and cardiovascular risk factors [1,4,8,19,26]. These studies support the hypothesis of a vascular role in the aetiopathogenesis of BPPV and its recurrence. Specifically, otoconial detachment from the otolith membrane might be facilitated by microvascular modification and ischemia, further enhanced by hypertensive peaks [4,54]. Furthermore, the blood supply to the inner ear is a terminal circulation, thus any occlusion of the AICA (anterior inferior cerebellar artery) or VBA (vertebrobasilar artery) can cause an ischemic event, leading to audio-vestibular disorders [1,19]. The vestibular system is degraded with age and as a result of changes caused by hypertension and atherosclerosis, resulting in progressive detachment of otoconia from the otolithic membrane [26]. Therefore, multiple systemic diseases increase the recurrence rate [1,4,19].

In this review, most of the studies found that patients with BPPV comorbid with hypertension had an increased recurrence rate of BPPV [1,4,8,18,19,26]. Tan et al. [26] divided the patients into two groups, a group of patients with idiopathic BPPV and hypertension and the second group of patients with idiopathic BPPV. They found a statistically significant difference in the recurrence rate, thus the presence of hypertension is significant for the prognosis of BPPV. De Stefano et al. [1] defined "groups of risk" in order to evaluate whether the combination of multiple conditions further increased the risk of recurrence and found that the combination of hypertension, diabetes, cervical osteoarthrosis and osteoporosis had the highest risk of relapse (HODo risk group). Zhu et al. [18] analyzed the clinical characteristics and risk factors for the recurrence of BPPV in different ages and found that hypertension and hyperlipidemia exhibit a higher risk of recurrence compared to age-matched patients without these diseases. Messina et al. [19] found that among patients with BPPV, 64.5% of patients with hypertension had recurrence; adding that cardiovascular risk factors expose the patients suffering from BPPV to a risk of relapse (OR > 2). Piccioti et al. [4] and Faralli et al. [25] also found that the presence of vascular factors increases the incidence of relapse. On the other hand, Sreenivas et al. [2] found that the presence of hypertension in patients with recurrence of BPPV was not statistically significant ($p = 0.085$). In the same line, Su et al. [3] and Babac et al. [15] did not find an association between recurrence of BPPV and cardiovascular disorders. Similarly, Wei et al. [24] did not detect a correlation between vascular comorbidities and recurrence commenting that this could be due to the short follow-up period of six months.

The role of vascular comorbidities in the recurrence of BPPV is still questionable. There are certain difficulties in quantifying clinical data, especially in observational studies, due to the diversity of comorbidities and the plurality of treatments. Moreover, the follow-up period in most of the studies does not provide the time to detect all events of recurrence. In addition, a lot of patients fail to attend follow-up visits or experience a transient recurrence with a rapid resolution of symptoms. However, it seems that hyperlipidemia and hypertension have a significant association with the recurrence of BPPV. Therefore, appropriate treatment of these conditions may be useful in limiting the frequency of recurrence.

*4.9. Migraine*

Migraine has long been associated with vertigo, with studies suggesting that patients suffering from migraine are two to three times more likely to suffer from vertigo, compared to the headache-free controls [55–57]. Moreover, migraine was found to be three times more common in patients with BPPV of an unknown cause than in those with BPPV secondary to trauma or surgical procedures [30]. The mechanisms by which this association arises are not well understood. One of the proposed theories suggests that migraine causes vasospasm of the labyrinthine arteries and the subsequent ischemic damage leads to the release of otoconia from the utricle [30]. Recurrent vasospasm is also associated with the oxidative stress of endothelial cells, which is a possible pathogenetic mechanism common to both migraine and BPPV [58,59]. Therefore, it is speculated that patients with migraines have a recurrent vascular damage in the inner ear that disposes to recurrent BPPV [30,55]. In addition, trigeminal nerve stimulation, an underlying pathophysiologic mechanism of migraine, induces fluid extravasation in the cochlea leading to the detachment of otoconia from the otolith organs [60]. Lastly, it has been reported that certain mutations in a $Ca^{2+}$ channel gene, detected in familial hemiplegic migraine, affect the ion channels of the brain as well as those found in the inner ear, causing imbalance of the resting potentials [30,61].

There are few articles in the literature that address the epidemiological relationship between migraine and the occurrence and recurrence of BPPV, despite the fact that there is a well-recognized association with vertigo. Ishiyama et al. [30] found increased recurrence rates (77%) in the BPPV with migraine group compared to 66% in the group of BPPV without migraine. Zhu et al. [18] in a large study analysis, also reported that BPPV recurrence was associated with migraine ($p = 0.005$). However, Hilton et al. [29], in a large BPPV cohort, compared the recurrence rates between the BPPV with migraine group and the BPPV without migraine group and found no significant difference (38.3% versus 32.1%). In relatively smaller studies, Babac et al. [15] Kansu et al. [7] and Brandt et al. [6] did not find a significantly higher recurrence of BPPV in patients with BPPV and migraine. It is worthwhile to mention the age distribution of patients with BPPV and migraine. In particular, Ishiyama et al. [30] showed that the age of onset in patients with BPPV without migraine was recorded mostly in older age groups, with a peak in the eighth decade. On the contrary, nearly half (47%) of the patients with onset of BPPV before the age of 50 years old had migraines. Similarly, Hilton et al. [29] found that patients over 60 years old had a lower likelihood of having concurrent BPPV and migraine, whereas younger age was independently associated with concurrent comorbidity of BPPV and migraine.

There is a complex relationship between BPPV and migraine due to the high prevalence of vertigo in migraine patients. Vestibular migraine has been recognized as one of the most common causes of recurrent vertigo occurring in migraine patients [62]. In several cases, vestibular migraine may be episodic and appears to be a BPPV reoccurrence, especially when the patients present with central positional nystagmus. Positional nystagmus is of central type and not due to BPPV when a) it has no latency and beats in a direction not aligned for the plane of a particular semicircular canal (e.g., no difference in the nystagmus vector with right versus left Dix-Hallpike), and b) there was no crescendo-decrescendo pattern to the nystagmus and lack of fatigability [62,63]. Distinguishing between the migraines and BPPV is crucial, because multiple maneuvers for misdiagnosed BPPV in a patient with migraines are uncomfortable, distressing and unnecessary if nystagmus is resulting from a migraine. In this case, the treatment should be targeted in the management of migraine episodes [62].

*4.10. Bilateral/Multicanal BPPV*

Bilateral and multiple-canal BPPV are less frequent forms of BPPV that typically require a larger number of maneuvers. Korres et al. [11] found increased recurrence rates in BPPV patients with bilateral canal involvement. Perez et al. [5] defined complex BPPV in cases of either BPPV affecting more than one canal or requiring a large number of maneuvers and found that these patients were at higher risk of recurrence. Moreover, they suggested that the labyrinths of patients with complex BPPV underwent inflammatory changes leading to recurrent episodes of BPPV [5]. Babac et al. [15], in a small group of patients with bilateral and multicanal BPPV, did not detect a negative impact of these factors on BPPV recurrence. Similarly, according to other studies [7,20], a significant correlation between bilateral/multicanal involvement of BPPV and BPPV recurrence was not found. Noticeably, the small number of patients suffering from bilateral/multicanal BPPV is a limitation of reaching reliable conclusions on the impact of these variables on BPPV recurrence, thus further investigation is required.

*4.11. Cervical Osteoarthritis (Spondylosis)*

Cervical spondylosis, also defined as osteoarthritis of the cervical spine, is a common age-related condition. More than 85% of people over the age of 60 are affected by cervical spondylosis [64]. It arises as a result of age-related dehydration of the nucleus pulposus and its collapse, causing bulging of the annulus fibrosus. As the disks dehydrate and shrink, signs of osteoarthritis develop, including bony projections along the edges of bones called osteophytes. These osteophytes cause cord space narrowing [64,65]. As it is reported, the vertebrobasilar circulation in patients with cervical spondylosis is insufficient [65,66]. Therefore, considering the fact that the blood supply to vestibulocochlear organ is an end artery, it is reasonable to assume that reduced blood flow to the labyrinth contributes to the dislodgement of otoconia from the macula of otolith organs [33]. In the literature, there is a deficit of studies examining the effects of cervical spondylosis on BPPV. De Stefano et al. [1] evaluated the relationship between recurrent episodes of BPPV and the most common comorbidities in the elderly population and found that the risk of relapsing BPPV in patients with cervical osteoarthritis increases 3 times; this association became statistically significant when related to the number of recurrences. On the contrary, Wei et al. [24] in a smaller study group with a relatively shorter follow-up period of 6 months, did not detect a correlation between cervical osteoarthritis and increased recurrence rates of BPPV. Li et al. [33] in a systematic review of the risk factor-associated recurrence of BPPV, found that cervical spondylosis, among other systemic diseases, could increase the recurrence of BPPV ($p < 0.05$).

It is possible that cervical spondylosis may favor the recurrence of BPPV. This could be explained by the fact that canalith repositioning procedure (CRP) on patients with dysfunction of the cervical spine is very difficult to be performed, thus leading to improper treatment or early recurrence of BPPV. Martelucci et al. [67] investigated the impact of reduced cervical mobility on CRP efficacy and suggested three pathophysiological mechanisms: (1) Debris could remain in the canal lumen and then return to the ampullary arm, causing the failure of the maneuver. (2) Part of debris could leave the canal while the rest could sprinkle in the endolymph and then accumulate again. Therefore, a transient regression of symptoms followed by an early relapse can occur. (3) The otoconial could relocate into the superior or horizontal semicircular canals, leading to a canal switch.

*4.12. Sleep Disorders*

Sleep disorders, especially insomnia, are associated with numerous physical and psychiatric health problems [68]. The pathophysiological link between BPPV and sleep disorders is still unclear. It is suggested that bad sleep leads the patients to multiple head movements during the night, therefore dispose them to a higher risk of BPPV relapse [3]. Other potential mechanisms include neuroendocrine dysfunction, caused by increased cortisol levels, as well as activation of inflammation of the nervous system, including vestibular neurons [69]. In addition, about 40% of individuals with insomnia have a comorbid psychiatric condition like anxiety and depression [69], which is known that may serve as the primary cause of vestibular symptoms as well as a risk factor for BPPV recurrence [70,71].

Only one study [3] analyzed the relationship between insomnia and BPPV recurrence; in this study, Su et al. [3] found that 30.4% of the participants in the recurrence group reported sleep disorders, the majority of which suffered from chronic insomnia and were under medication. Respectively, in the non-recurrence group, 13.2 % exhibited sleep disorders. The difference between the two groups was found to be significant.

## 5. Limitations

There are several limitations in our review. First of all, there was a high degree of heterogeneity between the studies. In particular, there were differences in the design of the studies such as duration of follow-up and cohort size. In addition, there was a diversity of the risk factors concerning diagnostic criteria of the comorbidities, quantification of their clinical data, as well as evaluation on disease control. Additionally, there was a small number of studies for some risk factors (bilateral/multicanal BPPV, cervical spondylosis, sleep disorders), which might have limited the reliability and validity of our results. Another important limitation was that most of the studies were retrospective studies, thus it was more difficult to elucidate causal relationships between the recurrence of BPPV and the risk factors. Last but not least, our review was a descriptive review and we did not assess the quality of the articles, nor did we use systematic review tools. Our intention was to avoid complex methods that in many cases are difficult to be interpreted by physicians and provide a clinical perspective on the recurrence of BPPV.

## 6. Conclusions

This comprehensive review evaluated some possible risk factors for BPPV recurrence as there is no general consensus in the literature concerning their significance. Our principal aim was to direct physician's attention to what factors should be assessed when encountering patients with BPPV. Therefore, a clinical practitioner should, first of all, take a good medical history. Patients with cardiovascular comorbidities, especially hyperlipidemia and hypertension, as well as patients with diabetes mellitus have an increased risk of BPPV recurrence. Thus, good control of these comorbidities should always be under consideration in these patients. In addition, osteoporosis and vitamin D deficiency should be probed when treating postmenopausal women with recurrent episodes of BPPV. Additionally, a typical blood test could be useful in order to provide information on a patient's lipidemic and glycemic profile as well as to reveal a possible vitamin D deficiency. Migraine and Meniere's disease have a complex relationship with BPPV; therefore, it is crucial for a physician to distinguish BPPV from these conditions in order to avoid unnecessary and distressing maneuvers. Trauma, advanced age and female gender do not seem to play an important role in BPPV recurrence, unless they are combined with other comorbidities, as mentioned above. Bilateral/multicanal BPPV, cervical spondylosis and sleep disorders are interesting, underestimated risk factors that need further investigation. In conclusion, identification of these risk factors contributes to the evaluation of BPPV patients, in order to establish a long-term prognosis, and helps physicians counseling patients regarding their expectations for the follow-up period.

In the future, more large-scale prospective studies are needed in order to clarify the role of these factors as well as pave the way for new therapeutic strategies.

**Author Contributions:** Conceptualization, G.P.; Methodology, I.S., P.B., P.K., G.G.D.; Investigation, data curation, and visualization, I.S., P.B., G.P.; Supervision, G.P.; Writing—original draft preparation, I.S. and G.P.; Writing—review and editing, I.S., P.K., G.P., G.G.D. All authors have read and agreed to the published version of the manuscript.

**Funding:** This research received no external funding.

**Institutional Review Board Statement:** Not applicable.

**Informed Consent Statement:** Not applicable.

**Data Availability Statement:** The data presented in this study are available upon request from the corresponding author.

**Conflicts of Interest:** The authors declare no conflict of interest.

## References

1. De Stefano, A.; Dispenza, F.; Suarez, H.; Perez-Fernandez, N.; Manrique-Huarte, R.; Ban, J.H.; Kim, M.B.; Strupp, M.; Feil, K.; Oliveira, C.A.; et al. A Multicenter Observational Study on the Role of Comorbidities in the Recurrent Episodes of Benign Paroxysmal Positional Vertigo. *Auris Nasus Larynx* **2014**, *41*, 31–36. [CrossRef] [PubMed]
2. Sreenivas, V.; Sima, N.H.; Philip, S. The Role of Comorbidities in Benign Paroxysmal Positional Vertigo. *Ear Nose Throat J.* **2021**, *100*, NP225–NP230. [CrossRef] [PubMed]
3. Su, P.; Liu, Y.C.; Lin, H.C. Risk Factors for the Recurrence of Post-Semicircular Canal Benign Paroxysmal Positional Vertigo after Canalith Repositioning. *J. Neurol.* **2016**, *263*, 45–51. [CrossRef]
4. Picciotti, P.M.; Lucidi, D.; De Corso, E.; Meucci, D.; Sergi, B.; Paludetti, G. Comorbidities and Recurrence of Benign Paroxysmal Positional Vertigo: Personal Experience. *Int. J. Audiol.* **2016**, *55*, 279–284. [CrossRef] [PubMed]
5. Pérez, P.; Franco, V.; Cuesta, P.; Aldama, P.; Alvarez, M.J.; Méndez, J.C. Recurrence of Benign Paroxysmal Positional Vertigo. *Otol. Neurotol.* **2012**, *33*, 437–443. [CrossRef]
6. Brandt, T.; Huppert, D.; Hecht, J.; Karch, C.; Strupp, M. Benign Paroxysmal Positioning Vertigo: A Long-Term Follow-up (6–17 Years) of 125 Patients. *Acta Otolaryngol.* **2006**, *126*, 160–163. [CrossRef] [PubMed]
7. Kansu, L.; Avci, S.; Yilmaz, I.; Ozluoglu, L.N. Long-Term Follow-up of Patients with Posterior Canal Benign Paroxysmal Positional Vertigo. *Acta Otolaryngol.* **2010**, *130*, 1009–1012. [CrossRef] [PubMed]
8. Kim, S.Y.; Han, S.H.; Kim, Y.H.; Park, M.H. Clinical Features of Recurrence and Osteoporotic Changes in Benign Paroxysmal Positional Vertigo. *Auris Nasus Larynx* **2017**, *44*, 156–161. [CrossRef] [PubMed]
9. Bhattacharyya, N.; Gubbels, S.P.; Schwartz, S.R.; Edlow, J.A.; El-Kashlan, H.; Fife, T.; Holmberg, J.M.; Mahoney, K.; Hollingsworth, D.B.; Roberts, R.; et al. Clinical Practice Guideline: Benign Paroxysmal Positional Vertigo (Update). *Otolaryngol.—Head Neck Surg.* **2017**, *156*, S1–S47. [CrossRef] [PubMed]
10. Del Rio, M.; Arriaga, M.A. Benign Positional Vertigo: Prognostic Factors. *Otolaryngol.—Head Neck Surg.* **2004**, *130*, 426–429. [CrossRef]
11. Korres, S.; Balatsouras, D.G.; Ferekidis, E. Prognosis of Patients with Benign Paroxysmal Positional Vertigo Treated with Repositioning Manoeuvres. *J. Laryngol. Otol.* **2006**, *120*, 528–533. [CrossRef] [PubMed]
12. Choi, S.J.; Lee, J.B.; Lim, H.J.; Park, H.Y.; Park, K.; In, S.M.; Oh, J.H.; Choung, Y.H. Clinical Features of Recurrent or Persistent Benign Paroxysmal Positional Vertigo. *Otolaryngol.—Head Neck Surg.* **2012**, *147*, 919–924. [CrossRef] [PubMed]
13. Yamanaka, T.; Shirota, S.; Sawai, Y.; Murai, T.; Fujita, N.; Hosoi, H. Osteoporosis as a Risk Factor for the Recurrence of Benign Paroxysmal Positional Vertigo. *Laryngoscope* **2013**, *123*, 2813–2816. [CrossRef]
14. Webster, G.; Sens, P.M.; Salmito, M.C.; Cavalcante, J.D.R.; dos Santos, P.R.B.; da Silva, A.L.M.; de Souza, É.C.F. Hyperinsulinemia and Hyperglycemia: Risk Factors for Recurrence of Benign Paroxysmal Positional Vertigo. *Braz. J. Otorhinolaryngol.* **2015**, *81*, 347–351. [CrossRef]
15. Babac, S.; Djeric, D.; Petrovic-Lazic, M.; Arsovic, N.; Mikic, A. Why Do Treatment Failure and Recurrences of Benign Paroxysmal Positional Vertigo Occur? *Otol. Neurotol.* **2014**, *35*, 1105–1110. [CrossRef]
16. Luryi, A.L.; Lawrence, J.; Bojrab, D.I.; LaRouere, M.; Babu, S.; Zappia, J.; Sargent, E.W.; Chan, E.; Naumann, I.; Hong, R.S.; et al. Recurrence in Benign Paroxysmal Positional Vertigo: A Large, Single-Institution Study. *Otol. Neurotol.* **2018**, *39*, 622–627. [CrossRef]
17. Nunez, R.A.; Cass, S.P.; Furman, J.M. Short- and Long-Term Outcomes of Canalith Repositioning for Benign Paroxysmal Positional Vertigo. *Otolaryngol. Neck Surg.* **2000**, *122*, 647–653. [CrossRef]
18. Zhu, C.T.; Zhao, X.Q.; Ju, Y.; Wang, Y.; Chen, M.M.; Cui, Y. Clinical Characteristics and Risk Factors for the Recurrence of Benign Paroxysmal Positional Vertigo. *Front. Neurol.* **2019**, *10*, 1190. [CrossRef]
19. Messina, A.; Casani, A.P.; Manfrin, M.; Guidetti, G. Survey Italiana Sulla Vertigine Parossistica Posizionale. *Acta Otorhinolaryngol. Ital.* **2017**, *37*, 328–335. [CrossRef] [PubMed]
20. Rhim, G. Il Serum Vitamin D and Recurrent Benign Paroxysmal Positional Vertigo. *Laryngoscope Investig. Otolaryngol.* **2016**, *1*, 150–153. [CrossRef] [PubMed]
21. Balatsouras, D.G.; Ganelis, P.; Aspris, A.; Economou, N.C.; Moukos, A.; Koukoutsis, G. Benign Paroxysmal Positional Vertigo Associated with Meniere's Disease: Epidemiological, Pathophysiologic, Clinical, and Therapeutic Aspects. *Ann. Otol. Rhinol. Laryngol.* **2012**, *121*, 682–688. [CrossRef]
22. Talaat, H.S.; Abuhadied, G.; Talaat, A.S.; Abdelaal, M.S.S. Low Bone Mineral Density and Vitamin D Deficiency in Patients with Benign Positional Paroxysmal Vertigo. *Eur. Arch. Oto-Rhino-Laryngol.* **2015**, *272*, 2249–2253. [CrossRef]
23. Yang, C.J.; Kim, Y.; Lee, H.S.; Park, H.J. Bone Mineral Density and Serum 25-Hydroxyvitamin D in Patients with Idiopathic Benign Paroxysmal Positional Vertigo. *J. Vestib. Res. Equilib. Orientat.* **2018**, *27*, 287–294. [CrossRef]
24. Wei, W.; Sayyid, Z.N.; Ma, X.; Wang, T.; Dong, Y. Presence of Anxiety and Depression Symptoms Affects the First Time Treatment Efficacy and Recurrence of Benign Paroxysmal Positional Vertigo. *Front. Neurol.* **2018**, *9*, 178. [CrossRef] [PubMed]
25. Faralli, M.; Ricci, G.; Molini, E.; Bressi, T.; Simoncelli, C.; Frenguelli, A.; Division, C.S. Paroxysmal Positional Vertigo: The Role of Age. *Acta Otorhinolaryngol. Ital.* **2006**, *26*, 25–31.
26. Tan, J.; Deng, Y.; Zhang, T.; Wang, M. Clinical Characteristics and Treatment Outcomes for Benign Paroxysmal Positional Vertigo Comorbid with Hypertension. *Acta Otolaryngol.* **2017**, *137*, 482–484. [CrossRef]

27. Prokopakis, E.; Vlastos, I.M.; Tsagournisakis, M.; Christodoulou, P.; Kawauchi, H.; Velegrakis, G. Canalith Repositioning Procedures among 965 Patients with Benign Paroxysmal Positional Vertigo. *Audiol. Neurotol.* **2013**, *18*, 83–88. [CrossRef] [PubMed]
28. Rashad, U.M. Long-Term Follow up after Epley's Manoeuvre in Patients with Benign Paroxysmal Positional Vertigo. *J. Laryngol. Otol.* **2009**, *123*, 69–74. [CrossRef] [PubMed]
29. Hilton, D.B.; Luryi, A.L.; Bojrab, D.I.; Babu, S.C.; Hong, R.S.; Santiago Rivera, O.J.; Schutt, C.A. Comparison of Associated Comorbid Conditions in Patients with Benign Paroxysmal Positional Vertigo with or without Migraine History: A Large Single Institution Study. *Am. J. Otolaryngol.—Head Neck Med. Surg.* **2020**, *41*, 102650. [CrossRef]
30. Ishiyama, A.; Jacobson, K.M.; Baloh, R.W. Migraine and Benign Positional Vertigo. *Ann. Otol. Rhinol. Laryngol.* **2000**, *109*, 377–380. [CrossRef] [PubMed]
31. Gordon, C.R.; Levite, R.; Joffe, V.; Gadoth, N. Is Posttraumatic Benign Paroxysmal Positional Vertigo Different from the Idiopathic Form? *Arch. Neurol.* **2004**, *61*, 1590–1593. [CrossRef]
32. Agrawal, Y.; Carey, J.P.; Della Santina, C.C.; Schubert, M.C.; Minor, L.B. Disorders of Balance and Vestibular Function in US Adults: Data from the National Health and Nutrition Examination Survey, 2001–2004. *Arch. Intern. Med.* **2009**, *169*, 938–944. [CrossRef] [PubMed]
33. Li, S.; Wang, Z.; Liu, Y.; Cao, J.; Zheng, H.; Jing, Y.; Han, L.; Ma, X.; Xia, R.; Yu, L. Risk Factors for the Recurrence of Benign Paroxysmal Positional Vertigo: A Systematic Review and Meta-Analysis. *Ear Nose Throat J.* **2020**, 0145561320943362. [CrossRef] [PubMed]
34. Vibert, D.; Kompis, M.; Häusler, R. Benign Paroxysmal Positional Vertigo in Older Women May Be Related to Osteoporosis and Osteopenia. *Ann. Otol. Rhinol. Laryngol.* **2003**, *112*, 885–889. [CrossRef] [PubMed]
35. Kutlubaev, M.A.; Xu, Y.; Hornibrook, J. Benign Paroxysmal Positional Vertigo in Meniere's Disease: Systematic Review and Meta-Analysis of Frequency and Clinical Characteristics. *J. Neurol.* **2021**, *268*, 1608–1614. [CrossRef] [PubMed]
36. Chen, J.; Zhang, S.; Cui, K.; Liu, C. Risk Factors for Benign Paroxysmal Positional Vertigo Recurrence: A Systematic Review and Meta-Analysis. *J. Neurol.* **2020**, 1–11. [CrossRef]
37. Lundberg, Y.W.; Zhao, X.; Yamoah, E.N. Assembly of the Otoconia Complex to the Macular Sensory Epithelium of the Vestibule. *Brain Res.* **2006**, *1091*, 47–57. [CrossRef]
38. Ross, M.D. Calcium Ion Uptake and Exchange in Otoconia. *Adv. Otorhinolaryngol.* **1979**, *25*, 26–33.
39. Preston, R.E.; Johnsson, L.G.; Hill, J.H.; Schacht, J. Incorporation of Radioactive Calcium into Otolithic Membranes and Middle Ear Ossicles of the Gerbil. *Acta Otolaryngol.* **1975**, *80*, 269–275. [CrossRef]
40. Vibert, D.; Sans, A.; Kompis, M.; Travo, C.; Mühlbauer, R.C.; Tschudi, I.; Boukhaddaoui, H.; Häusler, R. Ultrastructural Changes in Otoconia of Osteoporotic Rats. *Audiol. Neurotol.* **2008**, *13*, 293–301. [CrossRef]
41. Thalmann, R.; Ignatova, E.; Kachar, B.; Ornitz, D.M.; Thalmann, I. Development and Maintenance of Otoconia: Biochemical Considerations. *Ann. N. Y. Acad. Sci.* **2001**, *942*, 162–178. [CrossRef] [PubMed]
42. Yamauchi, D.; Nakaya, K.; Raveendran, N.N.; Harbidge, D.G.; Singh, R.; Wangemann, P.; Marcus, D.C. Expression of Epithelial Calcium Transport System in Rat Cochlea and Vestibular Labyrinth. *BMC Physiol.* **2010**, *10*, 1. [CrossRef] [PubMed]
43. Takemura, T.; Sakagami, M.; Nakase, T.; Kubo, T.; Kitamura, Y.; Nomura, S. Localization of Osteopontin in the Otoconial Organs of Adult Rats. *Hear. Res.* **1994**, *79*, 99–104. [CrossRef]
44. Mikulec, A.A.; Kowalczyk, K.A.; Pfitzinger, M.E.; Harris, D.A.; Jackson, L.E. Negative Association between Treated Osteoporosis and Benign Paroxysmal Positional Vertigo in Women. *J. Laryngol. Otol.* **2010**, *124*, 374–376. [CrossRef]
45. Parham, K.; Leonard, G.; Feinn, R.S.; Lafreniere, D.; Kenny, A.M. Prospective Clinical Investigation of the Relationship between Idiopathic Benign Paroxysmal Positional Vertigo and Bone Turnover: A Pilot Study. *Laryngoscope* **2013**, *123*, 2834–2839. [CrossRef] [PubMed]
46. Jeong, S.H.; Kim, J.S.; Shin, J.W.; Kim, S.; Lee, H.; Lee, A.Y.; Kim, J.M.; Jo, H.; Song, J.; Ghim, Y. Decreased Serum Vitamin D in Idiopathic Benign Paroxysmal Positional Vertigo. *J. Neurol.* **2013**, *260*, 832–838. [CrossRef]
47. Yamauchi, D.; Raveendran, N.N.; Pondugula, S.R.; Kampalli, S.B.; Sanneman, J.D.; Harbidge, D.G.; Marcus, D.C. Vitamin D Upregulates Expression of ECaC1 MRNA in Semicircular Canal. *Biochem. Biophys. Res. Commun.* **2005**, *331*, 1353–1357. [CrossRef] [PubMed]
48. Talaat, H.S.; Kabel, A.M.H.; Khaliel, L.H.; Abuhadied, G.; El-Naga, H.A.E.R.A.; Talaat, A.S. Reduction of Recurrence Rate of Benign Paroxysmal Positional Vertigo by Treatment of Severe Vitamin D Deficiency. *Auris Nasus Larynx* **2016**, *43*, 237–241. [CrossRef]
49. Angeli, R.D.; Lavinsky, L.; Dolganov, A. Alterations in Cochlear Function during Induced Acute Hyperinsulinemia in an Animal Model. *Braz. J. Otorhinolaryngol.* **2009**, *75*, 760–764. [CrossRef]
50. Yoda, S.; Cureoglu, S.; Yildirim-Baylan, M.; Morita, N.; Fukushima, H.; Harada, T.; Paparella, M.M. Association between Type 1 Diabetes Mellitus and Deposits in the Semicircular Canals. *Otolaryngol.—Head Neck Surg.* **2011**, *145*, 458–462. [CrossRef] [PubMed]
51. Paula Serra, A.; de Carvalho Lopes, K.; Dorigueto, R.S.; Freitas Ganança, F. Blood Glucose and Insulin Levels in Patients with Peripheral Vestibular Disease. *Braz. J. Otorhinolaryngol.* **2009**, *75*, 701–705. [CrossRef]

52. D'Silva, L.J.; Staecker, H.; Lin, J.; Sykes, K.J.; Phadnis, M.A.; McMahon, T.M.; Connolly, D.; Sabus, C.H.; Whitney, S.L.; Kludinga, P.M. Retrospective Data Suggests That the Higher Prevalence of Benign Paroxysmal Positional Vertigo in Individuals with Type 2 Diabetes Is Mediated by Hypertension. *J. Vestib. Res. Equilib. Orientat.* **2016**, *25*, 233–239. [CrossRef] [PubMed]
53. Liu, M.; Pereira, F.A.; Price, S.D.; Chu, M.J.; Shope, C.; Himes, D.; Eatock, R.A.; Brownell, W.E.; Lysakowski, A.; Tsai, M.J. Essential Role of BETA2/NeuroD1 in Development of the Vestibular and Auditory Systems. *Genes Dev.* **2000**, *14*, 2839–2854. [CrossRef] [PubMed]
54. Von Brevern, M.; Radtke, A.; Lezius, F.; Feldmann, M.; Ziese, T.; Lempert, T.; Neuhauser, H. Epidemiology of Benign Paroxysmal Positional Vertigo: A Population Based Study. *J. Neurol. Neurosurg. Psychiatry* **2007**, *78*, 710–715. [CrossRef] [PubMed]
55. Bruss, D.; Abouzari, M.; Sarna, B.; Goshtasbi, K.; Lee, A.; Birkenbeuel, J.; Djalilian, H.R. Migraine Features in Patients With Recurrent Benign Paroxysmal Positional Vertigo. *Otol. Neurotol.* **2021**, *42*, 461–465. [CrossRef] [PubMed]
56. Vuković, V.; Plavec, D.; Galinović, I.; Lovrenčić-Huzjan, A.; Budišić, M.; Demarin, V. Prevalence of Vertigo, Dizziness, and Migrainous Vertigo in Patients with Migraine. *Headache* **2007**, *47*, 1427–1435. [CrossRef] [PubMed]
57. Kuritzky, A.; Ziegler, D.K.; Hassanein, R. Vertigo, Motion Sickness and Migraine. *Headache J. Head Face Pain* **1981**, *21*, 227–231. [CrossRef]
58. Güçlütürk, M.T.; Ünal, Z.N.; Ismi, O.; Çimen, M.B.Y.; Ünal, M. The Role of Oxidative Stress and Inflammatory Mediators in Benign Paroxysmal Positional Vertigo. *J. Int. Adv. Otol.* **2016**, *12*, 101–105. [CrossRef]
59. Neri, M.; Frustaci, A.; Milic, M.; Valdiglesias, V.; Fini, M.; Bonassi, S.; Barbanti, P. A Meta-Analysis of Biomarkers Related to Oxidative Stress and Nitric Oxide Pathway in Migraine. *Cephalalgia* **2015**, *35*, 931–937. [CrossRef]
60. Vass, Z.; Steyger, P.S.; Hordichok, A.J.; Trune, D.R.; Jancsó, G.; Nuttall, A.L. Capsaicin Stimulation of the Cochlea and Electric Stimulation of the Trigeminal Ganglion Mediate Vascular Permeability in Cochlear and Vertebro-Basilar Arteries: A Potential Cause of Inner Ear Dysfunction in Headache. *Neuroscience* **2001**, *103*, 189–201. [CrossRef]
61. Ophoff, R.A.; Terwindt, G.M.; Vergouwe, M.N.; Van Eijk, R.; Oefner, P.J.; Hoffman, S.M.G.; Lamerdin, J.E.; Mohrenweiser, H.W.; Bulman, D.E.; Ferrari, M.; et al. Familial Hemiplegic Migraine and Episodic Ataxia Type-2 Are Caused by Mutations in the Ca2+ Channel Gene CACNL1A4. *Cell* **1996**, *87*, 543–552. [CrossRef]
62. Lempert, T.; von Brevern, M. Vestibular Migraine. *Neurol. Clin.* **2019**, *37*, 695–706. [CrossRef] [PubMed]
63. Argaet, E.C.; Bradshaw, A.P.; Welgampola, M.S. Benign Positional Vertigo, Its Diagnosis, Treatment and Mimics. *Clin. Neurophysiol. Pract.* **2019**, *4*, 97–111. [CrossRef]
64. Kelly, J.C.; Groarke, P.J.; Butler, J.S.; Poynton, A.R.; O'Byrne, J.M. The Natural History and Clinical Syndromes of Degenerative Cervical Spondylosis. *Adv. Orthop.* **2012**, *2012*, 393642. [CrossRef]
65. Bayrak, I.K.; Durmus, D.; Bayrak, A.O.; Diren, B.; Canturk, F. Effect of Cervical Spondylosis on Vertebral Arterial Flow and Its Association with Vertigo. *Clin. Rheumatol.* **2009**, *28*, 59–64. [CrossRef] [PubMed]
66. Li, Y.; Peng, B. Pathogenesis, Diagnosis, and Treatment of Cervical Vertigo. *Pain Physician* **2015**, *18*, E583–E595.
67. Martellucci, S.; Attanasio, G.; Ralli, M.; Marcelli, V.; de Vincentiis, M.; Greco, A.; Gallo, A. Does Cervical Range of Motion Affect the Outcomes of Canalith Repositioning Procedures for Posterior Canal Benign Positional Paroxysmal Vertigo? *Am. J. Otolaryngol.—Head Neck Med. Surg.* **2019**, *40*, 494–498. [CrossRef] [PubMed]
68. Fernandez-Mendoza, J.; Vgontzas, A.N. Insomnia and Its Impact on Physical and Mental Health. *Curr. Psychiatry Rep.* **2013**, *15*, 418. [CrossRef]
69. Shih, C.P.; Wang, C.H.; Chung, C.H.; Lin, H.C.; Chen, H.C.; Lee, J.C.; Chien, W.C. Increased Risk of Benign Paroxysmal Positional Vertigo in Patients with Non-Apnea Sleep Disorders: A Nationwide, Population-Based Cohort Study. *J. Clin. Sleep Med.* **2018**, *14*, 2021–2029. [CrossRef]
70. Bronstein, A. (Ed.) *Oxford Textbook of Vertigo and Imbalance*; Oxford University Press: London, UK, 2013; ISBN 9780199608997.
71. Eckhardt-Henn, A.; Dieterich, M. Psychiatric Disorders in Otoneurology Patients. *Neurol. Clin.* **2005**, *23*, 731–749. [CrossRef]

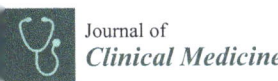

Article

# Video Head Impulse Test (vHIT): Value of Gain and Refixation Saccades in Unilateral Vestibular Neuritis

George Psillas [1,\*], Ioanna Petrou [1], Athanasia Printza [1], Ioanna Sfakianaki [1], Paris Binos [2], Sofia Anastasiadou [1] and Jiannis Constantinidis [1]

[1] 1st Otolaryngology Department, School of Medicine, Faculty of Health Sciences, Aristotle University of Thessaloniki, AHEPA Hospital, Stilponos Kyriakidi St., 546 36 Thessaloniki, Greece; petrouio@hotmail.gr (I.P.); nan@med.auth.gr (A.P.); g_sfakianaki@yahoo.com (I.S.); anastasiadousof23@gmail.com (S.A.); janconst@otenet.gr (J.C.)

[2] Department of Rehabilitation Sciences, Cyprus University of Technology, Limassol 3036, Cyprus; paris.binos@cut.ac.cy

\* Correspondence: psill@otenet.gr; Tel.: +30-2310-994-762; Fax: +30-2310-994-916

**Abstract:** The aim of this study was to evaluate gain and refixation saccades (covert and overt) using a video head impulse test (vHIT) in the horizontal and vertical planes in patients after the onset of unilateral acute vestibular neuritis (AVN). Thirty-five patients were examined in the acute stage of AVN and at follow-up (range, 6–30 months); a control group of 32 healthy subjects also participated. At onset, the mean gain was significantly lower on the affected side in all of the semi-circular canal planes, mainly in the horizontal canal plane, and saccades (covert and overt) were more prevalent in the horizontal compared to the vertical canal planes. Multi-canal affection occurred more frequently (80% for gain, 71% for saccades) than isolated canal affection. At follow-up, which ranged from 6 to 30 months, the gain was recovered in all of the canals (anterior in 50%, horizontal in 42.8%, and posterior canal in 41.1% of cases), while covert and overt saccades were reduced in the horizontal and vertical planes. However, covert saccades were still recorded in a greater proportion (69%) than overt saccades (57%) in the horizontal plane and at a lower rate in the vertical planes. The compensatory mechanisms after AVN mainly involve the horizontal canal, as the refixation saccades—especially covert ones—were more frequently recorded in the horizontal than vertical canals.

**Keywords:** video head impulse test; saccades; vestibular gain; vestibular neuritis; vestibuloocular reflex; semicircular canal

## 1. Introduction

Acute vestibular neuritis (AVN) is a clinical condition characterized by acute, prolonged vertigo of peripheral origin with nausea and vomiting followed by a period of unsteadiness [1]. AVN accounts for 3.2–9% of patients visiting a dizziness center and has an incidence of 3.5 per 100,000 population [2]. The leading theory for the etiology of AVN is viral inflammation processes, with the herpes simplex virus being most commonly implicated [3].

AVN involves both the superior and inferior vestibular nerves and may affect them separately. The superior vestibular nerve innervates the horizontal or lateral semi-circular canal (HC), the anterior or superior canal (AC), and the utricle of the labyrinth, while the inferior vestibular nerve innervates the posterior or inferior canal (PC) and the saccule.

The vestibulo–ocular reflex (VOR) is an important reflex that aims to ensure gaze stability to provide stable vision during rapid head rotations [4]. This is assessed by asking a patient to maintain their gaze on a target while an operator applies unpredictable and abrupt but small head turns in the horizontal and vertical planes [5,6]. If the VOR function is intact, the subject maintains fixation on the target during head rotations by generating eye movements that are equal and opposite to the rotation of the head; however, if their

VOR function is deficient (i.e., during AVN with unilateral reduced horizontal or vertical canal function), the eyes of the patient can fail to fix on the target, and the patient must make corrective refixation saccades (eye movements) back to the target. The saccades that can be detected by the operator following the end of the head movements are known as overt saccades, while those that occur during the head impulses are known as covert saccades [4–6]. Covert saccades are invisible to the clinician; fortunately, the video head impulse test (vHIT) can recognize covert saccades and measure the VOR gain [7]. The VOR gain is the ratio of the size of the slow-phase eye movement response to the size of the passive head movement stimulus, which is decreased in peripheral vestibular disorders [8]. Thus, the vHIT allows for objective analysis of VOR gain, VOR gain asymmetry (analogous to caloric canal paresis), and refixation saccades of all six semi-circular canals [9].

In this study, we aim to prospectively evaluate the VOR gain and refixation saccades (covert and overt) in AVN from the acute stage to the follow-up (ranging from 6 to 30 months). Although previous studies have assessed, through the use of vHIT, the VOR gain in the horizontal and vertical semi-circular canals in patients suffering from AVN [10–13], there has been no study analyzing the VOR gain and refixation saccades for AVN in both the horizontal and vertical planes.

## 2. Materials and Methods

Thirty-five patients, including 28 men and 7 women (age range, 24–77 years; mean age, 52.25; SD, ±13.23 years), participated in our study. The patients were admitted consecutively after diagnosed with acute vestibular neuritis (AVN), according to the following criteria [1,10]: (a) sudden rotatory vertigo lasting more than 24 h (accompanied by nausea and vomiting), (b) unidirectional horizontal-torsional spontaneous nystagmus towards the unaffected side, (c) a positive Unterberger test, where the patient was asked to undertake stationary stepping for one minute with their eyes closed and a positive test was indicated by rotational movement of the patient towards the side of the lesion, (d) unilateral affection, and (e) normal hearing.

The exclusion criteria were age under 18 years old, pregnancy, auditory or neurological disorders, history of psychiatric disorder, patients suffering from diabetes, patients with neck stiffness, a history of taking CNS depressants, excessive blinking, and a history of recent eye surgery. All patients were treated with intravenous corticosteroids during their stay at the hospital and, on discharge, they performed a vestibular rehabilitation program for 3 weeks. We had a long-term follow-up period (mean, 14.37; SD, ±7.69 months) that ranged from 6 to 30 months.

In addition, all of patients were required to complete the Greek version of the Dizziness Handicap Inventory (DHI) questionnaire (25 questions) during the acute phase and at the follow-up examination. For each item, the following scores were assigned: no = 0, sometimes = 2, yes = 4. A DHI score of 16–35 points indicates mild disability, 36–53 points indicates moderate disability, and more than 54 points indicates severe disability [14]. Pre- and post-treatment would have to differ by at least 18 points (95% CI for a true change) before the interaction could be said to have effected a significant change in a self-perceived handicap [15].

### 2.1. Control Group

The control group consisted of 32 healthy adults, including 13 men and 19 women (age range, 22–74 years; mean age, 45.18; SD, ±15.15 years), who were evenly distributed in all age groups. None of them had any history of vestibular, auditory, and/or neurological disorders.

Written informed consent was obtained from all subjects participating in this study. This study was approved by the ethics committee of the Aristotle University of Thessaloniki.

## 2.2. vHIT

vHIT was performed on all subjects using an EyeSeeCam system (Interacoustics, Middelfart, Denmark) at the time of the initial presentation, within 10 days of the onset of symptoms, and was repeated at the follow-up visit. All six semi-circular canals were evaluated. The system consists of a pair of lightweight goggles with a high-speed camera for recording eye movements and a sensor that measures head velocity. Participants were instructed to fixate on a target on the wall 1.2 m away, while the examiner stood behind them and performed ten unpredictable, low amplitude (10–20°) head impulses for all three canal planes (horizontal, right anterior/left posterior, left anterior/right posterior) and for each side; in general, the horizontal head velocities were higher (150–250 °/s) than the vertical head velocities (50–150 °/s). For the horizontal plane, the examiner placed their hands on the patient's jaw while, for the vertical plane, the dominant hand was placed on the top of the head and the other under the chin. For the right/left horizontal canal plane, horizontal head turns were performed to each side, always starting from the center (Figure 1). For the right anterior/left posterior canal testing, the subject turned 45° to the left and the impulses were delivered by either rotating the head forward or backward (always asking the patient to fixate on the target) while, for the left anterior/right posterior canal testing, the subject turned 45° to the right and the impulses were delivered by rotating the head either forward or backward.

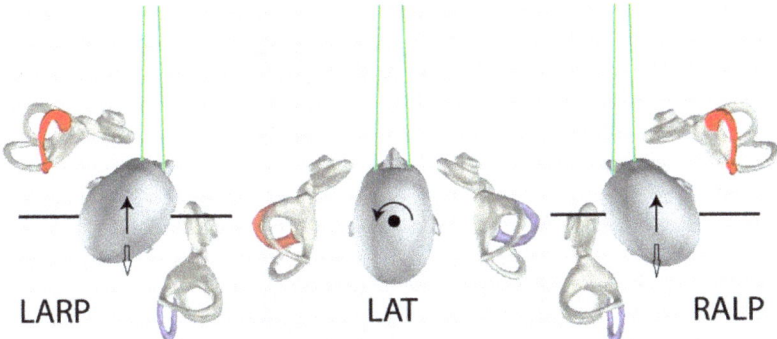

**Figure 1.** In the middle, affected HC (horizontal canal) plane, the head movements (circle black arrow) for left affected (red) HC/contralateral unaffected right (purple) HC, as viewed from above. On the left, affected AC (anterior canal) plane, the head movements (black arrow) for left affected (red) AC/contralateral unaffected right (purple) posterior canal (PC). On the right, affected PC plane, the head movements (white arrow) for left affected (purple) PC/contralateral unaffected right (red) AC. Inversely, on the left, affected PC plane, the head movements (white arrow) for right affected (purple) PC/contralateral unaffected left (red) AC. On the right, affected AC plane, the head movements (black arrow) for right affected (red) AC/contralateral unaffected left (purple) PC (with the permission of Curthoys IS). LARP: left anterior & right posterior canal, LAT: lateral or horizontal canals, RALP: right anterior & left posterior canal.

Each examined plane was described as: (a) Affected HC plane as affected HC/contralateral unaffected HC plane, (b) affected AC plane as affected AC/contralateral unaffected PC plane, and (c) affected PC plane as affected PC/contralateral unaffected AC plane (Figure 1).

The system's software calculates the VOR gain as the ratio of eye to head peak velocity from the average of head impulses and gain asymmetry (%) between the affected and unaffected canals for each plane, according to the following equation: $GA = ((Gc - Gi)/(Gc + Gi)) \times 100\%$, where GA: gain asymmetry, Gi: gain for ipsilateral canal and Gc: gain for contralateral canal. The EyeSeeCam system uses the regression method for VOR gain and gain asymmetry, which allows for graphical data analysis over the entire velocity range of head impulses; following the test completion, it provides the average regression plot slope (a best-fit line through data points at different head velocities with accompanying gain values). The instantaneous median VOR at 60 ms was used for measuring the horizontal gain. A perfect VOR gain is a gain of 1.0 (eye movement is exactly equal and opposite to head movements); while a VOR gain lower than 0.80 has been proposed as cut-point between normal and abnormally low VOR gain [16]. The gains measured in each plane are referred to as HC gain, AC gain, and PC gain, respectively. Depending on which ear was involved, the gain of the affected and the unaffected side was compared to the gain of the right and left ear of the healthy subjects (control group), respectively.

Pathological saccades were considered in a patient when their peak velocity was >100 °/s and their repeatability was observed in more than 50% of total impulses for each plane. The presence of pathological saccades in each plane was described as HC overt or covert saccades, AC overt or covert saccades, and PC overt or covert saccades, accordingly (Figure 2). In our study, the frequency of pathological saccades was counted in each patient for all the canals and the incidence of patients with pathological saccades was also calculated.

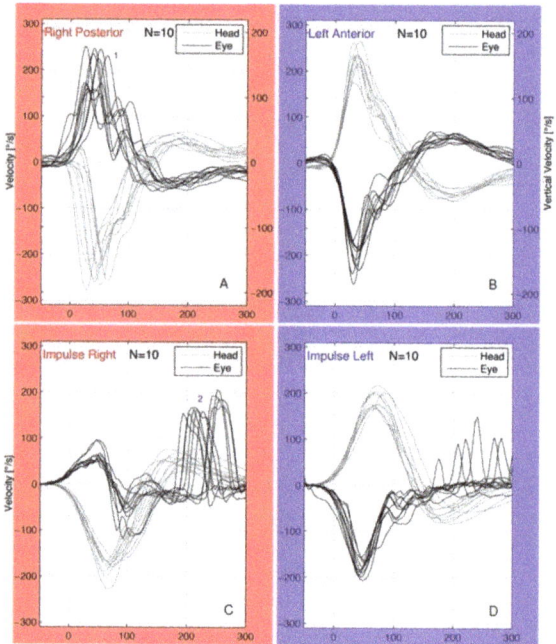

**Figure 2.** Patient with right acute vestibular neuritis (**A**,**B**) and affected posterior canal (PC) plane: pathological covert saccades (1) were present in the right PC (**A**). Covert saccades occurred during the head impulses and their peak velocity was more than 100 °/s; no saccades were observed in the left unaffected anterior canal (**B**). Patient with right acute vestibular neuritis (**C**,**D**) and affected horizontal canal (HC) plane: pathological overt saccades (2) were present in the right HC (**C**) following the end of the head movements; the saccades found in the left HC (**D**) were not pathological (peak velocity <100 °/s, repeatability <50% of total impulses).

## 3. Statistical Analysis

Continuous variables are reported as mean and standard deviation, after being checked for regularity with the Kolmogorov–Smirnov test. Categorical variables were reported to as frequencies and relative frequencies (%). Student's $t$-test (for two categories) or one-way ANOVA (for three or more categories) were used to compare the mean values of the continuous variables, with respect to the categories of a qualitative variable. Bonferroni correction was used for post hoc analysis. Pearson's correlation coefficient was also used to investigate the correlations between continuous variables. In all cases, we considered the results to have statistical significance when the $p$-values were less than 0.05. The SPSS v.25.0 software (IBM Corp., Armonk, NY, USA) was used for statistical analysis.

## 4. Results

In the 35 patients with AVN, at the acute stage, the mean gain was significantly lower (compared to control group) on the affected side in all of the canal planes, but mainly in the horizontal canal plane (Table 1). In the HC plane, the gain was abnormal in 28 (80%) out of 35 patients while, at the follow-up, the gain was normal in 12 (42.8%) out of 28 patients. In the AC plane, the gain was also abnormal in 28 (80%) out of 35 patients while, at the follow-up, the gain was normal in a greater proportion (50%, 14/28). In the PC plane, the gain was abnormal at a lower rate, compared to the other canals (48.5%, 17/35) while, at the follow-up, the gain was normal in 7 (41.1%) out of 17 patients. Interestingly, on the unaffected side, the mean gain at acute stage was found to be smaller than that of the control group in all the canal planes (Table 1). Moreover, according to vHIT measurements on the affected side, the gain improved at the follow-up in all the canal planes, but significantly in the HC ($p < 0.01$) and AC ($p < 0.001$) canal planes, respectively (Table 1). On the affected side, the mean gain asymmetry was decreased at the follow-up in all of the canal planes, but was more significant in the affected AC/unaffected PC planes (Table 2).

**Table 1.** Gain values of vHIT in vestibular neuritis at the acute stage and follow-up during head movements towards the affected and unaffected side, respectively, in horizontal (HC), posterior (PC) and anterior (AC) plane (see also Figure 1). *** $p < 0.001$, ** $p < 0.01$, * $p < 0.05$. SD: standard deviation, C.I.: confidence interval.

| Gain | | Mean ± SD | Significance | 95% C.I. for Mean |
|---|---|---|---|---|
| Affected HC | Acute stage<br>Follow-up<br>Control | 0.54 ± 0.36<br>0.77 ± 0.31<br>0.86 ± 0.19 | Acute—control ***<br>Acute—follow-up ** | 0.41–0.67<br>0.66–0.88<br>0.80–0.93 |
| Unaffected HC | Acute stage<br>Follow-up<br>Control | 0.84 ± 0.36<br>0.98 ± 0.32<br>1.10 ± 0.28 | Acute—control ** | 0.72–0.97<br>0.86–1.09<br>1.00–1.20 |
| Affected AC | Acute stage<br>Follow-up<br>Control | 0.64 ± 0.16<br>0.83 ± 0.15<br>0.78 ± 0.10 | Acute—control *<br>Acute—follow-up *** | 0.62–0.74<br>0.77–0.88<br>0.74–0.82 |
| Unaffected AC | Acute stage<br>Follow-up<br>Control | 0.79 ± 0.16<br>0.84 ± 0.18<br>0.90 ± 0.10 | Acute—control * | 0.73–0.85<br>0.77–0.90<br>0.86–0.94 |
| Affected PC | Acute stage<br>Follow-up<br>Control | 0.78 ± 0.17<br>0.83 ± 0.16<br>0.87 ± 0.12 | Acute—control * | 0.72–0.84<br>0.77–0.89<br>0.83–0.92 |
| Unaffected PC | Acute stage<br>Follow-up<br>Control | 0.77 ± 0.15<br>0.85 ± 0.14<br>0.86 ± 0.10 | Acute—control * | 0.72–0.83<br>0.80–0.90<br>0.82–0.90 |

**Table 2.** Gain asymmetry values of vHIT in vestibular neuritis at the acute stage and follow-up in the affected horizontal canal (HC), posterior canal (PC) and anterior canal (HC) plane. * $p < 0.05$.

| Gain Asymmetry | | Mean ± SD | Significance | 95% C.I. for Mean |
|---|---|---|---|---|
| Affected HC | Acute stage | 17.86 ± 28.50 | | 8.07–27.65 |
| | Follow-up | 9.83 ± 21.10 | | 2.58–17.08 |
| | Control | 12.81 ± 10.78 | | 8.92–16.7 |
| Affected AC | Acute stage | 7.80 ± 11.16 | | 3.97–11.63 |
| | Follow-up | 1.60 ± 8.45 | Acute—Follow-up * | −1.30–4.50 |
| | Control | 5.97 ± 6.31 | | 3.69–8.24 |
| Affected PC | Acute stage | 0.46 ± 11.42 | | −3.47–4.38 |
| | Follow-up | 0.11 ± 11.13 | Follow-up—control * | −3.71–3.94 |
| | Control | 5.94 ± 5.32 | | 4.02–7.86 |

Initially, the incidence of pathological covert saccades in all planes (94% in the HC, 57% in the AC, and 31% in the PC plane) was somewhat higher than that of overt saccades (86%, 49% and 26%, respectively); see Table 3. At the follow-up examination, the occurrence of covert saccades was significantly decreased in the HC (94% vs. 69%; $p < 0.05$) and AC planes (57% vs. 17%; $p < 0.01$). Similarly, the overt saccades were also significantly reduced in the HC (86% vs. 57%; $p < 0.05$) and AC planes (49% vs. 11%; $p < 0.01$). At the follow-up, regarding the total rate of covert and/or overt saccades for each canal plane, a relatively high incidence of saccades (90%) was found in the HC, compared to in the other canal planes (Table 3).

**Table 3.** Incidence of pathological covert and overt saccades during vHIT in patients suffering from vestibular neuritis at the acute stage and follow-up affected side. HC: horizontal canal plane, AC: anterior canal plane, PC: posterior canal plane. *** $p < 0.001$, ** $p < 0.01$, * $p < 0.05$.

| Affected Side | Covert | | | | | Overt | | | | | Total (Covert and/or Overt Saccades) | | | | |
|---|---|---|---|---|---|---|---|---|---|---|---|---|---|---|---|
| | Acute Stage | | Follow-Up | | | Acute Stage | | Follow-Up | | | Acute Stage | | Follow-Up | | |
| | N | % | N | % | p-Value | N | % | N | % | p-Value | N | % | N | % | p-Value |
| HC | 33 | 94% | 24 | 69% | * | 30 | 86% | 20 | 57% | * | 34 | 97% | 28 | 90% | |
| AC | 20 | 57% | 6 | 17% | ** | 17 | 49% | 4 | 11% | ** | 24 | 69% | 8 | 23% | *** |
| PC | 11 | 31% | 5 | 14% | | 9 | 26% | 5 | 14% | | 13 | 37% | 6 | 17% | |

At the acute stage, based on either gain values or incidence of saccades, the number of patients with multi-canal affection was greater than that with isolated canal affection (Table 4). More specifically, in terms of gain, 80% (28/35) showed multi-canal affection vs. 14% (5/35) for isolated canal affection. In terms of saccades (overt and covert), 71% (25/35) showed multi-canal affection vs. 28.5% (10/35) for isolated canal affection. Regarding gain values, the HC was involved in 28 patients, the AC in 28 patients, and the PC in 17 patients; notably, in two patients suffering from AVN, the gain was normal in all the canals. Refixation saccades were registered in the HC plane of 34 patients, in the AC plane of 24 patients, and in the PC plane of 13 patients (Table 4).

Table 4. Isolated and multi-canal involvement according to vHIT parameters (gain, covert saccades, and overt saccades) at the acute stage of vestibular neuritis (affected side). HC: horizontal canal plane, AC: anterior canal plane, PC: posterior canal plane.

|  | Isolated Canal Involvement | | | Multi-Canal Involvement | | | | | |
| --- | --- | --- | --- | --- | --- | --- | --- | --- | --- |
|  | HC | AC | PC | HC + AC | HC + PC | AC + PC | HC + AC + PC | Normal | Total |
| Gain | 2 | 2 | 1 | 12 | 2 | 2 | 12 | 2 | 35 |
| Saccades | 10 | - | - | 12 | 1 | 1 | 11 | - | 35 |

According to the DHI (acute stage), 5 (14.2%) patients had mild disability, 12 (34.2%) had moderate disability, and 18 (51.4%) patients had severe disability; the mean total DHI was 52.17 ± 13.23. At the follow-up, almost all the patients presented a normal DHI score, except for 5 (14.2%) patients who had mild disability; the mean total DHI was 7.94 ± 9.52. In the initial stage, the gain values and the gain asymmetry of each semi-circular canal on the affected and unaffected sides were not statistically correlated with the DHI measurements. At the follow-up, no statistical correlations were performed, as all of the DHI scores were below 35 and no clinical significance was expected.

## 5. Discussion

According to our results, the majority of patients (80%) with AVN had lower VOR gain in the HC and AC planes, compared to the PC plane (48.5%). The cause of this high affection of both HC and AC planes could be attributed to anatomical particularities of the bony channel of the superior vestibular nerve, as it is seven times longer, narrower, and has much more spicules along its course, compared to that of the inferior vestibular nerve; this makes the superior vestibular nerve more susceptible to compressive injury and ischemia [17].

In the period after AVN, a progressive restoration of the semi-circular canal gain was observed in our patients, mainly regarding the HC and AC gain (Table 1). A central compensation process, based on synaptic and neuronal plasticity, has been reported to be responsible for the gain improvement across all the canal planes [18]. Central mechanisms have also been implicated in the upregulation of the unaffected side [19]; at the acute stage, our lower gain values were effectively compensated as, otherwise, the lack of disinhibitory input through commissural pathways would cause a greater gain reduction at higher accelerations on the unaffected side [19]. The gain asymmetry decreased on the affected side, mainly in the affected AC/unaffected PC plane (Table 2). However, Allum and Honegger [20] reported that the mean gain asymmetry change between onset and 5 weeks was greater ($p < 0.001$) in the horizontal canal plane (from 36.9% to 19.4%) than in the other planes.

Although it has been reported that 3–6 months are necessary to observe a stabilization of the gain [21], a time of more than one year and a half may be required for higher horizontal head velocities [22]. In our study, our follow-up period was extended up to 30 months, and we found that the gain was best recovered in the affected AC plane (50%) compared to in the affected HC (42.8%) and PC (41.1%) planes. Büki et al. [23] showed that normal HC gain occurred in 55%, AC gain in 38%, and PC gain in 38% of 40 patients, supporting the idea that vertical canals recover less effectively. Furthermore, Magliulo et al. [13] reported that the PC gain was better normal in 42.1% (8/19), HC gain in 37.1% (13/35), and AC gain in 25.8% (8/31). The discrepancy between these findings could be attributed to the short-term follow-up of the two abovementioned studies: two months [23] and three months [13], respectively.

Despite the fact that the VOR gain was not fully recovered in all cases, the majority of patients returned to their daily living activities. The question was how, after AVN, can inadequate recovery of slow phase eye velocity compensate for the VOR deficit to natural head accelerations. Previous studies [8,24] have suggested that the presence of refixation saccades may play a very important role in stabilizing the gaze in space during head rotations. In patients with unilateral vestibular loss, these saccades may act to minimize the effect of the dynamic VOR deficit, and could also be considered as part of a compensatory mechanism to overcome the loss of peripheral vestibular function [4]. In our study, at the acute stage, the saccades were more obviously detected in the HC plane (covert 94%, overt 86%, mixed 97%; Table 3), compared to in vertical canal planes. It has been demonstrated [25] that averaged VOR speed gains were greater in the HC plane, compared to those of vertical canals, in normal subjects; therefore, it is possible that the saccade recordings are better produced during head rotational accelerations on the horizontal plane.

As mentioned previously, no other report in the literature has assessed the refixation saccades for AVN in the vertical planes. According to our results (Table 4), at the follow-up, both covert and overt saccades—especially those on the affected AC plane—were significantly reduced in all of the planes. It is worth noting that, in long-term re-examination, HC covert saccades were recorded at a greater proportion in our patients, compared to HC overt saccades (69% vs. 57%). Fu et al. [5] also registered, six months after AVN 87% covert vs. 59% overt saccades. It has been reported [6] that, as vestibular compensation is promoted, there is an evolution in the saccade pattern from overt to covert saccades. However, a higher percentage of overt compared to covert frequency has been observed 15 days after AVN (54.6% overt vs. 13.3% covert) [4], 87% overt vs. 43% covert at 1 month after AVN [26], and 73.4% overt vs. 14.7% covert at 4 months after AVN [27]. The role of covert and overt saccades after AVN has not yet been clarified. It has been proposed that covert saccades may contribute to the compensation of inadequate VOR response and to symptom-associated recovery [5]. Conversely, a high prevalence of overt saccades has been related to a worse prognosis after acute AVN [28]. Wettstein et al. [29] reported that patients suffering from AVN and higher percentage of covert saccades had better dynamic visual acuity; on the contrary, patients with few covert saccades and/or high amplitude of cumulative overt saccades had poor dynamic visual acuity. Navari et al. [27] supported the idea that residual disability after acute unilateral vestibulopathy was related with lower high-velocity VOR gain, increased gain asymmetry, and increased overt saccades number and amplitude. It seems that the presence of covert saccades is more essential for the vestibular compensation process and would faster facilitate the recovery, taking into account that almost all of our patients had a favorable outcome after AVN.

Due to the clinical application of the vHIT, the interpretation of the results was based on the gain value, which was used to determine whether the vestibular function could be classified as either normal or pathological. It has also been reported that it is advisable to check both gain and refixation saccades when performing vHIT to detect vestibular hypofunction [26]. However, patients suffering from vestibular disorders in which the gain was normal on vHIT testing have been reported, where only the presence of refixation saccades indicated the existence of peripheral vestibulopathy [30]. Thus, the occurrence of saccades could be more reliable than the gain value for the evaluation of vestibular function [31]. Two of our patients with AVN showed normal gain in all canals, raising a question regarding the pathophysiology of this disease; however, both of these patients showed refixation saccades (Table 4). Unlike the gain results (Table 4), and based on the saccade findings, there was no AC- or PC-isolated AVN, but more HC-isolated AVN (10 cases).

According to our results, multi-canal affection occurred more frequently (80% for gain, 71% for saccades) than isolated canal affection (see Table 4). Thus, at least two canals were usually implicated in the pathogenesis of AVN. We have retrieved reports that assessed the semi-circular canal involvement (horizontal and verticals) through vHIT in patients suffering from AVN, and found five studies measuring the gain in these canals (but not the presence of saccades). Multi-canal affection was reported in 60% [11], 62.5% [27], 68.9% [12], 75% [10], and 80% of cases [13], respectively; in almost all of these studies, both the HC and AC gain, or the gain of all three canals (HC + AC + PC), were more frequently found to be abnormal. However, only sporadic cases with isolated horizontal or anterior canal AVN have been described in the literature [10,23]. It seems that, in most AVN cases, the damage is extensive rather than selective; as, for example, both superior and inferior vestibular nerve AVN is more frequent than superior or inferior vestibular nerve AVN alone [10,13,27].

The DHI is the most widely used self-reported measurement of patients with dizziness [32]. Our long-term mean total DHI after AVN was 7.94, indicating a complete recovery. Other studies assessing long-term DHI results after AVN have presented comparable values, such as 12.51 (follow-up: 5.3 y) [33] and 18.3 (follow-up: 3 y) [11]. In our study, at the acute stage, no statistically significant correlation between the vHIT parameters and the DHI values was found. Similarly, Riska et al. [4] also did not find a significant difference in DHI score as a function of saccade group (DHI score: 48 for covert, 47 for overt, 54 for mixed saccades) less than one month after AVN. Patel et al. [11] reported that 10% of their patients, 3–36 months after AVN, showed DHI scores more than 35, but they did not find a correlation between ipsilesional high velocity VOR gain or gain asymmetry of the single or combined HC, AC, and PC with the DHI scores. However, Manzari et al. [6] observed a statistical correlation between the HC gain and DHI values six weeks after AVN. Fu et al. [5] compared two groups of patients at 6 months after UVN—28 patients without or with mild disability (according to DHI) to 19 patients with moderate to severe disability—and reported that the proportion of patients with presence of covert saccades in the first group was significantly higher than that in the latter group.

## 6. Conclusions

In the relatively long follow-up period after AVN, the vHIT gain was found to be increased on the affected side in all of the three semi-circular canals, mainly in those innervated by the superior vestibular nerve (i.e., HC and AC canals). The vHIT gain was recovered in all canals, and both covert and overt saccades were reduced in all the canal planes—notably, they were more significantly in the affected AC/unaffected PC plane. The compensatory mechanisms after AVN mainly involved the HC, as the refixation saccades—especially the covert compared to overt saccades—were more frequently detected in the HC plane than in the vertical canal planes. In AVN, multi-canal affection occurred more frequently than isolated semi-circular canal affection, indicating that the vestibular nerve damage is usually more extensive than selective.

**Author Contributions:** Conceptualization, G.P.; methodology, G.P., I.P. and A.P.; investigation, data curation, and visualization, G.P., I.P. and S.A.; project administration, I.S.; resources, P.B.; supervision, G.P. and J.C.; writing—original draft preparation, G.P. and I.P.; writing—review and editing, G.P. and I.P. All authors have read and agreed to the published version of the manuscript.

**Funding:** This research did not receive any specific grant from funding agencies in the public, commercial, or not-for-profit sectors.

**Institutional Review Board Statement:** Not applicable.

**Informed Consent Statement:** Informed consent was obtained from all subjects involved in the study.

**Data Availability Statement:** The data presented in this study are available upon request from the corresponding author.

**Conflicts of Interest:** The authors declare no conflict of interest.

## References

1. Strupp, M.; Brandt, T. Vestibular neuritis. *Semin. Neurol.* **2009**, *5*, 509–519. [CrossRef] [PubMed]
2. Kim, J.S. When the room is spinning: Experience of vestibular neuritis by a neurotologist. *Front. Neurol.* **2020**, *11*, 157. [CrossRef] [PubMed]
3. Himmelein, S.; Lindemann, A.; Sinicina, I.; Horn, A.K.E.; Brandt, T.; Strupp, M.; Hüfner, K. Differential involvement during latent herpes simplex virus 1 infection of the superior and inferior divisions of the vestibular ganglia: Implications for vestibular neuritis. *J. Virol.* **2017**, *91*, e00331-17. [CrossRef] [PubMed]

4. Riska, K.M.; Bellucci, J.; Garrison, D.; Hall, C. Relationship between corrective saccades and measures of physical function in unilateral and bilateral vestibular loss. *Ear Hear.* **2020**, *41*, 1568–1574. [CrossRef]
5. Fu, W.; He, F.; Wei, D.; Bai, Y.; Shi, Y.; Wang, X.; Han, J. Recovery pattern of high-frequency acceleration vestibulo-ocular reflex in unilateral vestibular neuritis: A preliminary study. *Front. Neurol.* **2019**, *10*, 85. [CrossRef] [PubMed]
6. Manzari, L.; Graziano, D.; Tramontano, M. The different stages of vestibular neuritis from the point of view of the video head impulse test. *Audiol. Res.* **2020**, *10*, 31–38. [CrossRef]
7. Halmagyi, G.M.; Curthoys, I.S.; Cremer, P.D.; Henderson, C.J.; Staples, M. Head impulses after unilateral vestibular deafferentation validate Ewald's second law. *J. Vestib. Res.* **1990–1991**, *1*, 187–197. [CrossRef]
8. MacDougall, H.G.; Curthoys, I.S. Plasticity during vestibular compensation: The role of saccades. *Front. Neurol.* **2012**, *3*, 21. [CrossRef]
9. MacDougall, H.G.; McGarvie, L.A.; Halmagyi, G.M.; Curthoys, I.S.; Weber, K.P. Application of the video head impulse test to detect vertical semicircular canal dysfunction. *Otol. Neurotol.* **2013**, *34*, 974–979. [CrossRef]
10. Taylor, R.L.; McGarvie, L.A.; Reid, N.; Young, A.S.; Halmagyi, G.M.; Welgampola, M.S. Vestibular neuritis affects both superior and inferior vestibular nerves. *Neurology* **2016**, *87*, 1704–1712. [CrossRef]
11. Patel, M.; Arshad, Q.; Roberts, R.E.; Ahmad, H.; Bronstein, A.M. Chronic symptoms after vestibular neuritis and the high-velocity vestibulo-ocular reflex. *Otol. Neurotol.* **2016**, *37*, 179–184. [CrossRef] [PubMed]
12. Bartolomeo, M.; Biboulet, R.; Pierre, G.; Mondain, M.; Uziel, A.; Venail, F. Value of the video head impulse test in assessing vestibular deficits following vestibular neuritis. *Eur. Arch. Otorhinolaryngol.* **2014**, *271*, 681–688. [CrossRef] [PubMed]
13. Magliulo, G.; Gagliardi, S.; Ciniglio Appiani, M.; Iannella, G.; Re, M. Vestibular neurolabyrinthitis: A follow-up study with cervical and ocular vestibular evoked myogenic potentials and the video head impulse test. *Ann. Otol. Rhinol. Laryngol.* **2014**, *123*, 162–173. [CrossRef]
14. Sestak, A.; Maslovara, S.; Zubcic, Z.; Vceva, A. Influence of vestibular rehabilitation on the recovery of all vestibular receptor organs in patients with unilateral vestibular hypofunction. *NeuroRehabilitation* **2020**, *47*, 227–235. [CrossRef] [PubMed]
15. Jacobson, G.P.; Newman, C.W. The development of the Dizziness Handicap Inventory. *Arch. Otolaryngol. Head Neck Surg.* **1990**, *116*, 424–427. [CrossRef] [PubMed]
16. Yilmaz, M.S.; Egilmez, O.K.; Kara, A.; Guven, M.; Demir, D.; Genc Elden, S. Comparison of the results of caloric and video head impulse tests in patients with Meniere's disease and vestibular migraine. *Eur. Arch. Otorhinolaryngol.* **2021**, *278*, 1829–1834. [CrossRef]
17. Gianoli, G.; Goebel, J.; Mowry, S.; Poomipannit, P. Anatomic differences in the lateral vestibular nerve channels and their implications in vestibular neuritis. *Otol. Neurotol.* **2005**, *26*, 489–494. [CrossRef]
18. Lacour, M.; Helmchen, C.; Vidal, P.P. Vestibular compensation: The neuro-otologist's best friend. *J. Neurol.* **2016**, *263* (Suppl. S1), S54–S64. [CrossRef]
19. Palla, A.; Straumann, D. Recovery of the high-acceleration vestibulo-ocular reflex after vestibular neuritis. *J. Assoc. Res. Otolaryngol.* **2004**, *5*, 427–435. [CrossRef]
20. Allum, J.H.J.; Honegger, F. Improvement of asymmetric vestibulo-ocular reflex responses following onset of vestibular neuritis is similar across canal planes. *Front. Neurol.* **2020**, *11*, 565125. [CrossRef]
21. Manzari, L.; Princi, A.A.; De Angelis, S.; Tramontano, M. Clinical value of the video head impulse test in patients with vestibular neuritis: A systematic review. *Eur. Arch. Otorhinolaryngol.* **2021**, *278*, 4155–4167. [CrossRef] [PubMed]
22. McGarvie, L.A.; MacDougall, H.G.; Curthoys, I.S.; Halmagyi, G.M. Spontaneous recovery of the vestibulo-ocular reflex after vestibular neuritis; Long-term monitoring with the video head impulse test in a single patient. *Front. Neurol.* **2020**, *11*, 732. [CrossRef] [PubMed]
23. Büki, B.; Hanschek, M.; Jünger, H. Vestibular neuritis: Involvement and long-term recovery of individual semicircular canals. *Auris Nasus Larynx* **2017**, *44*, 288–293. [CrossRef] [PubMed]
24. Schubert, M.C.; Zee, D.S. Saccade and vestibular ocular motor adaptation. *Restor. Neurol. Neurosci.* **2010**, *28*, 9–18. [CrossRef]
25. Cremer, P.D.; Halmagyi, G.M.; Aw, S.T.; Curthoys, I.S.; McGarvie, L.A.; Todd, M.J.; Black, R.A.; Hannigan, I.P. Semicircular canal plane head impulses detect absent function of individual semicircular canals. *Brain* **1998**, *121*, 699–716. [CrossRef]
26. Yang, C.J.; Cha, E.H.; Park, J.W.; Kang, B.C.; Yoo, M.H.; Kang, W.S.; Ahn, J.H.; Chung, J.W.; Park, H.J. Diagnostic value of gains and corrective saccades in video head impulse test in vestibular neuritis. *Otolaryngol. Head Neck Surg.* **2018**, *159*, 347–353. [CrossRef]
27. Navari, E.; Cerchiai, N.; Casani, A.P. Assessment of vestibulo-ocular reflex gain and catch-up saccades during vestibular rehabilitation. *Otol. Neurotol.* **2018**, *39*, e1111–e1117. [CrossRef]
28. Cerchiai, N.; Navari, E.; Sellari-Franceschini, S.; Re, C.; Casani, A.P. Predicting the outcome after acute unilateral vestibulopathy: Analysis of vestibulo-ocular reflex gain and catch-up saccades. *Otolaryngol. Head Neck Surg.* **2018**, *158*, 527–533. [CrossRef]
29. Wettstein, V.G.; Weber, K.P.; Bockisch, C.J.; Hegemann, S.C. Compensatory saccades in head impulse testing influence the dynamic visual acuity of patients with unilateral peripheral vestibulopathy1. *J. Vestib. Res.* **2016**, *26*, 395–402. [CrossRef]
30. Perez-Fernandez, N.; Eza-Nuñez, P. Normal gain of VOR with refixation saccades in patients with unilateral vestibulopathy. *J. Int. Adv. Otol.* **2015**, *11*, 133–137. [CrossRef]
31. Korsager, L.E.; Faber, C.E.; Schmidt, J.H.; Wanscher, J.H. Refixation saccades with normal gain values: A diagnostic problem in the video head impulse test: A case report. *Front. Neurol.* **2017**, *8*, 81. [CrossRef]

32. Mutlu, B.; Serbetcioglu, B. Discussion of the dizziness handicap inventory. *J. Vestib. Res.* **2013**, *23*, 271–277. [CrossRef]
33. Mandalà, M.; Nuti, D. Long-term follow-up of vestibular neuritis. *Ann. N. Y. Acad. Sci.* **2009**, *1164*, 427–429. [CrossRef]

MDPI  
St. Alban-Anlage 66  
4052 Basel  
Switzerland  
Tel. +41 61 683 77 34  
Fax +41 61 302 89 18  
www.mdpi.com

*Journal of Clinical Medicine* Editorial Office  
E-mail: jcm@mdpi.com  
www.mdpi.com/journal/jcm

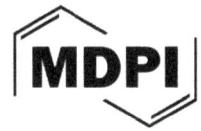

www.ingramcontent.com/pod-product-compliance
Lightning Source LLC
LaVergne TN
LVHW070637100526
838202LV00012B/831